Issues in
Women's
Occupational
Health

Invisible

La santé des
travailleuses

Edited by/
Sous la direction de

Karen Messing
Barbara Neis
Lucie Dumais

gynergy
books

Printed and bound in Canada using union labour by:
Imprimerie Gagné Ltée

*gynergy books acknowledges the generous support of
the Canada Council.*

Published by:
gynergy books
P.O. Box 2023
Charlottetown, P.E.I.
Canada, C1A 7N7

Canadian Cataloguing in Publication Data
Main entry under title:
Invisible

In English and French.
Includes bibliographical references.
ISBN 0-921881-37-1

1. Women — Employment — Health aspects. 2. Industrial
hygiene — Canada. 3. Occupational diseases. I. Messing, Karen.
II. Neis, Barbara, 1952- . III. Dumais, Lucie, 1960- .
IV. Title: Invisible: la santé des travailleuses

HD6067.2.C2158 1995   331.4'25   C95-950204-1

Contents

1 Making Risks Visible in Women's Jobs/ Rendre visibles les risques du travail des femmes

175 Making Issues Visible to Researchers/ Rendre les enjeux visibles aux milieux de recherche

Introduction

"All the authorities were male and it was simple for a male to identify that, 'Oh yeah, there's a guard gone on the saw, therefore you replace it.' It's really simple, they just do that. But when it comes to facing a problem that women have, they couldn't identify it as a health and safety issue — or they *wouldn't*."

— Judy Vanta,
Occupational Health and Safety Committee,
Newfoundland Federation of Labour, at the Colloquium on
Social, Physical and Technical Barriers to the Safe Integration
of Women in the Workplace.

Occupational health problems of working women are difficult for employers, scientists, decision makers — even workers themselves — to see. Women workers tell us that their struggles — to have simple repairs made to dangerous office equipment, to find stools upon which to perch during off hours at the bank, to remove dust-catching carpets at primary schools — are met with incredulity and even mockery. The invisibility of women's occupational health problems arises partly from attitudes towards women's "natural" work. Daycare workers lifting children, waitresses carrying heavy trays or check-out cashiers lifting bottles of milk and juice are somehow not "handling manual materials" in the same sense as stevedores loading boxes are, even though the total weight handled each day in each job may be very similar.

In the same way, it is sometimes hard to recognize double shifts or night shifts when they are viewed as part of women's "natural" work. Working at night disrupts the body's circadian rhythms and can lead to sleep disturbances and eventually to health problems. Because of the stressful nature of night work, lawmakers in many countries have argued over whether women are tough enough to be allowed to work night shifts. Women have only recently been allowed to take industrial night shift jobs in Europe. But female hospital staff and other health care workers continued to work nights during all the heated debate and no one suggested that they should stop. Furthermore, when the night shift and the double shift are unpaid, legislators do not consider them when setting standards. There are no regulations or even guidelines to limit the length or the combined chemical and ergonomic exposures of women's total domestic and professional work day.

Scientific procedures and policy standards that have been developed in relation to men's jobs may be "blind" to the risks in women's jobs. When the occupational health and safety law was passed in 1979 in Quebec, employment sectors were ranked according to their priority for the implementation of prevention efforts. The criteria used to rank these sectors were the numbers of compensated work accidents and health problems in each sector, and the findings of a literature survey done in 1978. Dangers for women's reproductive processes, the largely unstudied (at that time) women's employment "ghettos" and work incompatible with family responsibilities did not enter into the calculation. Although this mechanism involved no explicit discriminatory procedures, it resulted in the near absence of women (only 15 percent) from the two groups for which prevention has been made fully available.[1]

In fact, sex-specific hazards do not seem to be regarded as legitimate occupational health risks when the sex to which they are specific is female. For example, in Quebec, about one-third of pregnant workers are re-assigned or given temporary leave because their jobs are incompatible with healthy pregnancy. In the popular press, this high proportion is presented as an indicator of abuse of the system rather than as a sign of the difficulties in women's jobs.[2] The construction employers' association has protested paying for this programme through workers' compensation, saying, "Being pregnant is not a work accident."[3] The Quebec Institute for Research in Occupational Health and Safety (IRSST) appears to share this view that dangers for pregnant women are not real occupational health hazards. In an aside on page 110 of their report, we learn that they exclude this category of hazards from their analysis of risks by employment sector with no explicit justification.[4]

Some reluctance on the part of government decision makers and employers to recognize the health risks in women's jobs seems to derive from fear that these problems are so pervasive that the slightest acknowledgement will result in a flood of claims. They are not necessarily wrong — when there is delay in recognizing risks, problems build up and accumulate. This has, in fact, happened with several hazards for women in the workplace. As well, the build-up continues if no prevention programme results from the recognition of the hazard. The programme established to remove pregnant women from dangerous workplaces contained no impetus to remove the hazards, since the problems are attributed to pregnancy and not to the workplace. Thus, the same businesses have become the scene of repeated pregancy leaves or reassignment. When, as often happens, the worker on leave is not replaced, co-workers and supervisors grow to resent the pregnant woman. A feeling develops that the pregnant women, not the employers, are abusing the system.

Similarly, women are blamed for the controversy surrounding video display terminals. These were introduced massively into women's workplaces without adequate safety testing for risks to pregnancy or osteo-articular problems. Women protested, but it took a long time before tests were done and corrective measures taken.

A final example of the consequences of delay in recognizing hazards in women's jobs can be seen in the current "epidemic" of cumulative trauma disorders (tendinitis, carpal tunnel syndrome, bursitis). These result from the repetitive work in many women's jobs on assembly lines and in offices. The extent of the problem, however, is not due to sudden recognition of the health risk, but rather to the previous delay in recognition and correction.

Women, including those of us who are feminists, may collude with attempts to conceal occupational hazards in our jobs because we are afraid any effect on our health may be taken to mean we are too "weak" to do the job. This is the reason why feminists have often argued with those who do research on the occupational hazards to healthy menstrual function. Feminists ask: Won't this research play into the hands of those who say women aren't fit to work? Despite a growing literature on the effects of working conditions such as heat, cold and chemical exposures on menstrual pain and regularity, the only reference to menstruation in the recent 214-page "state of the art review" by a team of American feminist occupational health experts consists of two pages of historical treatment of the compatibility of the menstrual cycle with leadership.[5] When women raise issues about the safety of our jobs, we may be afraid to hear questions about whether women should be in the workplace at all.

This book is an attempt to start a process which will substitute intelligent inquiry for denial and refusal to recognize women's occupational health problems. The contributors to this volume believe that it is in the interest of women workers to describe as carefully and fully as possible the risks found in women's jobs, especially those that are specific, or relatively specific, to women's bodies. Experience has taught us that trying to conceal difference does not prevent discrimination.

Given the widespread notion that women's work is harmless, we thought it important to begin the book with a series of chapters about occupational health problems in specific workplaces. Barbara Neis' article on asthma in crab-processing plants in Quebec and Newfoundland gives a portrait of a pervasive health problem while allowing us to understand some of the political issues involved in recognizing women's occupational health problems in the troubled Newfoundland economy. Nicole Vézina's paper on ergonomic analysis of sex-typed jobs in food processing and Susan Stock's study of musculoskeletal problems in a small daycare centre show how jobs that appear natural for women give rise to pain and physical problems. Other papers, like Janet Sprout and Annalee Yassi's chapter on occupational health in the service sector, and Ellen Balka's investigation of the effects of technological evolution on telephone operators, paint a broader portrait of stressful situations in workplaces with large numbers of women. Finally, the chapters by Vivienne Walters and Lynn Skillen on the health service sector reveal the problem of recognizing hazards in professions in which caring for others results in an accumulation of emotional and physical difficulties.

Many researchers exploring women's occupational health have produced methodological challenges to "gender-blind" analyzes and procedures. The book's second section presents some responses to these challenges through action-oriented research. Karen Messing separates out questions of biology, gender and working conditions in occupational health studies. Catherine Teiger, an ergonomist, has used an analysis of the work process to enable researchers and workers to recognize some hidden components in women's jobs and together to find ways to reduce mental and physical fatigue. Lucie Dumais raises issues that arise in collaborations between sociologists, occupational health specialists and union representatives, based on her experience in examining the social origins of occupational problems. Donna Mergler, who participated in a committee on workplace effects on mental health and became involved in a debate on how to analyze data by gender, gives us her proposal in this section. And Danièle Kergoat, a pioneer in the recognition of the sexual division of labour in France, concludes the section with a historical perspective on the difficult process by which women's concerns are being integrated into the sociology of labour.

The book's third and final section presents experiences with public policy regarding women's occupational health. Katherine Lippel, a specialist in law, has compared the decisions given to women with those given to men by the Quebec Occupational Health and Safety Commission in cases involving compensation for stress-related disability. Her analysis reveals how differently those responsible for compensation see and treat women and men and their jobs. Nicolette Carlan, the head of a provincial health and safety panel, describes the difficulties experienced by the panel when they tried to gather information on women's occupational health for policy purposes. Joan Stevenson, a specialist in biomechanics, demonstrates how details in pre-employment strength testing procedures can make them unfair to women applicants and less than useful in predicting who can do a job safely. Dorothy Wigmore, a longtime union researcher and activist, has gathered a great deal of information about how violence against women workers has been and should be dealt with in the workplace. Joan Eakin has uncovered many of the health and safety problems of women in small workplaces — a topic of special interest, since women are over-represented in these workplaces. The section, and the book, concludes with a look towards the future by Pat Armstrong, who examines the implications for women and men of changes in the job market.

The content of this book reflects a variety of approaches to women's occupational health; we believe it is very important to profit from many disciplines. Historically, important contributions to the study of women's occupational health have been made by physicians,[6] chemists[7] and sociologists.[8] In this volume, social scientists provide important analyzes of the sexual and social division of labour (Armstrong, Eakin, Kergoat, Walters), women's relation to technology (Balka) and social questions preventing the recognition of occupational health hazards (Carlan, Lippel, Neis). They also ask broader questions about the definition of problems and solutions in occupational health (Dumais). These issues are fundamental to understanding why women are assigned to certain jobs and to developing social, as well as technical, solutions. It is in this context, set by the social scientists, that medical scientists, biologists and ergonomists (Mergler, Messing, Skillen, Sprout, Stevenson, Stock, Teiger, Vézina, Wigmore and Yassi) discuss the interactions of women's minds and bodies with their work sites.

Despite our various backgrounds and approaches to our research, the defining characteristic of the contributors to this book is our commitment to the improvement of women's working conditons. We strive to provide accurate analyses, not only for the pleasure of doing research, but also to help orient action in the workplace. For this reason, we invited policy makers and occupational health intervenors in unions and management to be with us as we discussed our papers.

Recently, following the Ontario Federation of Labour conference on women's occupational health, we received a letter from a metal worker that expresses many of the problems confronted by women workers. It reads:

> I have filed a claim for vibration destruction in my knees due to working full shifts on a vibrating floor. The suggestion has been made that perhaps due to my age the calcium level or lack of it in my legs is responsible and perhaps a woman of my age should not have been put down there ... There are at present no female doctors on the review boards for the Workers' Compensation Board to bring the required balance to any of their decisions. By the time a female fights her way through the maze of male advocates who don't believe her anyhow and then is confronted by these "old boys" she has begun to doubt her own just claim ...
> — Ms. Carrie Chenier, United Steelworkers of America

We are adamant that women workers like Ms. Chenier will not always have to accept that their health and safety problems are their own fault simply because they are not young men. As we meet and talk with women workers, we can see that they are already changing the focus and orientation of the prevention and compensation systems for health and safety. We continue our research in the hope that we, too, can contribute to this process.

Karen Messing
Barbara Neis
Lucie Dumais

NOTES

1. The causes and the consequences of this exclusion for women workers are more fully explained in: CINBIOSE, *Quand le travail léger pèse lourd: Vers une nouvelle approche en prévention dans les emplois des femmes*, (Montreal: Centre pour l'étude des interactions biologiques entre la santé et l'environnement, 1995), report presented to the Women's Committees of the Centrale des Enseignantes et des Enseignants du Québec, the Confédération des Syndicats Nationaux and the Fédération des Travailleurs et Travailleuses du Québec.

2. For example, see: Beaulieu, C., "Les travailleuses enceintes perdent leur El Dorado," *Le Devoir* (29 July 1988).

3. Blanchard, S., "Les entrepreneurs en construction exigent la révision de la «coûteuse» CSST," *Le Devoir* (28 February 1992), p. A3.

4. Hébert, F., *L'inégalité des risques affectant la sécurité des travailleurs par secteur*

d'activité en 1986. (Montreal: IRSST, 1994).

5. Headapohl, D. M. (ed.), "Occupational Medicine: Women Workers," *Occupational Health: State of the Art Reviews* 8, 4, pp. 800-1.

6. Hamilton, Alice, *Exploring the Dangerous Trades*, (Boston: Little, Brown, 1943).

7. Stellman, Jeanne, *Women's Work, Women's Health*, (New York: Pantheon, 1978).

8. Hochschild, Arlie R., *The Managed Heart*, (Berkeley: University of California Press, 1983).

Introduction

Les personnes en autorité étaient toutes des hommes et il était facile pour un homme de comprendre que «ah oui, il manque un protecteur à la scie», alors on le remplace. C'est vraiment simple; ils le font. Mais quand il s'agissait d'un problème rencontré par les femmes, ils n'arrivaient pas à le définer comme étant un enjeu de santé et de sécurité, et ils ne le faisaient pas.

— Judy Vanta,
Comité de santé et sécurité au travail, Newfoundland Federation of Labour,
lors de l'atelier sur les barrières sociales, physiques et techniques à
l'intégration sécuritaire des femmes en milieu de travail.

Les problèmes de santé des femmes au travail semblent être difficiles à percevoir pour les employeurs, les scientifiques, les décideurs, voire les travailleuses elles-mêmes. Certaines d'entre elles nous ont raconté, par exemple, comment leurs batailles pour corriger légèrement de l'équipement de bureau dangereux, ou pour trouver un tabouret où s'asseoir pendant les pauses à la banque ou encore pour enlever des tapis qui ramassaient la poussière dans une école primaire, ont été accueillies par l'incrédulité ou la moquerie.

Cette invisibilité provient en partie des attitudes envers le travail «naturel» des femmes. Une travailleuse en garderie qui soulève un enfant, une serveuse de restaurant qui porte des plateaux chargés ou une caissière qui manipule des contenants de lait et de jus ne sont pas perçues comme des manutentionnaires, au même titre que les débardeurs qui transportent des caisses, même si le poids total manipulé dans une journée peut être similaire. De même, certaines personnes ont du mal à reconnaître le travail de nuit lorsque celui-ci est perçu comme inhérent au travail «naturel» des femmes. On sait que travailler la nuit dérègle le rythme circadien et peut engendrer des troubles du sommeil et, à la longue, des problèmes de santé. À cause de ce caractère pénible du travail de nuit, les législateurs de plusieurs pays ont longuement discuté de la résistance des femmes et de la pertinence d'autoriser leur présence dans les emplois de nuit. En Europe, l'accès des femmes aux emplois industriels de nuit n'a ainsi été autorisée que tout récemment. Pourtant, alors même que ce débat faisait rage, le personnel hospitalier et les autres travailleuses de la santé travaillaient déjà la nuit sans que personne ne semble s'en offusquer!

Quand ces emplois de nuit ou ces doubles emplois ne sont pas rémunérés, les législateurs n'en tiennent pas compte dans l'établissement des normes. Ainsi, lorsqu'il s'agit de limiter la durée ou le niveau des expositions chimiques ou des contraintes ergonomiques, aucune législation ni recommandation ne combine la double journée de travail des femmes, professionnelle et domestique.

Les procédures scientifiques et les normes recommandées, parce qu'elles ont été développées à partir d'emplois masculins, peuvent être insensibles aux risques spécifiques des emplois féminins. Quand le Québec a adopté sa Loi sur la santé et la sécurité au travail, en 1979, les secteurs d'emploi ont été classés selon leur priorité, en termes de prévention. Les critères utilisés pour cette classification ont été le nombre d'accidents et de problèmes de santé qui ont reçu compensation, ainsi qu'une étude de documents menée en 1978. Les dangers pour le système reproducteur des femmes, les problèmes spécifiques des ghettos d'emploi féminins (largement sous-étudiés à l'époque) et les problèmes de conciliation entre le travail et les responsabilités familiales n'ont donc pas été pris en compte dans l'établissement des priorités. Bien que la procédure choisie n'ait pas été explicitement discriminatoire, elle a conduit à une quasi absence des femmes dans les deux catégories d'emplois pour lesquels la prévention est le plus accessible (elles y forment 15 p. 100 de la main-d'oeuvre).[1]

En fait, les risques spécifiques à un sexe ne semblent pas être considérés comme des problèmes légitimes de santé au travail ... si le sexe dont il est question est féminin. Au Québec par exemple, environ un tiers des travailleuses enceintes bénéficient de réaffectations ou de congés temporaires parce que leur travail est incompatible avec une saine grossesse. Dans la presse grand public, cette forte proportion est souvent présentée comme la preuve d'un abus du système et non comme un signe d'un haut niveau de problèmes dans les emplois des femmes.[2] L'Association des entrepreneurs en construction a d'ailleurs protesté contre le fait que ce programme relève de la Commission de santé et sécurité du travail, soutenant que: «être enceinte n'est pas un accident de travail.»[3] L'Institut de recherche en santé et sécurité du travail (IRSST) du Québec semble partager ce point de vue à l'effet que les dangers pour les femmes enceintes ne sont pas de vrais risques professionnels, puisqu'il a exclu cette catégorie de risques de son analyse des problèmes de santé par secteurs d'emploi, sans fournir la moindre justification (le fait n'est indiqué qu'en à-côté, en page 110 du rapport).[4]

De la part des employeurs et des décideurs gouvernementaux, la réticence à reconnaître les facteurs de risques pour la santé des travailleuses semble provenir de leur crainte qu'il s'agisse de problèmes si communs que la moindre reconnaissance pourrait entraîner un déluge de réclamations. Ils n'ont pas entièrement tort. Quand on retarde à reconnaître des risques, les problèmes s'accumulent et s'amplifient. Ce fut le cas de nombreux problèmes de santé des travailleuses. Les problèmes s'amplifient plus encore si aucun programme de prévention n'est mis en place, même après reconnaissance du risque. Par exemple, le programme de retrait préventif de la femme enceinte exposée à un danger ne comporte aucune mesure incitative pour éliminer ce danger puisqu'on a attribué les problèmes à la grossesse et non pas au travail. Ainsi, les mêmes milieux font l'objet de demandes répétées de retrait ou de réaffectation. Quand la travailleuse n'est pas remplacée, ce qui arrive souvent, les collègues et les superviseurs en veulent à la femme enceinte. On commence à penser que ce sont les femmes qui abusent, et non l'employeur.

De la même façon, on blâme les femmes pour l'inquiétude qui a surgi autour des terminaux à écran cathodique. Ceux-ci furent introduits massivement dans les postes de travail des femmes sans vérification préalable des risques pour la grossesse ou pour les problèmes ostéo-articulaires. Les femmes ont protesté, mais il a fallu longtemps avant que les études ne soient faites et des mesures correctives ne soient proposées.

L'actuelle «épidémie» de lésions attribuables au travail répétitif (tendinites, bursites, syndromes du canal carpien) offre un autre exemple des effets du retard dans la prise de conscience des dangers des emplois féminins. Ces problèmes sont la conséquence du caractère répétitif des gestes dans de nombreux emplois traditionnels des femmes, notamment aux chaînes de montage ou dans les emplois de bureau. Le caractère aigu que prend aujourd'hui ce problème n'est pas dû au seul fait qu'on ait reconnu ce risque, mais au fait qu'on ait autrefois tardé à le reconnaître et à mettre en place les correctifs.

Certaines femmes, y compris des féministes, se sont faites complices des tentatives pour camoufler les risques associés aux emplois des femmes, de peur que la reconnaissance des problèmes de santé soit utilisée pour prouver que les femmes sont trop «faibles» pour ces travaux. C'est pour cette raison que certaines féministes ont souvent contesté, par exemple, les recherches sur les effets du travail sur le cycle menstruel; elles se demandent encore si ces recherches ne serviront pas de munition à ceux qui affirment que les femmes ne sont tout simplement pas faites pour le travail. Malgré une documentation de plus en plus abondante sur les effets des conditions de travail comme la chaleur, le froid ou les produits chimiques sur les douleurs menstruelles et sur la régularité du cycle, une récente «mise à jour» de 214 pages, produite par une équipe américaine d'expertes féministes en santé au travail, n'a fait qu'une seule référence aux menstruations: un traitement historique de deux pages sur la question de la compatibilité entre le cycle menstruel et le leadership.[5] Quand des femmes soulèvent des questions sur la sécurité de nos emplois, nous craignons que cela ne remette en cause la place des femmes sur le marché du travail.

Le présent ouvrage s'enscrit dans un processus de reflexion qui ménera à des études sérieuses pour remplacer l'actuel déni et le refus de reconnaître les problèmes des travailleuses. Nous croyons, ainsi que toutes celles qui ont contribué à cette publication, qu'il en va de l'intérêt des travailleuses de décrire avec autant de soin que possible les risques associés aux emplois qu'elles occupent en grande partie, et les risques qui sont associés exclusivement ou principalement aux caractéristiques biologiques et physiques des femmes. Notre expérience nous a montré que le fait de taire les différences entre les sexes ne protège pas contre la discrimination.

Compte tenu de la croyance largement répandue, que le travail des femmes est inoffensif, nous croyons qu'il est important de commencer notre démonstration par une série de chapitres traitant de problèmes de santé propres à divers milieux de travail. L'article de Barbara Neis sur l'asthme dans des usines de traitement de crabes au Québec et à Terre-Neuve trace le portrait d'un problème de santé commun, tout en nous permettant de comprendre les enjeux politiques liés à la reconnaissance de tels problèmes de santé des travailleuses dans le contexte de l'économie chancelante de Terre-Neuve. Le texte de Nicole Vézina sur l'analyse ergonomique des postes divisés selon le sexe dans l'industrie de la transformation alimentaire, et celui de Susan Stock sur l'application de l'épidémiologie et de l'ergonomie dans l'étude des problèmes ostéo-articulaires dans une petite garderie, montrent comment les tâches qui semblent pourtant naturelles pour les femmes engendrent néaumoins des problèmes physiques et de la douleur. D'autres articles, comme le chapitre de Janet Sprout et Annalee Yassi sur les problèmes de santé dans le secteur des services, ou celui de Ellen Balka sur les effets des changements technologiques sur les opératrices de téléphone, esquissent un tableau plus général des situations de stress dans les environnements où travaillent un grand nombre de femmes. Les chapitres de Vivienne Walters et de Lynn Skillen sur le secteur de la santé nous présentent des professions où le soin accordé aux autres résulte en une accumulation de problèmes d'ordre affectif ou physique, avec d'énormes difficultés à faire reconnaître ces risques.

Plusieurs équipes de recherches travaillant dans ce domaine de la santé des travailleuses ont entrepris une remise en question méthodologique des procédures et analyses qui ne tiennent pas compte du genre. La seconde partie de ce livre, sur les enjeux de la recherche-action, présente quelques réponses à ces remises en question. Karen Messing établit la distinction entre les questions d'ordre biologique, les questions de genre et de conditions de travail dans les études sur la santé au travail. Catherine Teiger, une ergonome, a utilisé l'analyse des processus de travail pour permettre aux chercheurs et aux chercheures, ainsi qu'aux travailleuses, de reconnaître certaines composantes méconnues du travail des femmes et de développer des approches qui puissent permettre de réduire la fatigue physique et mentale. À partir de son expérience dans l'étude des origines sociales des problèmes au travail, Lucie Dumais soulève des questions relevant de l'analyse interdisciplinaire, concernant la collaboration entre sociologues, spécialistes de la santé au travail et syndicalistes. Lors des travaux d'un comité sur les effets du travail sur la santé mentale, Donna Mergler a été au coeur d'un débat sur le mode d'analyse des données selon le sexe; sa position méthodologique est présentée ici. Danièle Kergoat, une pionnière dans la reconnaissance de la division sexuelle du travail en France, termine cette section avec une perspective historique sur le processus difficile qui conduit à l'intégration des préoccupations des femmes dans la sociologie du travail.

La dernière partie porte sur les expériences en matière de politiques publiques, dans le secteur de la santé au travail des femmes. Katherine Lippel, spécialiste en droit, a comparé les décisions de la Commission sur la santé et la sécurité du travail du Québec et celles du tribunal d'appel, concernant les demandes de compensation relatives à des situations de stress, pour les hommes et pour les femmes. Son analyse révèle à quel point les situations de travail des hommes et des femmes sont perçues différemment par les responsables de la compensation. Nicolette Carlan, directrice d'un comité provincial en santé et sécurité au travail, décrit les difficultés rencontrées par ce comité, lorsqu'il a tenté de colliger l'information sur les problèmes de santé des travailleuses, afin de permettre la mise en place de nouvelles mesures. Joan Stevenson, spécialiste en biomécanique, démontre comment certains détails dans les tests pré-embauche de la force physique, rendent ces tests injustes envers les femmes, et guère utiles pour prédire qui pourra effectuer le travail de manière sécuritaire. Dorothy Wigmore, chercheure et militante syndicale de longue date, a réuni beaucoup d'information sur les approches utilisées et requises pour traiter de la violence contre les travailleuses. Eakin a mis en évidence des façons différentes d'aborder les problèmes de santé et de sécurité dans les milieux de travail de petite taille, ce qui est d'un grand intérêt ici dans la mesure où les femmes sont largement sur-représentées dans ces petites unités. Cette partie et la publication se terminent sur une note prospective, alors qu'Armstrong examine les effets des transformations dans le marché du travail pour les femmes et pour les hommes.

Le contenu de ce livre reflète une diversité d'approches parce que nous croyons qu'il est très important de profiter de l'apport de plusieurs disciplines. Historiquement, des médecins[6], des chimistes[7] et des sociologues[8] ont contribué de façon importante à l'étude des problèmes de santé des travailleuses. Dans ce volume, des spécialistes des sciences sociales fournissent des analyses de première importance sur la division sexuelle et sociale du travail (Armstrong, Eakin, Kergoat, Walters), sur la relation des femmes avec la technologie (Balka) et sur les dimensions sociales qui empêchent la reconnaissance des facteurs de risque pour la santé des travailleuses (Carlan, Lippel, Neis). Elles posent aussi des questions plus générales sur la définition des problèmes et l'élaboration des solutions dans le domaine de la santé au travail (Dumais). Ces réflexions sont essentielles si l'on veut comprendre pourquoi les femmes sont assignées à certaines tâches, et si l'on veut développer des solutions sociales autant que techniques à leurs problèmes de santé. C'est dans le contexte ainsi défini par les sciences sociales que les chercheures en sciences médicales, en biologie et en ergonomie (Mergler, Messing, Skillen, Sprout, Stevenson, Stock, Teiger, Vézina, Wigmore et Yassi) peuvent ensuite discuter les interactions entre le corps des femmes, leur esprit, et leur environnement de travail.

Ce qui caractérise les femmes qui ont collaboré à ce livre, c'est leur volonté d'améliorer la condition des travailleuses. Nous espérons fournir des analyses précises non seulement pour le plaisir de mener des recherches de haute qualité, mais aussi pour orienter l'action, dans les milieux de travail. Pour cette raison, nous avons invité des décideurs en matière de santé au travail et des responsables syndicaux et patronaux à se joindre à nous quand nous avons discuté de nos articles.

Récemment, à la suite d'une conférence sur la santé des travailleuses de la Fédération du travail de l'Ontario, nous avons reçu une lettre d'une travailleuse en métallurgie qui décrivait plusieurs problèmes rencontrées par ces travailleuses:

J'ai rempli une réclamation pour la destruction de mes genoux sous l'effet des vibrations, parce que je travaille de longues heures sur un plancher qui vibre. On m'a suggéré que, à cause de mon âge, le niveau de calcium ou son insuffisance dans mes jambes, pouvait être en cause et que, peut-être, une femme de mon âge ne devrait pas être envoyée ici ... Présentement, il n'y a, dans les comités de révision du Bureau de compensation des travailleurs, aucune femme médecin qui puisse contrebalancer n'importe quelle de leurs décisions. Avant qu'une femme réussisse à mener sa bataille à travers une panoplie d'avocats mâles qui ne la croient pas, de toute façon, pour être ensuite confrontée à ces «old boys», elle commence à douter de la justesse de sa réclamation ...

— Mme Carrie Chenier, Métallurgistes Unis d'Amérique

Nous espérons qu'un jour les travailleuses comme Mme Chenier n'auront plus à accepter la responsabilité de leurs problèmes de santé et de sécurité ... sous prétexte qu'elles ne sont pas de jeunes hommes. Selon ce que nous entendons lors de nos rencontres avec des travailleuses, elles sont déjà en train de changer les priorités et les orientations des systèmes de prévention et de compensation, en matière de santé et sécurité au travail. Nous espérons que nos recherches contribueront à maintenir ce processus de changement.

Karen Messing
Barbara Neis
Lucie Dumais

NOTES

1. Les causes et conséquences de cette exclusion des travailleuses des premiers groupes prioritaires de la CSST sont analysées plus en détail dans: CINBIOSE, *Quand le travail léger pèse lourd. Vers une nouvelle approche en prévention dans les emplois des femmes*, (Montréal, Centre pour l'étude des interactions biologiques entre la santé et l'environnement, 1995), rapport présenté aux Comités de la condition féminine de la Centrale des enseignantes et des enseignants du Québec, de la Confédération des syndicats nationaux et de la Fédération des travailleurs et des travailleuses du Québec.

2. Lire, par exemple: Beaulieu, C., «Les travailleuses enceintes perdent leur El Dorado», *Le Devoir* (le 29 juillet 1988).

3. Blanchard, S., «Les entrepreneurs en construction exigent la revision de la «coûteuse» CSST», *Le Devoir* (le 28 février 1992), p. A3

4. Hébert, F., *L'inégalité des risques affectant la sécurité des travailleurs par secteur d'activité en 1986*, (Montréal: IRSST, 1994).

5. Headapohl, D.M. (éd.), "Occupational Medicine: Woman Workers," *Occupational Health: State of the Art Reviews* 8, 4 (1993), pp. 800-1.

6. Hamilton, Alice, *Exploring the Dangerous Trades*, (Boston: Little, Brown, 1943).

7. Stellman, Jeanne, *Women's Work, Women's Health*, (New York: Pantheon, 1978).

8. Hochschild, Arlie R., *The Managed Heart*, (Berkeley: University of California Press, 1983).

Making Risks Visible in Women's Jobs

Rendre visibles les risques du travail des femmes

Barbara Neis

Can't Get My Breath
Snow Crab Workers' Occupational Asthma

Utilisant une approche comparative d'études de cas de l'asthme du crabe des neiges à Terre-Neuve et au Labrador et au Québec, cet article vise à améliorer notre compréhension des dangers du travail menaçant la santé respiratoire des femmes. La majorité des travailleurs de l'industrie du crabe sont des femmes, et la plupart des travailleurs atteints par la maladie de l'asthme semblent être des femmes. L'analyse se base sur des données de première main recueillies par observations et par entretiens à Terre-Neuve et au Labrador, alors qu'au Québec on a plutôt réalisé une revue de littérature complétée par des entretiens téléphoniques. Bien que les premières recherches sur l'asthme du crabe des neiges aient été effectuées à Terre-Neuve, il y a eu peu de débats publics ou de recherches sur la question. Les institutions (gouvernements, entreprises) ont agi en fonction de cas particuliers plutôt que par mesure de prévention. Il y a peu de professionnelles de la santé ayant une formation adéquate dans le domaine de l'asthme comme maladie professionnelle pour desservir les travailleuses présentant des symptômes. Celles qui sont atteintes par la maladie continuent de travailler, fondant leur décision sur le fait que la saison de travail est courte; elles absorbent des médicaments pendant cette période. Très peu de travailleuses ont reçues une compensation. En comparaison, au Québec, les institutions ont rapidement réagi à la découverte de la maladie en faisant de la prévention et de la recherche. Cela semble avoir réduit considérablement le nombre de personnes atteintes de la maladie. Dans les deux provinces, l'industrie de la pêche au crabe a connu une expansion depuis la crise des pêcheries de fonds. Cela a augmenté le nombre de travailleuses exposées à des risques en même temps que les possibilités d'emplois alternatifs baissaient. En résulte une hausse du nombre de travailleuses qui, malgré leurs symptômes, continuent de travailler et sont réticentes à rapporter leurs problèmes de santé aux autorités publiques.

This article uses a comparative case study of snow crab workers' asthma in Newfoundland and Labrador and Quebec to contribute to our understanding of occupational threats to women's respiratory health. A majority of snow crab processing workers are women and women appear to predominate among workers with snow crab asthma symptoms. The article draws on primary data collected through observation and interviews in Newfoundland and Labrador and, for the Quebec case, a review of research reports and publications, updated with phone interviews. Although some of the first research on snow crab asthma was carried out in Newfoundland, there has been little public reocgnition of this occupational disease and no organized effort to either study it or minimize incidence. Institutional response has taken the form of secondary rather than primary prevention and workers with symptoms appear to have limited access to health professionals with adequate training in occupational asthma. Affected workers often continue to work, relying on the seasonality of the industry and medication to manage their symptoms. Few have access to Workers' Compensation benefits for time loss or disability. In contrast, institutional response to the discovery of snow crab asthma in Quebec included research and primary prevention-related initiatives. These appear to have significantly reduced incidence in that province. Snow crab processing has expanded in both provinces since the collapse of the groundfish stocks. Resulting reduced employment alternatives may be contributing to increased under-reporting and "managing" with medication among crab processing workers in both provinces.

INTRODUCTION

The threat organic allergens and chemical irritants pose to women's occupational health appears to be one of the many areas of women's work where substantive research is lacking (Messing, 1991). I have argued elsewhere that fish processing workers in Newfoundland and Labrador are exposed to a broad spectrum of work-related health risks (Neis, 1994). Research confirms that similar risks exist in other provinces and countries (Messing and Reveret, 1983; Baldursson, 1984; Plouffe et al., 1989). The percentage of female fish processing workers varies significantly from place to place and sector to sector. One sector that has a particularly high percentage of female workers is snow crab processing[1] (Dave Lewis, Personal Communication; Equipe de Santé, 1983). Snow crab occupational asthma (OA) represents a significant threat to the occupational health of these workers.

Although data on the incidence of snow crab OA by gender are elusive, existing research suggests that a majority of sufferers from this occupational disease are women (Malo et al., 1992). Thousands of women in Atlantic Canada work processing snow crab and the numbers are on the increase. In the early 1980s, there were an estimated 1,083 crab processing workers in Quebec (Equipe de Santé, 1984). This number may have increased with the recent opening of new crab processing plants on the Lower North Shore. In Newfoundland and Labrador, the first dedicated snow crab production lines were established as early as 1971-72 (Department of Fisheries and Oceans, 1992). Crab production increased from 2.4 million kilograms in 1986 to 6.3 million kilograms in 1992. By 1993, there were an estimated 4,025 crab processing workers in the province (personal communication, Policy Analyst, Provincial Department of Fisheries). There are also some snow crab processing workers in New Brunswick.

By focusing on snow crab workers' OA, this paper contributes to our knowledge of occupational threats to women's respiratory health. A review of the literature on OA identified no research primarily concerned with the gender-related impacts of this occupational disease. One study noted that while a family doctor's diagnosis of asthma is an important indicator of OA, after 40 years of age, the label "asthmatic" is more likely to be applied to women than to men with similar symptoms (Dodge and Burrows, 1980). In other words, there appears to be a "diagnostic bias" related to gender among physicians. Research on socioeconomic impacts of OA has found that women may be more likely than men to report unemployment and limitation in everyday activities (Venables et al., 1989). Some research exists on different forms of crab OA. A recent American study of primarily female, blue crab processing workers found a "healthy worker effect" (i.e. a tendency for workers with respiratory symptoms to leave their jobs) but noted that this effect was limited among older, skilled black female workers with few employment alternatives (Mundt, 1990). Research on snow crab asthma has noted that women are overrepresented among the studied population with crab asthma, whereas men are overrepresented among the studied population with red cedar asthma making it difficult to separate the effects of agents from those of gender (Malo et al., 1992). Findings from research among snow crab processing workers on the Magdalen Islands and in the Gaspé region are not broken down by sex (Auger et al., 1984). I have encountered no research that has examined the relationship between OA and pregnancy.

This paper draws on the general literature on OA as well as literature specific to snow crab OA to discuss causes, symptoms, diagnosis, incidence, socioeconomic impacts, prevention and compensation. The analysis, developed around a comparative case study of crab workers' OA in Quebec and Newfoundland and Labrador, will explore some of the social, regulatory and technical factors that influence not only incidence, but also prevention and compensation for workers.

Data for the comparative case study are drawn from two sources: published Quebec research carried out in the 1980s, which was updated using phone interviews with researchers and medical professionals; and research in Newfoundland and Labrador that was carried out in 1993 and 1994. This research involved observations in four crab plants combined with interviews with workers, management, and medical and occupational health professionals.[2] Because the Newfoundland and Labrador research was interview-based and did not include diagnoses of crab workers' OA, the summary of these research findings refers to workers with "asthma-like" symptoms. Where diagnoses are mentioned, these refer to diagnoses by local medical professionals independent of the research.

SNOW CRAB OA
Causes and Symptoms

Asthma involves a reversible obstruction of the air passages resulting in difficult breathing. "During an attack of asthma, air is easily inhaled, but not easily exhaled. The result is that with each inhalation, more air is trapped in the lungs, which become overstretched. Asthmatic people require visible effort to breathe. With the narrowing of the airways, the simple act of breathing becomes very difficult" (Bertolini, 1987:1). Illness and death due to asthma appear to be on the increase at a global level. There is also evidence that it is underdiagnosed and undertreated (Hargreave et al., 1990).

Occupational asthma (OA) is any asthma that is work-related. Definitions of OA depend in part on how they are being used (Merchant, 1990). A relatively simple definition is "an asthmatic syndrome caused by exposure to specific occupational agents such as chemicals, fumes and dusts," some of which are well-recognized and others obscure (Smith, 1990:1007). OA is the most common occupational respiratory ailment in developed countries (Malo and Cartier, 1993). It has now displaced asbestosis and silicosis, associated with traditional male occupations like mining, from their position of dominance within this category (Malo, 1990; Malo and Cartier, 1993). Over 300 causal agents for OA have been identified (Chan-Yeung, 1990).

OA can have immunologic or nonimmunologic origins. Allergic asthma is immunologic and involves a bodily response to alien substances or microbes that results in the production of antibodies. Although normally good, antibodies can respond in a wrong way, causing asthma and other allergies. Nonimmunologic or irritant-induced OA may occur after acute exposure to a significant concentration of gas or a fume. This is generally referred to as Reactive Airways Disease Syndrome (RADS). Irritant-induced asthma may also occur after repeated exposure to an industrial chemical (Bertolini, 1987; Malo and Cartier, 1993). Snow crab OA is known to have immunologic origins although one relatively early study raised the possibility that it might have a nonimmunologic dimension. Guillot (1984) noted that some snow crab workers experience irritation in the upper respiratory tract and that crab OA appears to be linked to several sources of exposure, including steam and warm, cooked crab. He found that the pH of water used to cook crab increased with cooking time. An analysis of this water found ammonia, trimethylamine, dimethylamine and methylamine. A number of other elements were also present at much lower concentrations including some aromatic amines such as pyridine.

One possibility, not discussed in the literature, is that there is a relationship between the irritant effect of exposure to the chemical irritants in the cooking water/steam and the development of crab asthma through sensitization to an allergen. Guillot's *in vitro* studies suggest that the chemicals might inhibit the capacity of the lungs to respond to attacks by foreign bodies and to remove dust particles penetrating the upper respiratory tract, thus allowing deeper penetration of allergens into the lung and increasing the risk of sensitization to the snow crab allergen. The irritant effects of the cooking water chemicals could be exacerbated by periodic exposure to high levels of other chemical irritants like ammonia and chlorine. This sometimes occurs in crab plants (Neis, 1994; Report, 1978).

There are two main classes of asthmatic reaction: immediate and non-immediate. Immediate asthmatic reactions come on in minutes and last one-and-one-half to two hours. The relationship to causal exposure is evident and can be reversed by bronchodilators and blocked by sodium cromoglycate but not by corticosteroids.

Non-immediate asthmatic reactions can take several forms. They can come on slowly after one hour and last about five; they can come on after several hours, peak at five to eight hours and last about a day; or they can come on in the early hours of the morning, recur without further exposure at the same time each night for several to many nights, and may not improve for some time after cessation of exposure. Immediate and non-immediate patterns of reaction can also occur together (Bertolini, 1987).

Sufferers with snow crab OA can have three different patterns of response: immediate, late and combined. Symptoms include attacks of difficult breathing, tightness of the chest, coughing, wheezing and other breathing sounds associated with air-flow obstruction. These symptoms are typically worse during working days and may wake sufferers at night, but improve when the workers are away from work. However, chest symptoms may persist when workers are exposed to irritants outside of work. Itchy and watery eyes, sneezing, stuffy and runny nose, and skin rashes are also often associated with crab workers' OA (Bertolini, 1989; Mundt, 1990). Some workers develop "leukocytosis and fever" which suggests that "either another type of immunologic response plays a role in these reactions or that the antibody response is not relevant in some workers" (Cartier et al., 1984:268). Other symptoms reported by some crab processing workers include sore throats and laryngitis.

Hughson (1992:707) argues that "[t]he inherent variability of OA and the importance of individual susceptibility make this a difficult subject for epidemiologic study ... More information is needed concerning the use of diagnostic tests, the frequency of OA, and the degree of risk associated with occupational exposures." The development and nature of OA is influenced by three main factors: (1) the immunological reactivity of the subject; (2) the nature of the causal agents; and (3) the circumstances of exposure. Predisposing factors include the level and duration of exposure, and the properties of the agents. They also include, however, such individual variations as the ability of some people to produce abnormal amounts of IgE antibodies. The effect of smoking is controversial (Malo et al., 1992). Some argue it has been shown to increase the risk of developing OA, with some suggestion that this smoking must take place at the time of exposure. Smoking may also shorten the interval between first exposure and the onset of sensitization (Burge, 1991). Chan-Yeung and Lam (1986:696) argue that "although smoking may increase the prevalence of sensitization, there is little evidence to suggest that smokers are more predisposed to asthma."

A recent retrospective study of workers with OA found that subjects exposed to snow crab antigens tend to develop symptoms after a longer period than those exposed to chemical allergens (Malo et al., 1992). Existing research suggests that snow crab OA may develop any time from a few weeks to several years after initial exposure, but most cases seem to develop in six to 12 months (Bertolini, 1989). As with all agents, continuous exposure and concentration of exposure lead to earlier development of symptoms.

Diagnosis

There are two basic steps to diagnosing OA: to establish the diagnosis of asthma; and then to establish that the asthma is the result of occupational exposure.

The questionnaire is the most basic tool used in both epidemiological surveys and individual assessments. Although the questionnaire is useful, biases can influence results, with possible exaggeration occurring where OA is well compensated and underreporting occurring where it is not (Malo and Cartier, 1993). It is extremely important that the questionnaire yield a careful occupational history that includes accounts of potential exposures at home, in the workplace and the community, and the pattern of asthma associated with these exposures (Merchant, 1990). The work environment history must include information on the materials handled by the worker and co-workers, symptoms, onset in relationship to materials, etc. It should also include questions documenting the full range of exposures and date of commencement of the asthma. It is important that the patient be assessed as soon as possible, and that the patient remain on the job until the diagnosis is confirmed.

So-called "objective measures" are considered necessary in diagnosing OA and assessing disability. For instance, airflow obstruction reversed by treatment with bronchodilators or steroids should be demonstrated. In the case of high molecular weight agents like the crab allergen, allergy skin tests might be appropriate. Objective measures should also include, where possible, specific challenge or exposure tests. Challenge tests should mimic the workplace concentration as closely as possible. A negative challenge test, while important, cannot exclude the diagnosis of OA because it may reflect prolonged absence from the workplace and reduced sensitivity to the agent. In addition, the asthma may be caused by another agent and "the method of a challenge test may not be correct for the particular offending agent. In the laboratory it is often very difficult to reproduce exactly the same process as in the workplace" (Chan-Yeung, 1990:817). Although the challenge test has been treated as the "gold standard" in confirming diagnosis, it is not suitable for subjects with moderate or severe airway obstruction or patients on drugs or with upper respiratory infection. Drugs should be discontinued 24 hours prior to challenge testing (Smith, 1990).[3]

Calculating Incidence

When possible, snow crab OA should be confirmed using objective confirmation of work-relatedness (DeWitte et al., 1994). The total number of cases of crab workers' OA is not known and incidence varies from plant to plant (Bertolini, 1989). The only research on snow crab OA that has achieved something akin to an ideal methodology was carried out in Quebec in the early 1980s. This research estimated the incidence of the disease at around 15 percent of workers after three years of exposure in two plants with poor enclosure of cooking pots, poor ventilation and exposure to warm crab meat (Cartier et al., 1984). A comparative study of crab, lobster and shrimp processing workers carried out in the same area and around the same time found a much higher incidence of respiratory symptoms among crab processing workers than among those working with the other crustaceans (Auger et al., 1984). The original intent of this latter study was to establish the incidence of respiratory problems among workers processing crustaceans (crab, lobster, shrimp) in the Magdalen Islands and the Gaspé region. However, researchers failed to contact all of the workers (Auger et al., 1984).[4]

Recent research suggests that in some plants in Newfoundland and Labrador, incidence levels could be as high today as those identified in Quebec in the early 1980s. As recommended by the Quebec researchers, cooking areas had been contained to varying degrees in four plants observed in 1993 and 1994. However, some workers in these plants have now been working with crab for up to 10 or 12 years (longer than in the Quebec research) and several plants have reported outbreaks of asthma-like symptoms among workers in recent years. These outbreaks coincided with technological and other changes that may have increased exposure to the allergen.

Incidence can be influenced by the level of concentration of the causal agent (Hughson, 1992; Malo and Cartier, 1993). It can vary between workplaces, partly because concentration and exposure are linked to processing techniques and technology: the same allergen may be more or less hazardous depending on the form of delivery. For example, allergens in steam, powder or aerosol form may be much more problematic than allergens in the form of dust or chemicals (Pepys, 1982; O'Hollaren, 1992). Prawn-induced OA symptoms increased dramatically when air jet technology was used to remove prawn from the shells but declined when a water jet system was introduced (Gaddie et al., 1980).

New uncontained technologies introduced in the 1990s into some crab processing plants in Newfoundland and Labrador may have increased exposure to the allergen in respirable form. These technologies include a rotating drum that automates removal of meat from the knuckles and shoulders using high pressure water jets. The drum is attached to a shaker that separates the meat fragments from the water. In two plants visited, the introduction of these technologies coincided with outbreaks of asthma-like symptoms in workers who claim to have been previously asymptomatic. In both cases, renovations associated with the introduction of these new technologies reduced ventilation. These technologies may be increasing the amount of the allergen that is solubilized in water. If ventilation is not adequate, this solubilized allergen could be accumulating in water vapour in the plant atmosphere.

The temperature of the crab meat has also been found to be associated with the incidence of OA-like symptoms (Forest et al., 1984). Meat should be cooled after cooking and kept cool during processing. If the water used in the drum and shaker is not cold enough, it can raise the temperature of the crab meat, thus increasing the risk of exposure to the allergen among workers. By speeding up production, new technologies can also increase severalfold the volume of crab processed on a shift and hence the volume of allergen passing through the plant. Workers in two plants where outbreaks have occurred described periods when mist was so thick in the plant you could hardly see the worker next to you. Similar conditions are reported to have existed in Quebec when the outbreaks occurred which prompted the early 1980s research (Chagnon, personal communication).

Exposure is related not only to technologies and to the volume of production, but also to the length of shifts and work weeks. In the 1990s, the quota system for managing crab harvesting in Newfoundland and Labrador seems to have contributed to a reduction in the length of the crab fishing season while prolonging shifts and work weeks. Workers in one plant reported 11 to 12 hour days, from 7:30 in the morning until 7:00 at night, with only two or three 15 minute breaks and a half hour lunch during the busiest weeks. Six day weeks were common.[5]

Estimates of incidence need to take account of the "healthy worker effect." As noted above, Mundt (1990) found that those with allergic symptoms were more likely to leave jobs than those who remained.[6] None of the existing studies of snow crab OA in either Newfoundland and Labrador or in Quebec have traced all former workers. Mundt (1990) also hypothesizes that factors other than health, including limited employment alternatives, can play a key role in asthmatic workers' reactions to their illness, particularly among marginal workers. Similar constraints may well apply among the primarily female snow crab processing workers in rural, single-industry communities in Atlantic Canada. A "healthy worker effect," if it exists among snow crab workers, may be most common among mobile, younger workers, and workers who have become so ill they are barred from the plant. During interviews in one community, several young people were reported to have found they became ill at the plant and to have failed to return because of this.[7] Several other older workers with severe asthma-like symptoms continued working at the plant, perhaps because of limited employment opportunities and a greater commitment (years and skill) to this particular form of employment and to their communities (home ownership and young children). In the two plants where it was possible to do more in-depth research, some who developed asthma-like symptoms were eventually forced to give up their jobs because of the symptoms. Evidence of a "healthy worker effect" suggests that incidence figures based on an examination of the workers who remain at work may underestimate the true incidence of this condition.

Research on incidence also needs to take into account other factors that might be influencing whether or not symptomatic workers remain in their jobs. In Newfoundland and Labrador, there is anecdotal evidence of employer intimidation and dismissal of workers with symptoms. Dr. Edstrom (chairperson of the 1978 Task Force) reports that when the study was completed, the plant owner told him that if he "didn't provide him with information about the individual patients who had this problem that he would fire all the staff and re-hire again." This information was not provided. In a phone interview, a worker at this plant reported that after the study, several workers were not called back to work. This evidence suggests that workers, particularly those in non-unionized plants, might be attempting to hide their symptoms from other workers, employers and perhaps local medical personnel for fear of losing their jobs. It also suggests that employers might be monitoring their workers for symptoms and failing to recall those they feel might end up applying for compensation at the start of new seasons.

Finally, drug usage by workers with asthma-like symptoms could be masking the prevalence of the disease, particularly if these drugs are not prescribed by local physicians. In both Newfoundland and Labrador and Quebec, some medical officers reported anecdotal evidence of inhaler or so-called "puffer" (bronchodilator) sharing among some workers and referred to workers who had gotten their "puffers" outside their communities (Chrétien, personal communication).

Socioeconomic and Health Effects of OA

Existing research has documented significant physical, mental and socio-economic effects of OA. Such effects include: continued symptoms and continued medication dependency after the elimination of exposure; hospital admission; depression; interference with sexual activity and marital relationship; unemployment; loss of income; and significant limitations on daily activities (Venables et al., 1989).

The long-term health consequences of OA require more research. There now exist several follow-up studies that suggest a majority of workers do not recover completely several years after removal from exposure (Chan-Yeung, 1987; 1990; Malo et al., 1992). This pattern cannot be explained by selectivity among follow-up patients. In some individuals, "exposure to the offending agents permanently alters the responsiveness of their airways" (Chan-Yeung, 1990:819). Lower susceptibility to long-term symptoms seems to be linked to earlier diagnosis and earlier removal. According to one recent study, older workers with longer duration of symptoms and longer duration of exposure prior to claim have the worst prognoses (Yassi, 1988).

The length of time required for improvement after cessation of exposure among workers with crab OA has been studied in Quebec (Malo et al., 1988). Follow up with these workers occurred at one, two and five years after they had left work; none of the subjects had been exposed to or eaten crab since the time of diagnosis. This study found that most subjects were still symptomatic of asthma at the time of the follow-up, but the authors noted that this finding is based on questionnaire results which may have been biased because subjects knew responses might be used for compensation. Crab workers who had worked for a longer time after the onset of symptoms were more likely to remain symptomatic than those who had left earlier (Hudson et al., 1985). In general, the prognosis for those with snow crab OA worsens with increased duration of exposure, increased duration of exposure after onset of symptoms, and increased severity of the asthma when they are removed (Malo and Cartier, 1993).

Workers may not be immune to the health effects of crab OA even after they quit their jobs. In one plant in Newfoundland and Labrador, two workers claimed they were so sensitized to the crab allergen that symptoms could be triggered by exposure to the clothes of family members who work in the plant. Cross-reactivity with other shellfish meant one woman could neither prepare nor consume seafood products encountered in her new workplace.

Chan-Yeung (1987;1990) notes that evidence of long-term symptoms raises the issue of compensation for permanent disability. On the basis of their follow-up study of workers with snow crab OA, Malo et al. (1988) concluded that: (1) compensation should be given to sujects with OA if permanent impairment and disability are documented; (2) the criteria for compensation should be need for medication and level of bronchial obstruction and hyperresponsiveness; (3) optimal timing for assessment for compensation would be two years after removal from work, when workers with OA tend to plateau.

The mental health consequences of continuing at a job that you feel is making you sick must also be considered. In Newfoundland and Labrador, crab processing workers with symptoms described collapsing on the job and ending up at the hospital; and having to go outside during their shift or on their break to breathe in and out in a struggle to get enough air. One woman said she began to cry when she could not get enough air and eventually had to go home. Another commented: "I guess I hated the thought of having to get up and go to work knowing you were going to get sicker and sicker every time you went in there." In a plant with several diagnosed cases, workers seemed fatalistic about the illness, believing that they would eventually develop it. This fear may translate, in some cases, into the belief that they have crab asthma despite contrary medical evidence. One source reports "mass hysteria" among otherwise asymptomatic workers during some outbreaks (Report, 1978).

Female workers in Newfoundland and Labrador are reported to time their pregnancies so that they will be pregnant while at work during the summers and have their births the following winter so they will have a few months to be with the baby before going back to work. The possible impact of pregnancy on susceptibility to snow crab OA, as well as possible effects of OA and OA medication on fetuses, needs to be explored. Pregnant women were excluded from research on snow crab asthma, so nothing is known about the possible relationship between maternal exposure and fetal exposure (Cartier, et al., 1984). Pregnancy could influence exposure, since pregnant women take in more air and hence more toxins (Messing, 1991:14). Exposure assessments are relatively loose in existing research — in most cases, exposure is linked to job category. Nothing appears to be known about the relationship between the intensity of work, exposure and risk. Pregnancy might also influence women's immunity, particularly in a population that is socioeconomically marginal and has poor nutrition. This could increase the risk of developing crab workers' OA.

The socioeconomic and other impacts of OA are significant. Twenty-eight percent of 154 claimants for OA in Ontario between 1975 and 1981 were granted a permanent disability award by Workers' Compensation. Seventy-seven percent of those with occupational respiratory allergies had left their employment and at least three quarters attributed the move to their allergic condition. Of those who left, only 57 percent eventually found work (Yassi, 1988). Venables et al. (1989:440) conclude that "[p]atients with occupational asthma are usually previously healthy young adults with families and financial commitments ... [It entails a major life change that] ... can lead to anxiety and depression which further increase the handicap." This life change often includes leaving a well-paying job where they have accumulated years of seniority and/or expertise (Yassi, 1988).

More research is needed on the socioeconomic consequences of snow crab OA. The impact of job loss can be devastating for workers living in small rural communities. One worker had given up her job at the plant three times before the local medical officer finally wrote a note forbidding the plant to rehire her. She was fortunate enough to find alternative work in the community but the wages are significantly lower and she finds she misses the company and camaraderie of the plant. Another woman, who had left the plant rather than "develop asthma" (she was already having symptoms and using a bronchodilator) was unemployed at the time of the interview. A third had started up a small sewing business but was finding it almost impossible to manage financially on the small income it generated. Loss of her income from the plant was a major blow to the household.

There are also socioeconomic impacts for workers who remain at their jobs. None of those interviewed in Newfoundland and Labrador were entitled to sick pay, and time off work could jeopardize their access to unemployment insurance (UI) earnings as well as reduce the amount they would receive on UI should they qualify. In a recent outbreak of asthma-like symptoms in one of the plants, the woman with the most severe case was reported to have been hospitalized on intravenous respiratory drugs and an oxygen mask for some weeks. She lost several weeks' work due to her symptoms and, as a result, was ineligible for UI.

The short-term and, for some, long-term costs of medication also must be noted. Most workers probably do not have health plans. This means they must pay for their own bronchodilators and steroids, which can cost over 20 dollars for Ventolin and as much as 90 dollars a month for the more expensive medications. In short, a diagnosis of OA can have considerable medical, personal, social and financial consequences (Dewitte et al., 1994).

Prevention

The negative impacts of OA highlight the importance of prevention. Venables (1992) argues that prevention can be grouped into primary, secondary and tertiary preventive activities. Primary prevention refers to controlling exposures; secondary prevention refers to detection of asthma early enough to minimize impairment and disability; and tertiary prevention refers to the provision of good quality medical care to patients with asthma.

Primary prevention, or controlling exposures, depends on recognition that there are two causal pathways to occupational asthma: exposure to a sensitizing agent; and heavy exposure to an inhaled irritant known to produce RADS "which can occur within minutes to hours after high-level exposure to pulmonary irritants and is characterized by recurrent attacks of bronchoconstriction thereafter" (Hughson, 1992:706; see also Smith, 1990).[8] Relatively little is known about irritant-induced asthma and many allergens are capable of being irritants (Pepys, 1982; Venables, 1992). The threshold limit values (TLVs) of exposure capable of sensitization are much lower and more difficult to establish for allergens than for irritants (Mathews, 1985). Some argue that setting TLVs and monitoring workers for symptoms doesn't work for allergens because: (1) there is no known "safe" level of exposure; (2) sensitization is irreversible; and (3) sensitization can be a crippling or even a fatal experience (Mathews, 1985: 369). Once sensitized, the amounts needed to elicit the response are small (Pepys, 1982: 534). This is why primary prevention is key.

Effective primary prevention is linked to the presence of an institutional basis for prompt and effective response to identification of the presence of an occupational health problem. There are at least 15 different measures that can be applied to primary prevention of occupational asthma: "elimination, substitution, isolation, enclosure, ventilation, process change, product change, housekeeping, dust suppression, maintenance, sanitation, work practices, personal protective devices, waste disposal practices, and administrative controls" (Venables, 1992:817). However, as Venables argues, in order for these to be applied, education, labelling, warning systems, environmental monitoring and management programmes need to be in place. Where substitution is not possible, as in the case of crab processing, levels of exposure and numbers of workers exposed can be reduced. This may require costly changes to workplace layouts, such as enclosing areas where contaminants are released. Personal protective equipment is the least useful form of prevention because it must be handled "obsessionally to prevent exposure during gowning up and de-gowning" (Burge, 1991:228). Protective equipment may work, but it needs to be assessed for each condition and workers need to be monitored closely for deterioration (Chan-Yeung, 1990). Personal protection is only really applicable with "highly motivated workers in high risk situations" (Burge, 1982-83:108).

Secondary prevention can be as limited as waiting for notification by a patient's general practitioner, or as active as detailed screening procedures. It depends on identifying the source of exposure, early diagnosis, prompt removal from exposure and screening others at risk. The Canadian Thoracic Society's Ad Hoc Committee on Occupational Asthma recently argued that first level prevention should be encouraged by provincial and federal occupational health and safety authorities, and that every effort should be made to identify industries with known causes of asthma and advise them of the risk to workers. They argued against reliance on periodic screening, pre-employment screening or measures of airway responsiveness (Ad Hoc, 1989:1032).

A COMPARISON STUDY OF SNOW CRAB OA IN QUEBEC AND IN NEWFOUNDLAND AND LABRADOR

The following section compares the institutional basis for prevention, diagnosis and compensation of snow crab OA in Quebec with that in Newfoundland and Labrador.

In Quebec, the Community Health Department of the Centre Hospitalier Hotel-Dieu de Gaspé used the mandate given such departments under Chapter 63 of the Occupational Health and Safety Act as the rationale for launching a multidisciplinary study of crab asthma in response to outbreaks among workers there in 1981 (Auger et al., 1984). They developed: a multiphase study intended to identify the nature of the health problem, its causes, incidence, and effective diagnosis; recommendations for changes in work places designed to minimize exposure; and a follow-up study to examine, on a plant-by-plant basis, the relationship between certain causal factors (including the temperature of crab meat at the saws, as well as plant design, lay-out and ventilation) and the presence of respiratory symptoms (Chagnon, et al., 1985). They also developed a protocol for medico-environmental surveillance related to crab asthma, although it is not clear whether this has been followed in recent years or whether the infrastructural support necessary for its implementation exists in all areas where crab are now processed.

In most cases, the recommendations of the Quebec research involved bringing production facilities in line with ventilation and other requirements already contained in Chapter 9 of Quebec's Law on agricultural products, marine products and foods (Province de Québec: 125 ff). Improved ventilation and cooling of the crab are reported to have been enough to stop the reappearance of symptoms in Quebec plants in the mid-1980s. A follow-up study found that respiratory symptoms were significantly less common in plants with these changes than in those without (Chagnon et al., 1985). The subsequent development of snow crab workers' asthma in a further eight workers may, however, reflect the persistence of problems (Cartier et al., 1986). It is possible that earlier higher level exposures were responsible in these cases. However, new cases are still developing. One doctor I interviewed attributed these new cases to new workers with a predisposition to crab asthma. Another suggested that the incidence of crab asthma is significantly higher than is reflected in current reports due to underreporting and workers avoiding doctors knowledgeable about the disease. He attributed new cases to working conditions rather than "predisposition."

Snow crab workers diagnosed with OA in Quebec are supposed to be treated as unfit for work in their current job, making them eligible for compensation. In 1984 and 1985, 50 cases were accepted by workers' compensation. Since that time, numbers have declined so that only four cases were accepted in 1986, 14 in 1987, six in 1988, none in 1990, two in 1991 and none in 1992 — for a total of 75 (Malo, personal communication).[9] The research from the early 1980s has played a role in increasing access to compensation among crab processing workers in Quebec (Fernande Molaison, 1988). The reduction in cases seems to be linked to more effective prevention. However, in a seasonal industry, compensation may be less adequate than the combined income from work and UI, particularly in the longer term, because disability earnings will be low and employment alternatives limited. As a result, some Quebec workers may be managing on medication rather than seeking compensation.

Dr. Chrétien, on the Lower North Shore, suggested that workers with crab asthma symptoms avoid him and go to other, less experienced doctors in order to get medication. They come to see him, he claimed, only when their asthma is so severe that they cannot continue to work and must apply for compensation. This doctor argues that fear of loss of employment, perhaps exacerbated by the current crisis in the fisheries, and in addition to a fairly prolonged and difficult compensation and medical screening process, may be contributing to a pattern of underreporting of symptoms in Quebec.

Recent research on all types of OA in Quebec found minimal differences in limitations and quality of life between those with OA and those with asthma, suggesting that the Quebec compensation system is functioning fairly well in this area (DeWitte et al., 1994; Malo et al., 1993). However, scrutiny of different categories of workers, including those employed in single industry communities, and a comparison of male and female workers, might have found some interesting variations between subgroups.

Snow crab OA appears to represent a major threat to the health of exposed workers in Newfoundland and Labrador, and because of the sexual division of labour and sexual segregation of work, women workers probably experience greater exposures than men. Sex segregation can mean that the occupational health risks confronting women are somewhat different from those confronting men and it can also limit the employment alternatives for women who need to change jobs in response to an occupational health problem.

As is often the case, the labour force in crab processing is largely sex-segregated, with women concentrated in a narrow range of jobs, such as tip rolling (removing meat from the leg tips) and packing, tied directly to processing. Men are more likely to work in discharge, storage, freezers and as butchers (removing the legs from the uncooked crab). In one Newfoundland plant with a number of workers with asthma-like symptoms, some symptomatic male workers had been moved into areas with lower levels of exposures. One female worker had also been moved into a lower exposure processing job and a second had been able to get clerical work in the office. However, none of the symptomatic women had been moved out into the unloading, storage or butchering areas where exposures in this plant appeared to be the lowest. Since the fishery crisis, work in this plant has become more sex-segregated as jobs formerly dominated by women have been taken over by men displaced from the fishery. In the job with what may be the highest exposures — the small, enclosed black light area where shell is separated from meat — all of the workers were women.

Although some of the first research in the world on snow crab OA appears to have been carried out in Newfoundland (Report, 1978) little has been done in the province since then to minimize this occupational health risk. Prevention is linked to research and public awareness. No full-fledged epidemiological research on the incidence of snow crab OA has been conducted in Newfoundland and Labrador. An early study of queen (an old name for "snow") crab processors described 17 cases of asthma and allergic rhinitis in a sample of 61 employees "who had reported illness following employment" (Report, 1978). Some of these workers had recently experienced short-term, high-level exposures to chlorine. A second Newfoundland-based study, published in 1986, identified four percent of the working population of the plant with asthmatic conditions linked to employment (Bokhout, 1986). There were methodological problems with both of these studies.

A search of Workers' Compensation records in 1993 produced only two compensated cases of allergy to seafood in Newfoundland and Labrador. These Workers' Compensation data do not provide an accurate picture of incidence in this province. Interviews with medical personnel revealed that they had some awareness of this occupational health risk and had diagnosed it in patients, but that they would rarely submit forms to Workers' Compensation. The Medical Care Plan (MCP) forms have no category for crab asthma so doctors use the category for "asthma" instead. In the case of Labrador, individual claims are not even filed with MCP. As a result, there is no centralized database from which an accurate understanding of the number of workers diagnosed with crab asthma could be garnered.

The 1978 Newfoundland Report appears to have resulted in no follow-up beyond improved ventilation in the particular plant concerned. The intent of this investigation was to resolve an acute situation, which it is reported to have done (Edstrom, personal communication). No steps appear to have been taken to ensure that a similar situation did not develop in other crab plants, or to follow up affected workers in order to define more precisely the cause of the asthmatic symptoms or to assess the effectiveness of the changes introduced. One consequence of this has been a pattern of outbreaks of asthma-like symptoms in newly renovated plants. These outbreaks may or may not be reported to the Department of Employment and Labour Relations. If they are reported, then some intervention, generally geared to improved ventilation and enclosure of the cooking area, seems to result. No attention appears to have been paid to the temperature of the crab meat (a factor identified as important in Quebec research). Newfoundland and Labrador has no legislative requirements related to this.

At present in Newfoundland and Labrador, there are no specific design requirements for crab plants (other than the general ones for fish processing) related to ventilation, layout, enclosure, etc.. While cooking areas are generally enclosed, the extent and effectiveness of the enclosure varies. Two plants that experienced recent outbreaks of what seems to have been crab asthma had just been renovated. Although these renovations reduced the level of ventilation, this did not prevent their reopening. New technologies are not examined from the perspective of their possible impact on the incidence and severity of crab OA, or their impact on the effectiveness of existing ventilation systems. Since there is no special standard for crab plant ventilation and since follow-up does not seem to entail thorough assessments of all plantworkers, it is unclear whether changes introduced in plants where intervention has occurred have, in fact, reduced the risk of OA. In some cases, workers have been offered protective masks. However, the only documented cases of this happening occurred after symptoms developed, and these preventive devices had not been tested for their effectiveness in relation to the causal agent(s).

Education and awareness are not only critical for effective prevention, but also required under the regulations of the Occupational Health and Safety Act in Newfoundland and Labrador. A number of problems with education and awareness related to crab asthma have emerged in recent research. For example, I documented two cases (from the mid-1980s and early 1990s) where new crab plant managers were unaware of the risk of crab asthma and were surprised by outbreaks among the worker population. Management in a third plant also appeared to know relatively little about this problem. In one case, a manager reported "getting in trouble" with the owners when she brought medical personnel into the plant in response to an outbreak of asthma-like symptoms in the working population.

Although there is no constant finding that a positive relationship exists between smoking and sensitization to the crab allergen, plant management in two plants seemed inclined to view those who smoke as particularly vulnerable to crab OA and to blame symptoms on smoking. In some cases, these views were shared by workers. One worker commented, for example, "most of the people who get sick smoke. I don't think the smoke and the crab mixes." A relatively high percentage of crab processing workers appears to smoke, and poorly ventilated lunchrooms mean that almost everyone is exposed to secondhand smoke during the brief breaks. Some workers who develop asthma-like symptoms report giving up smoking because of their symptoms. Limited knowledge concerning crab OA, in combination with government-promoted anti-smoking campaigns, seems to be contributing to a perception that respiratory symptoms are related to smoking rather than work and that smoking rather than work-related exposures to crab is responsible for individual vulnerability to crab OA. As noted above, there is not strong support for this in the literature.

Workers in the plants studied in Newfoundland and Labrador appeared to have some knowledge about crab asthma but their knowledge was not always accurate. In one plant, some reported believing that co-workers had brought their sensitivity to crab to the plant, until an outbreak among workers with several years' experience had caused them to alter this view. Information on crab asthma had been communicated to the workers in a relatively systematic way by management in only one of the four plants we visited. This communication happened after an outbreak occurred, not before. Several workers admitted to managing on medication during the processing season. Most of these workers said that at the end of the season, the "puffers would go up in the cupboard" until the following year. However, some workers were having to use their bronchodilators year-round, an indication that they may have developed chronic asthma symptoms that will persist when they give up their jobs at the plant. Workers seemed generally unaware of the significant risk that if exposures continued, crab OA might develop into a chronic disability that would persist after they left their jobs. The above evidence suggests some employers are in violation of Section 5 of the Newfoundland and Labrador Occupational Health and Safety Act, not only by providing unsafe workplaces but also by failing to ensure that workers and supervisors are "made familiar with health or safety hazards that may be met by them in the workplace" (Government of Newfoundland, 1990).

There have been important gains in understanding about OA in the past decade, but in Newfoundland and Labrador, as elsewhere, this knowledge has not generally been well communicated to the primary caregivers who first encounter clients and provide the majority of treatment (Merchant, 1990), or to inspectors who are responsible for prevention. Evidence from interviews with medical personnel and members of the hygiene section of the Department of Employment and Labour Relations in Newfoundland and Labrador suggests that, until recently, when department and medical personnel assumed their positions they were not necessarily familiar with the literature on crab OA and its implications for diagnosis, treatment and workplace modifications. In rural areas, where turnover in medical personnel is often high, new personnel entering crab processing communities may still be unaware of this risk to occupational health.

Pepys (1982) calls for the creation of specialized referral centres for patients and cooperation between industry and clinical investigators. Chan-Yeung (1990:820) argues: "The management of patients with occupational asthma requires the full cooperation of management, union, and the compensation boards, or similar agencies." Neither such clinics nor such full cooperation exist in Newfoundland and Labrador.

In many areas of Newfoundland and Labrador, it appears to be common practice among medical professionals to prescribe Ventolin bronchodilators in combination with an inhaled steroid to crab processing workers with asthma-like symptoms. The possible long-term health consequences of continued exposure for crab workers with OA needs to be considered when assessing the appropriateness of prescribing medications and allowing them to return to work. Such practices take pressure off the government to introduce appropriate preventive legislation, and take pressure off the employer to clean up the workplace and find jobs without exposures for affected workers (Burge, 1991). I also documented a few cases where medical professionals have required their workers to give up their jobs apparently without helping them to apply for compensation. When medication is accompanied by a failure to file for compensation, this ensures that the worker and the Medical Care Plan are covering the financial and health costs of crab workers' OA, instead of employers. Failure to report might also jeopardize workers' ability to qualify for Workers' Compensation in the future when medications become ineffective. The potential side effects of asthma medications (in the case of women, both for them and for their fetuses, should they become pregnant) as well as the need for careful, individualized treatment regimes (Hargreave et al., 1990) and full information on both the part of the physician and the patient also need to be considered. If workers are attempting to mask their symptoms out of fear of being laid off or declared unfit for work, this will make effective, safe treatment more difficult. Doctors might be more likely to pursue the option of compensation for workers if they had knowledge of and ready access to a specialized clinic with the facilities for diagnosing OA within the province.[10]

In Newfoundland and Labrador, lack of access to compensation, limited knowledge about OA on the part of medical professionals and the absence of clear standards for enclosure and ventilation within crab processing plants suggest that the current system for preventing, responding to, treating and compensating crab workers with OA is highly inadequate.

CONCLUSION

OA is one of many occupational health risks that confront women in their workplaces. To date, much of the research on OA has concentrated on men's occupations. When it has examined occupations dominated by women, this research has generally failed to explicitly address the gendered dimensions of this threat to occupational health.

The social, regulatory and technical barriers to occupational health confronted by the women who work in crab plants have received little attention. Although one of the first studies on snow crab OA appears to have been carried out in Newfoundland in the 1970s, relatively little research has been done since (Report, 1978). Research from Quebec suggests that snow crab OA represents a major threat to the occupational health of these primarily female workers. This research, carried out in the early 1980s, contributed both to our general understanding of the incidence, causes and long-term consequences of this occupational disease, as well as to reduced risk and improved access to compensation in that province. However, it did not directly address issues related to the gender of these workers and has not been updated to address the possible impacts of changes within the industry, as well as within the wider economy of rural communities that might be influencing the incidence and prevention of crab OA.

This paper has identified a range of social, technical and other factors that have contributed to the risk of developing snow crab OA. Risks appear to be greater in Newfoundland and Labrador than in Quebec because of a combination of limited research and lack of primary prevention. Once workers are sensitized, they require much cleaner workplaces. For this reason, primary prevention must be top priority. In both Quebec and Newfoundland and Labrador it is arguable that the current fisheries crisis, in combination with already existing limits on employment opportunities for women (both within fish processing and in their wider communities), have created a context within which protests from workers will be muted and women (and men) will strive to continue working despite significant risks to their long-term health. At the same time, new technologies may be increasing exposures to the crab allergen. Proactive research and intervention related to this occupational health problem are called for. Workers who have lost their jobs or must leave their places of work because they have developed snow crab OA need to be diagnosed and assessed. They require access to compensation and either nonexposure work in their former workplace or training for new employment and possibly relocation assistance.

Further research is required to establish the incidence of this disease in a range of crab plants generating different products and using different technologies. The possible role of chemical irritants in the development of asthma symptoms needs to be investigated further. Detailed research on socioeconomic impacts is also required, as well as further research on the reasons for the failure of both medical professionals and the Newfoundland and Labrador government to adopt a preventive approach to this occupational health problem. All of this research must be gender-informed.

ACKNOWLEDGEMENTS

Research for this paper was partially funded by a Challenge Grant from Human Resources Development, a seed grant from the Vice President's Research Fund at Memorial University and by Memorial University's Undergraduate Assistance programme. Jennifer Rooney and Victoria Silk worked as Research Assistants on the project. Consultations with Sharon Buehler and Bonnie James helped in the development of the research. Lucie Dumais and Victoria Silk offered useful comments on drafts. I am currently developing a larger, more detailed report on this research for submission to the Institute of Social and Economic Research at Memorial University, St. John's. This research would not have been possible without the willing participation of workers and management in several communities and medical professionals in both Quebec and Newfoundland and Labrador. I take full responsibility for any errors or omissions.

NOTES

1. Estimates from Newfoundland and Labrador and Quebec suggest women make up approximately 70 percent of crab processing workers (Dave Lewis, Newfoundland Department of Fisheries, personal communication, 1983).

2. Although four plants were observed, the level of observation varied significantly among plants. In two cases, observation involved a plant tour and brief interviews with management. In the third case, several interviews with plant workers and former plant workers with OA like symptoms were carried out. In the fourth case, I spent several days observing plant activities, engaged in informal discussions with plant workers on their jobs and in the lunch room, and interviewed management, local medical personnel and current and former plantworkers with OA like symptoms.

3. The Ad Hoc Committee on Occupational Asthma of the Standards Committee, Canadian Thoracic Society (1989), recently argued that inhalation challenges were not necessary for workers exposed to a known cause of occupational asthma and in whom a demonstrated relation between changes in airflow obstruction and airway responsiveness and exposure at work had been found. Where challenge tests are not available, suitable, or pose too significant a risk, Chan-Yeung (1990) recommends serial measures of lung function at work and home.

4. This project attempted to locate former workers, but data from the project are not broken down into current vs. former worker categories. Researchers also did not track either all workers or all former workers (Auger et al., 1984).

5. Recent changes in the Newfoundland and Labrador product mix could, however, reduce risks confronting workers in the future. During the past two years good markets for shell-on products and changes in government regulations have contributed to a significant decline in meat production in many plants. Shell-on products are sometimes processed in an area separated from the cooking and meat production area where ventilation is superior. In one plant, workers moved from the meat processing area to the shell-on processing area reported fewer symptoms. Shell-on products probably involve less exposure to the allergen.

6. Skin test results and questionnaires were the methods used in this research and reported allergic symptoms did not correlate well with skin test results. Some of those who stayed had crab asthma.

7. These workers were from other communities and could not be traced at the time of this research.

8. In Britain and Quebec, irritant-induced asthma is excluded from the category "occupational asthma" (Malo et al., 1992). In the U.S., definitions may include asthma exacerbated by work (Venables, 1992).

9. There were reported to be four in 1994 (Chagnon, personal communication).

10. One doctor said that he felt he could not make a certain diagnosis in the case of crab asthma and did not want to risk jeopardizing the future employment options of his patients without such a diagnosis.

REFERENCES

Ad Hoc Committee on Occupational Asthma of the Standards Committee, Canadian Thoracic Society. "Occupational Asthma: Recommendations for Diagnosis, Management and Assessment of Impairment." *Canadian Medical Association Journal* 1,40 (1989). pp. 1029-32.

Auger, Roland, D. Smola, J-M. Tardif, F-L Forest and M. Chagnon. *Projet crustacés Phase II: Rapport Final*. Département de Santé Commnautaire de Gaspé, 1984.

Baldursson, B.E. "Work Stress in Fishing Transformation Plants." *Special Publication Canadian Journal of Fisheries and Aquatic Sciences* 72 (1984). pp. 26-9.

Bertolini, Renzo. *Asthma: a Summary of the Occupational Concern.* Hamilton, Ontario: Canadian Centre for Occupational Health and Safety, 1987.

— *Crab Workers' Asthma: A Summary of the Occupational Health Concern.* Hamilton, Ontario: Canadian Centre for Occupational Health and Safety, 1989.

Bokhout, Martin. "The Crab Lung Syndrome." *Focus on Community Health* 2, 4 (1986). pp. 1-3.

Burge, Paul Sherwood. "The Prevention of Occupational Asthma." *European Journal of Respiratory Diseases*, Supplement 126 (1982/83). pp. 107-10.

— "New Developments in Occupational Asthma." *British Medical Bulletin* 48, 1 (1991). pp. 221-30.

Cartier, A., J-L. Malo, F. Forest, M. Lafrance, L. Pineau, J-J. St-Aubin and J-Y Dubois. "Occupational Asthma in Snow Crab-processing Workers." *Journal of Allergy and Clinical Immunology* 74, 3 (1984). pp. 261-9.

Cartier, André, Jean-Luc Malo, Heberto Ghezzo, Marjorie McCants and Samuel B. Lehrer. "IgE Sensitization in Snow Crab-processing Workers." *Journal of Allergy and Clinical Immunology* 78, 2 (1986) pp. 344-8.

Chagnon, Marie, Daniel Smolla and Jean-Marc Tardif. *Projet crustacés: Phase III*. Abridged Report. Département de Santé Communautaire, Centre Hospitalier Hotel-Dieu de Gaspé, 1985.

Chan-Yeung, Moira. "Pulmonary Perspective: Evaluation of Impairment/Disability in Patients with Occupational Asthma." *American Review of Respiratory Disease* 135 (1987). pp. 950-1.

— "A Clinician's Approach to Determine the Diagnosis, Prognosis, and Therapy of Occupational Asthma." *The Medical Clinics of North America* 74, 3 (1990). pp. 811-22.

Chan-Yeung, M., and S. Lam. "State of the Art — Occupational Asthma." *American Review of Respiratory Disease* 137 (1986). pp. 686-703.

Department of Fisheries and Oceans (DFO). "Newfoundland Crab Fishery: Management Options for the 1992 Fishery." A Draft Discussion Paper prepared for the Special Regional Crab Advisory Committee Meeting, St. John's (March 3-4,

1992).

Dewitte, J-D., M. Chan-Yeung and J-L Malo. "Medicolegal and Compensation Aspects of Occupational Asthma." *European Respiratory Journal* 7 (1994). pp. 969-80.

Dodge, Russell, and Benjamin Burrows. "The Prevalence and Incidence of Asthma and Asthma-like Symptoms in a General Population Sample." *American Review of Respiratory Disease* 122 (1980). pp. 567-75.

Équipe de santé au travail. *Projet crustacés: Rapport final.* Département de Santé Communautaire, Centre Hospitalier Hotel-Dieu de Gaspé, 1983.

Faculty of Medicine, Memorial University. *Report of the Task Force to Investigate Respiratory Complaints at the Jason Crab Factory in Bareneed, Newfoundland.* St. John's, NF: Memorial University, July 25, 1978.

Fernande Molaison, Pêcheries Gagnon et Turbide, Inc. *Décisions de la Commission d'Appel en Matière de Lésions Professionnelles (C.A.L.P.)*, 1988. pp. 722-4.

Forest, F.L., R. Auger and J-M Tardif. "Respiratory Problems Associated with the Processing of Shellfish in Eastern Canada." *Special Publication Canadian Journal of Fisheries and Aquatic Sciences* 72 (1984). pp. 8-9.

Gaddie, John, Joseph Legge, James A. Friend and Thomas Reid. "Pulmonary Hypersensitivity in Prawn Workers." *Lancet* (Dec. 20/27, 1980). pp. 1350-3.

Guillot, Jean-Guy. "Vapeurs de crabe." *Interface* (mars/avril, 1984). pp. 27-32.

Government of Newfoundland. *An Act Respecting Occupational Health and Safety in the Province.* St. John's, NF: Office of the Queen's Printer, 1990.

Hargreave, Frederick E., J. Dolovich and M. T. Newhouse. "The Assessment and Treatment of Asthma: A Conference Report." *Journal of Allergy and Clinical Immunology* 85, 6 (1990). pp. 1098-111.

Hudson, P., A. Cartier, L. Pineau, M. Lafrance, J. J. St-Aubin, J. Y. Dubois and J. L. Malo. "Follow-up of Occupational Asthma Caused by Crab and Various Agents." *Journal of Allergy and Clinical Immunology* 76, 5 (1985). pp. 682-8.

Hughson, William G. "Epidemiologic Considerations in Occupational Asthma." *Immunology and Allergy Clinics of North America* 12, 4 (1992). pp. 697-710.

Malo, Jean-Luc. "Compensation of Occupational Asthma in Quebec." *CHEST* 98, 5 (November Supplement, 1990). pp. 236S-9S.

Malo, Jean-Luc, André Cartier, Heberto Ghezzo, Monique Lafrance, Marjorie McCants and Samuel B. Lehrer. "Patterns of Improvement in Spirometry, Bronchial Hyperresponsiveness, and Specific IgE Antibody Levels After Cessation of Exposure in Occupational Asthma Caused by Snow-crab Processing." *American Review of Respiratory Disease* 138 (1988). pp. 807-12.

Malo, Jean-Luc, Heberto Ghezzo, Carlos D'Aquino, Jocelyne L'Archeveque, André Cartier and Moira Chan-Yeung. "Natural History of Occupational Asthma: Relevance of Type of Agent and Other Factors in the Rate of Development of Symptoms in Affected Subjects." *Journal of Allergy and Clinical Immunology* 90 (1992). pp. 937-44.

Malo, Jean-Luc, and André Cartier. "Occupational Reactions in the Seafood Industry." *Clinical Reviews in Allergy* 11, 2 (1993). pp. 223-40.

Malo, Jean-Luc, L-P. Boulet, J-D. Dewitte, A. Cartier, J. L'Archeveque, J. Coté, G.

Bédard, S. Boucher, F. Champagne, G. Tessier, A-P. Contandriopoulos, E. Juniper and G. Guyatt. "Quality of life of subjects with Occupational Asthma." *Journal of Allergy and Clinical Immunology* 91, 6 (1993). pp. 1121-7.

Mathews, John. *Health and Safety at Work: Australian Trade Union Safety Representatives Handbook.* Sydney: Pluto Press, 1985.

Merchant, James. "Priorities for the Management of Environmental and Occupational Asthma." *CHEST* 98, 5 (1990). pp. 146S-7S.

Messing, Karen. *Occupational Safety and Health Concerns of Canadian Women: A Background Paper.* Ottawa: Women's Bureau, Labour Canada, 1991.

Messing, Karen, and J-P Reveret. "Are Women in Female Jobs for Their Health? A Study of Working Conditions and Health Effects in the Fish-processing Industry in Quebec." *International Journal of Health Services* 13, 4 (1983). pp. 635-47.

Mundt, K. "Immuno-Epidemiology of Crab-Induced Occupational Allergies." Ph.D. dissertation. University of North Carolina, 1990.

Neis, Barbara. "Occupational Health and Safety of Women Working in Fish and Crab Processing in Newfoundland and Labrador." *Chronic Diseases in Canada* 15, 1 (1994). pp. 6-11.

O'Hollaren, Mark T. "Occupational Asthma Due to High Molecular Weight Allergens." *Immunology and Allergy Clinics of North America* 12, 4 (1992). pp. 795-816.

Pepys, Jack. "Occupational Asthma: An Overview." *Journal of Occupational Medicine* 24, 7 (1982). pp. 534-7.

Plouffe, G, N. Vézina and D. Mergler. "Le froid, facteur contributif aux maux de dos dans une usine de transformation de poissons congelés." *Proceedings of the 22nd Annual Meeting of the Human Factors Association of Canada* (1989). pp. 179-83.

Province de Québec. *Loi sur les produits agricoles, les produits marins et les aliments.* Québec: Province de Québec. Chapter 9, pp. 125-39.

Smith, Dorsett D. "Medical-Legal Definition of Occupational Asthma." *CHEST* 98 (1990). pp. 1007-11.

Venables, K.M., A.G. Davison and A.J. Newman Taylor. "Consequences of Occupational Asthma." *Respiratory Medicine* 83 (1989). pp. 437-40.

Venables, K.M. "Preventing Occupational Asthma." *British Journal of Industrial Medicine* 49 (1992). pp. 817-9.

Yassi, Annalee. "Health and Socioeconomic Consequences of Occupational Respiratory Allergies: A Pilot Study Using Workers' Compensation Data." *American Journal of Industrial Medicine* 14 (1988). pp. 291-8.

Nicole Vézina, Julie Courville,
Lucie Geoffrion

Problèmes musculo-squelettiques, caractéristiques des postes des travailleurs et des postes des travailleuses sur une même chaîne de découpe de dinde

Repetitive strain injuries affecting male and female workers in the food sector in Quebec are increasing. The present study examines work on a conveyor belt in a poultry processing factory where labour is divided on a gender basis. The study objectives were to: (1) characterize and compare men's and women's jobs; (2) compare health profiles by gender; and (3) understand each gender's reluctance to accept the other's jobs. The men's jobs require strength, know-how and a well-sharpened knife. The women's jobs require precision, speed and quality work. Static postures mean that women get cold on some jobs. Seventy percent of male workers reported no physical pain. In contrast, 41 percent of female workers reported pain resulting in either absence, medication or consultation of a doctor. It is suggested that the persistent sexual division of labour in this factory is due to job constraints — including meticulousness and precision of execution — and work organization as well as to gendered representations of work. Women report that men's jobs require "too much physical effort" while men judge women's jobs as "too boring." In conclusion, the possible consequences of the desegregation of jobs for workers' health is questioned since men's jobs appear to stretch to the limit their physical abilities and women's jobs "wear them down."

Dans le secteur agro-alimentaire au Québec, le nombre de lésions musculo-squelettiques dues au travail répétitif (LATR) est grandissant et affecte autant les hommes que les femmes. La présente étude fut faite sur une chaîne de découpe de dinde, dans une usine de transformation de volaille, où il existe une division sexuelle du travail. Trois objectifs furent visés: caractériser et comparer les postes d'hommes et les postes de femmes; comparer l'état de santé des deux groupes; mieux comprendre la réticence de chacun des deux groupes à occuper les postes de travail de l'autre. Aux postes d'hommes, on exerce de la force et on a besoin de savoir-faire et d'un couteau bien affilé. Les postes de femmes se caractérisent surtout par le besoin de précision, de vitesse et de qualité de coupe. À certains de ces postes de femmes, le refroidissement dû au statisme est plus grand. Parmi les hommes, 70 p.100 ne rapportent aucun site de douleurs, alors que 41 p.100 des femmes ont des douleurs qui les ont amenées à s'absenter, prendre des médicaments ou consulter un médecin. On tente d'expliquer la persistance de la division sexuelle en fonction de facteurs tels que les contraintes respectives des postes, l'organisation du travail, des caractéristiques telles que la minutie et la précision, et une représentation sexuée du travail (les femmes disant devoir déployer «trop» d'efforts physiques sur certains postes, alors que les hommes décrivent d'autres postes comme «trop ennuyants»). On se demande finalement quelles seraient les conséquences d'une éventuelle désexisation des postes du point de vue de la santé au travail, dans la mesure où les postes actuels des hommes sont «limitants», et ceux des femmes, «usants».

PROBLÉMATIQUE

La fréquence des problèmes musculo-squelettiques liés au travail répétitif[1] est de plus en plus élevée parmi des travailleuses telles que les caissières de supermarché, les couturières, les codeuses, les ouvrières de l'électronique, etc. (Hünting et al., 1981; Laville et al., 1985; Ryan, 1989; Hinnen et al., 1992). On reconnaît, dans ces secteurs d'emploi, différents facteurs de risque qui pourraient contribuer au développement de ce type de lésions: cycles de travail courts, précision et répétitivité des gestes, espace restreint, mobilité réduite, posture contraignante, absence de micropauses, etc. (Kilbom et al., 1986). Il s'agit souvent de caractéristiques typiques du travail féminin.

Le secteur agro-alimentaire est maintenant reconnu au Québec pour la fréquence élevée et grandissante des lésions musculo-squelettiques qu'on y retrouve. Dans les abattoirs et les usines de transformation de la viande et de la volaille, le travail est très parcellisé et souvent effectué à des chaînes qui n'offrent pas la possibilité de contrôler son rythme de travail. L'utilisation du couteau nécessite de la précision et de la dextérité. Les facteurs de risque mentionnés plus haut se retrouvent donc dans les usines de porc et de boeuf, où le travail est effectué exclusivement par des hommes. Dans les abattoirs de volaille cependant, la main-d'oeuvre est mixte. Dans un cas comme dans l'autre, la prévalence des problèmes musculo-squelettiques aux membres supérieurs est alarmante (Armstrong et al., 1982; Viikari-Juntura, 1983; Toulouse et al., 1992; Patry et al., 1993; Courville et al., 1994).

Les abattoirs et usines de transformation du porc et du boeuf constituent sûrement une chasse gardée masculine, mais il apparaît évident que les contraintes physiques à plusieurs postes de ces entreprises représentent des barrières très difficiles à franchir par les travailleuses. Dans les abattoirs et usines de transformation de la volaille, les hommes et les femmes occupent souvent des postes différents, les travailleuses occupant les postes à la chaîne alors que les travailleurs se trouvent en bout de ligne (Mergler et al., 1987; Messing et al.,1983). Dans l'étude qui fait l'objet de cette présentation, la situation est très différente et la répartition des postes entre les hommes et les femmes à une même chaîne de découpe de la dinde a tout particulièrement attiré notre attention.

Notre présence dans cette usine de transformation de la volaille fait suite à une demande des représentants syndicaux et patronaux de l'entreprise qui faisaient face à un taux d'accidents très élevé. L'étude a été menée da façon paritaire avec le comité de santé-sécurité qui s'était fixé pour objectif premier la diminution de la fréquence des problèmes musculo-squelettiques. En effet, en 1988, on retrouvait, dans les registres officiels de l'entreprise, l'enregistrement de 179 accidents et maladies professionnelles, soit un taux d'accidents de 74,9 par 100 employés. À la suite d'une analyse des accidents, deux départements sont ressortis très nettement avec des fréquences élevées d'accidents: le département de découpe de poulets sur cônes et le département de dépeçage de dindes. À la découpe du poulet, les 18 hommes et femmes font rotation aux 20 minutes sur les 6 postes de la chaîne. Au dépeçage de la dinde, les 27 travailleurs et travailleuses se sont répartis les 15 postes de travail à la chaîne, de telle sorte que l'on peut reconnaître deux circuits de rotation, celui des hommes et celui des femmes. C'est cette chaîne de découpe de la dinde qui a été choisie pour faire l'objet de la présente étude. En effet, en plus de la fréquence des problèmes musculo-squelettiques, les contremaîtres rencontraient à cette chaîne des difficultés d'implantation de la nouvelle politique de l'usine visant à augmenter la polyvalence des personnes sur l'ensemble des postes de leur département. Cette nouvelle mesure devait augmenter la flexibilité des travailleurs et des travailleuses, ce qui devait faciliter la gestion du personnel. Plusieurs tentatives avaient donc été faites au département de la découpe de dinde afin que les hommes apprennent le travail aux postes des femmes et que les femmes puissent accomplir le travail aux postes des hommes. Mais ces tentatives se sont soldées par un échec: autant les hommes que les femmes ne voulaient occuper les postes de l'autre groupe.

Nos objectifs ont d'abord été de tenter de caractériser et de comparer les postes d'hommes et les postes de femmes, ensuite de faire un portrait comparatif de l'état de santé des deux groupes, et enfin, de mieux comprendre la réticence de chacun des deux groupes à occuper les postes de travail de l'autre. Cela dans le but de mieux comprendre le développement des problèmes musculo-squelettiques chez les travailleurs et les travailleuses et l'impact sur la santé de la division sexuelle du travail.

MÉTHODOLOGIE

Dans cette usine de transformation de la volaille, au moment de l'étude, environ 240 personnes sont employées, dont 27 travaillent de façon régulière à la chaîne de découpe de la dinde. Les données qui ont permis d'obtenir un portrait de la population travaillant à cette chaîne et un tableau comparatif des perceptions des travailleurs et des travailleuses à leurs postes de travail ont été obtenues par des entretiens individuels. Afin de préciser l'importance et les circonstances des accidents, leurs dossiers d'accidents ont été analysés de janvier 1986 à décembre 1992. La description des opérations et des contraintes de chacun des postes de travail a été possible grâce à des observations sur le terrain et sur vidéo. Finalement, des rencontres de discussion avec des travailleurs, des travailleuses et des contremaîtres sur l'ensemble des résultats obtenus a permis d'approfondir notre compréhension de la situation de travail analysée.

Les entrevues individuelles

Toutes les personnes travaillant régulièrement à la chaîne de découpe de dinde sont interrogées individuellement à l'aide d'un questionnaire comprenant des questions ouvertes et fermées. À la suite d'un prétest auprès de six sujets, certaines questions sont reformulées. Ce prétest permet aussi aux trois personnes effectuant les entrevues d'uniformiser leur méthode. Les rencontres durent en moyenne 90 minutes et les répondants et répondantes sont libérés de leur travail pour y participer.

Le questionnaire permet de recueillir des informations sur les points suivants: les caractéristiques individuelles, l'histoire professionnelle, les postes occupés en rotation régulière ou occasionnelle, les difficultés physiques et mentales rencontrées au travail en général, la tenue vestimentaire, les outils utilisés et l'affilage des couteaux. L'évaluation de chacun des postes occupés sur une base régulière se fait par les répondants et répondantes sur des points spécifiques: la cadence, la précision, la force, la posture, le couteau, les gants, la température corporelle, la température des mains. Le niveau de difficulté est précisé suivant cette échelle: aucune difficulté, un peu difficile, difficile, très difficile. On demande également quels postes sont les plus appréciés et lesquels sont détestés, ainsi que les raisons des préférences.

Des schémas corporels sont utilisés pour indiquer les sites de fatigue à la fin de la journée de travail et les sites de douleur pendant l'accomplissement du travail. Il s'agit de la fatigue et de la douleur ressenties au cours de la dernière semaine de travail. Une autre série de questions permet d'apprécier le niveau de gravité des douleurs ressenties (persistance de la douleur, consultation médicale, médication, perte de capacité et de jouissance de la vie). Des questions concernant la grossesse et les menstruations sont également posées aux travailleuses. La dernière partie du questionnaire apporte des renseignements sur les responsabilités familiales.

Les registres d'accidents

Les dossiers d'accidents de 26 des 27 personnes interrogées ont été analysés de janvier 1986 à décembre 1992. Un seul travailleur n'a pas donné son consentement permettant l'accès à son dossier. Les rapports contiennent des informations sur les circonstances de l'accident, le type d'accident, le site de la lésion et le nombre de jours de travail perdus.

Les observations des postes de travail

Lors des observations préliminaires, chaque poste de la chaîne a été filmé pendant 10 minutes de côté et de face, simultanément, à l'aide de deux caméras vidéo. Les opérations, les postures et les mouvements effectués à chacun des postes avaient alors été décrits de façon sommaire. À la suite de l'analyse du questionnaire, cinq postes sont ciblés comme étant plus à risque et plusieurs travailleurs et travailleuses sont alors filmés à chacun de ces postes. Ces derniers enregistrements ont servi plus tard à l'analyse plus systématique des contraintes liées à ces postes. Dans le cadre de la présente communication, les observations servent à caractériser et à comparer les postes de travail.

Les rencontres de discussion

Trois rencontres ont été organisées, lesquelles se voulaient, à l'origine, des rencontres collectives, mais l'entreprise n'a pu libérer que deux personnes pour chacune de ces rencontres. Un premier entretien a été réalisé avec deux travailleuses, un deuxième avec deux travailleurs et un troisième entretien a eu lieu avec deux contremaîtres. Ces rencontres visaient à augmenter notre compréhension de la situation de travail. Elles avaient pour but d'obtenir les réactions de ces personnes face aux résultats observés et d'avoir des réponses aux questions soulevées par l'analyse des résultats. Chaque entretien a duré environ deux heures au cours desquelles les thèmes suivants ont été abordés: les exigences des postes de travail, l'interrelation entre les postes, l'aménagement de la chaîne, les outils, la formation reçue, les exigences de précision et le contrôle de qualité. Avec les contremaîtres, l'historique de ce département, l'origine de la division sexuelle du travail ainsi que la marge de manoeuvre des contremaîtres ont également été discutés. Il s'agissait d'entretiens semi-dirigés.

RÉSULTATS
Caractéristiques personnelles de la population étudiée

Davantage de femmes (N=17) que d'hommes (N=10) travaillent à la chaîne de découpe de dinde. L'âge moyen des deux groupes se situe autour de la trentaine avec un minimum et un maximum de 25 et 36 ans chez les femmes, de 22 et 41 ans chez les hommes (tableau 1). Notons une différence de 10 centimètres entre la taille moyenne des femmes et celle des hommes, et une différence de 14 kilogrammes, en moyenne, pour le poids.

Tableau 1   Caractéristiques personnelles des travailleurs et des travailleuses de la chaîne de découpe de dindes

Caractéristiques personelles	Femmes (N=17) Moyenne + écart-type	Hommes (N=10) Moyenne + écart-type
Age (années)	29 + 4	32 + 6
Ancienneté dans l'usine (années)	5 + 1	7 + 4
Ancienneté sur la chaîne de dinde	4 + 1	5 + 4
Taille (cm)	167 + 4	177 + 6
Poids (kg)	60 + 10	74 + 7

Bien que les travailleurs aient une ancienneté moyenne, dans l'usine, plus importante de deux ans que celle des travailleuses, la différence n'est que d'un an pour l'ancienneté sur la chaîne de découpe de dinde. La figure 1 montre cependant que la répartition du nombre d'années d'ancienneté à la chaîne de découpe de dinde est différente si l'on compare les deux groupes. La moitié des hommes ont en effet trois ans et moins d'ancienneté et l'autre moitié a six ans et plus d'ancienneté, alors que plus de 80 p.100 des femmes ont de quatre ans à six ans d'ancienneté. Les travailleuses forment donc un groupe assez homogène en ce qui concerne l'ancienneté alors que le groupe des hommes se partage entre les anciens et les nouveaux.

Figure 1 Ancienneté des femmes et des hommes sur la chaîne de découpe de dindes

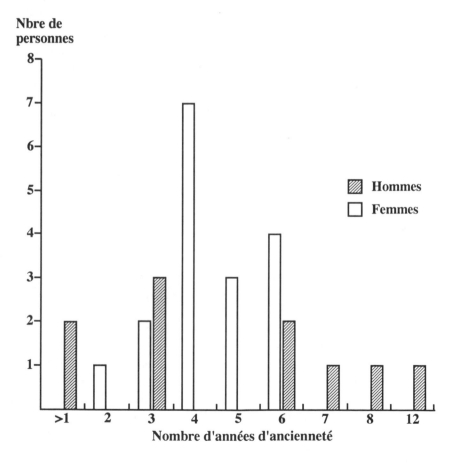

Portrait général de la chaîne de découpe de dinde

La volaille transformée dans cette usine provient de différents abattoirs de la région. Il s'agit donc de poulets et de dindes déjà éviscérés, nettoyés et refroidis. Selon les normes d'Agriculture Canada, l'intérieur des volailles ne doit pas s'élever au-dessus de 4° C pendant la transformation. Les salles de découpe sont refroidies et la température ambiante ne doit pas dépasser 12° C.

Selon l'historique obtenu des contremaîtres, il y a 16 ans la chaîne de découpe de dinde était telle qu'on la connaît: une chaîne en mouvement munie de crochets auxquels est suspendue la volaille. Au début, la chaîne fonctionnait à 125 dindes à l'heure et les personnes qui dépeçaient faisaient également le parage du morceau de chair enlevé. La cadence a augmenté graduellement à 225 puis, 250 pour passer à la cadence actuelle de 300 dindes à l'heure qui remonte maintenant à six ans.

On retrouve à la figure 2 une représentation schématique de la chaîne de découpe de dinde. Celle-ci comporte 15 postes de travail occupés en rotation. À ces postes, on peut ajouter le poste d'emballage des boîtes de cinq kilogrammes et le poste de remplacement pour les toilettes. Ces postes sont occupés de façon inégale par les travailleurs et travailleuses. Par exemple, le poste de remplacement est occupé par chacun pour une journée entière, environ une fois par deux semaines, alors que l'emballage est souvent utilisé pour l'assignation temporaire.[2] Nous limiterons donc notre description aux 15 postes de la chaîne.

Description de chacun des postes de travail de la chaîne de découpe de dinde

Les dindes mêlées à de la glace sont d'abord transvidées dans un grand bac situé au début de la chaîne. Au premier poste, la personne saisit la dinde dans le bac et la soulève pour l'enfiler sur une tige munie de crochets. Il s'agit du poste de l'*accrochage*. Les dindes les plus lourdes peuvent peser plus de 25 kilogrammes. Les dindes sont ensuite entraînées par la chaîne à un niveau plus élevé. Les 11 prochains postes de la chaîne se situent en effet sur une plate-forme de métal (postes 2 à 12). Les morceaux de dinde dépecés à ces postes sont déposés sur des tapis roulants qui circulent sous la chaîne. Ils sont ainsi entraînés vers la table de parage (postes 13 à 15).

La *coupe des ailes* correspond au deuxième poste. Cette tâche est exécutée par deux personnes, l'une coupant les ailes gauches et l'autre, les ailes droites. Chaque aile doit être détachée au niveau de l'épaule et une partie doit être désossée. La chair de l'aile sera déposée sur le tapis roulant alors que les os et la peau seront lancés dans un bassin situé devant la chaîne.

Figure 2   Représentation schématique de la chaîne de découpe de dindes

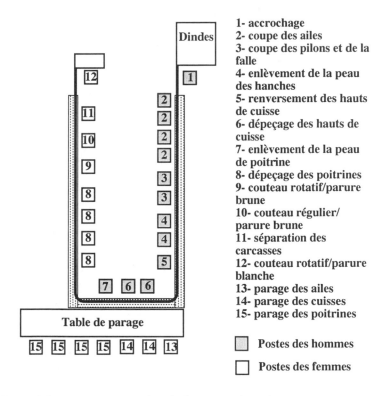

1- accrochage
2- coupe des ailes
3- coupe des pilons et de la falle
4- enlèvement de la peau des hanches
5- renversement des hauts de cuisse
6- dépeçage des hauts de cuisse
7- enlèvement de la peau de poitrine
8- dépeçage des poitrines
9- couteau rotatif/parure brune
10- couteau régulier/parure brune
11- séparation des carcasses
12- couteau rotatif/parure blanche
13- parage des ailes
14- parage des cuisses
15- parage des poitrines

☐ Postes des hommes
☐ Postes des femmes

Le troisième poste est celui de la *coupe des pilons et de la falle*. Deux travailleurs occupent ce poste et coupent les deux pilons et la falle (peau pendant au niveau du cou) d'une dinde sur deux. Les morceaux sont lancés dans des récipients. Au quatrième poste, la *peau des hanches est enlevée* par deux personnes qui saisissent soit le côté gauche, soit le côté droit. La peau est coupée le long du dos, tirée vers le bas et lancée dans un bassin.

On *renverse les hauts de cuisse* au cinquième poste. Une seule personne apprête les deux cuisses de toutes les dindes. Après avoir coupé les tendons à l'aide du couteau, il s'agit de désarticuler l'os de la cuisse en la renversant vers l'arrière d'un coup sec. Ces *hauts de cuisse sont ensuite dépecés* au sixième poste. Une personne apprêtera les côtés gauches et une autre personne, les côtés droits. À ce poste, on coupe au niveau de l'articulation pour détacher l'os de la cuisse, on enlève la chair de la cuisse, puis l'os est lancé dans un bassin et la chair déposée sur le tapis roulant. La *peau de la poitrine doit ensuite être enlevée*. Une seule personne occupe ce septième poste.

On passe ensuite au *dépeçage de la poitrine*. À ce huitième poste, plusieurs opérations doivent être effectuées pour détacher complètement la poitrine du bréchet. Quatre personnes sont assignées à ce poste, deux pour les poitrines gauches et deux pour les poitrines droites. Les poitrines sont lancées sur le tapis roulant. Au neuvième poste, une personne enlève la *parure brune à l'aide d'un couteau rotatif*. La parure brune correspond aux morceaux de chair brune que l'on retrouve sur les os du dos de la dinde. Au dixième poste, une autre personne enlève la *parure brune mais avec un couteau ordinaire*.

On procède ensuite à la *séparation des carcasses*. Une seule personne se trouve à cet onzième poste. Elle doit couper de chaque côté de la carcasse et ensuite tirer vers le bas afin de séparer la carcasse en deux. Elle doit ensuite détacher et renverser la fourchette. Cette partie de la carcasse est déposée dans un bassin pour la personne située au poste suivant. L'autre partie de la carcasse est détachée de la chaîne et lancée dans un autre récipient. Au douzième poste, c'est à l'aide d'un couteau rotatif qu'une personne enlève la *parure blanche* restant sur les carcasses.

Les trois derniers postes ne se situent pas sur la plate-forme, mais plus bas, sur le plancher de ciment. C'est à ces postes que l'on effectue le parage des différents morceaux déposés sur les tapis roulants soit *les ailes* (poste 13), *les hauts de cuisse* (poste 14) et *les poitrines* (poste 15). Le parage consiste à nettoyer ces morceaux des surplus de gras, de la peau, des parcelles d'os ou de cartilage et des caillots de sang. On doit saisir les morceaux qui circulent sur les tapis roulants et effectuer le parage sur une table à l'aide d'un couteau. Une personne s'occupe du parage des ailes, deux personnes parent les hauts de cuisse et trois, les poitrines.

Distribution des hommes et des femmes sur les différents postes de la chaîne

Bien que l'entreprise souhaite que toutes les personnes travaillant sur cette chaîne puissent occuper tous les postes en rotation, on peut reconnaître deux séries de postes qu'occupent en rotation deux groupes de personnes différentes. Il s'agit en fait d'une «sexisation» des postes puisque l'un des groupes est constitué surtout d'hommes et l'autre groupe presque exclusivement de femmes. Les hommes occupent les postes 1 à 7, et les femmes les postes 8 à 15 (figure 2). En reconstituant l'historique avec les contremaîtres, nous avons appris que la «sexisation» des postes date du tout début de la chaîne (1976). Elle aurait été instaurée par le contremaître de l'époque. Selon ce dernier, certains emplois devaient être confiés aux hommes et d'autres aux femmes. Il préférait placer des femmes aux postes de finition et de parage. Il assignait les femmes au dépeçage des poitrines à cause des exigences de précision et de qualité. Les poitrines de dinde représentent en effet le morceau de choix de la volaille.

Il y a quelques années certaines femmes ont commencé à se plaindre de se retrouver toujours aux postes de parage et ont demandé d'apprendre le travail effectué aux postes des hommes. De son côté, l'employeur a mis de l'avant une nouvelle mesure concernant l'augmentation de la polyvalence de ses employés afin de faciliter sa gestion. Chaque personne de la chaîne de découpe de dinde fut donc sollicitée pour apprendre les opérations à faire aux postes qu'elle ne connaissait pas, mais cette mesure n'amena pas les résultats escomptés. La plupart des femmes, à la suite de leur apprentissage aux postes des hommes, ne voulaient plus y retourner. Toutes ont invoqué la même raison: les postes des hommes sont physiquement trop durs. Du côté des hommes, la résistance était encore plus grande puisque les travailleurs les plus anciens ont même refusé de recevoir une formation aux postes des femmes. Les travailleurs ont exprimé différents motifs pour expliquer leur réticence à occuper les postes féminins: deux trouvent que les postes des femmes sont plus ennuyeux, deux considèrent que ça va trop vite et deux autres que ça donne mal dans le dos. Un autre croit que le travail demande trop de précision et enfin le seul travailleur qui occupe les postes de femmes se plaint du «zigonnage». Trois travailleurs n'ont pas donné de raison.

Au tableau 2, on peut constater que les femmes ont davantage développé de polyvalence que les hommes, puisqu'au moment des entrevues individuelles, non seulement quatre femmes vont régulièrement du côté des hommes, mais quatre autres travailleuses s'y rendent de façon occasionnelle. Une seule femme, cependant, n'est pas régulière aux postes féminins. Il faut mentionner qu'aucune femme n'occupe le premier poste de la chaîne correspondant à l'accrochage de la volaille. Il semble que ce poste soit considéré trop lourd par toutes les femmes. Le seul travailleur qui occupe régulièrement les postes de femmes remplace depuis quelques mois une travailleuse en congé de maternité. Celui-ci n'avait aucune expérience antérieure sur la chaîne de découpe de dinde. C'est délibérément que le contremaître a choisi un homme pour la remplacer afin d'inciter les hommes à apprendre les opérations des postes de femmes.

Tableau 2 Occupation régulière ou occasionnelle des postes d'hommes et des postes de femmes selon le sexe

	Travailleuses N=17		Travailleurs N=10	
	Régulier	**Occasionnel**	**Régulier**	**Occasionnel**
Postes des femmes	16	1	1	0
Postes des hommes	4	4	9	0

Répétitivité et rotation

Bien que la vitesse de traitement de la chaîne puisse varier entre 225 et 300 volailles à l'heure, la vitesse régulière est de 300 dindes à l'heure. Une nouvelle dinde est donc accrochée à la chaîne à toutes les 12 secondes. La longueur des cycles de travail d'un poste à l'autre peut cependant être différente puisque plusieurs personnes peuvent se trouver au même poste (figure 2). Par exemple, quatre personnes font le dépeçage des poitrines. Chacune a donc 24 secondes pour couper la poitrine gauche ou droite d'une dinde sur deux. Par contre, au parage des ailes, une seule travailleuse fait toutes les ailes. Elle n'a donc que six secondes pour parer chaque aile. Au parage des poitrines, le cycle est de 18 secondes. Pour tous les autres postes, le cycle est de 12 secondes.

La rotation des postes semble dater de plusieurs années puisque déjà il y a 10 ans, la rotation s'effectuait à toutes les heures. Elle est passée aux demi-heures il y a six ans et, deux ans plus tard, aux quinze minutes. Cette rotation d'un poste à l'autre à l'intérieur de chacun des groupes s'effectue aux 15 minutes pour les postes qui se situent sur la plate-forme (postes 2 à 12). Il est à noter qu'aux postes où l'on retrouve plusieurs personnes, le temps passé à exécuter le même type d'opérations est plus long. Par exemple, comme il y a quatre travailleuses au dépeçage des poitrines, elles passeront quatre fois 15 minutes, soit une heure complète, à exécuter les mêmes opérations.

Au premier poste de la chaîne, l'accrochage, la rotation se fait à l'heure. Chacun des hommes de la chaîne ira donc passer une heure par jour à l'accrochage. Aux six postes de la table de parage, il y a rotation aux deux heures avec le groupe de travailleuses qui est sur la plate-forme. Ainsi, au cours d'une journée de travail, un groupe de huit femmes peut commencer sur la plate-forme en faisant une rotation aux 15 minutes aux huit postes. Après la pause, six de ces femmes descendent à la table de parage et y demeurent jusqu'au lunch. Elles retourneront aux postes de la plate-forme pour l'après-midi. Lorsque les travailleuses sont à la table de parage, la rotation entre les trois postes est laissée à leur discrétion. On y observe peu de rotation.

Figure 3   Pourcentage du temps passé à chacun des postes occupés par des hommes

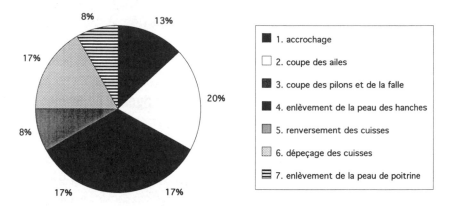

Figure 4   Pourcentage du temps passé à chacun des postes occupés par des femmes

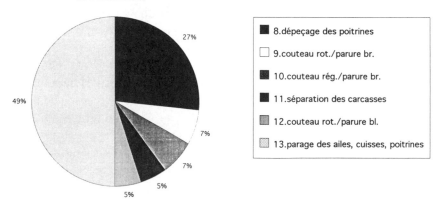

Sur les figures 3 et 4, on retrouve le pourcentage de temps passé par les travailleurs et les travailleuses à chacun des postes. Ces pourcentages ont été obtenus en calculant le temps passé à chacun des postes sur une période de deux jours en suivant la rotation normale des hommes et celle des femmes à leurs postes respectifs. On constate que les femmes consacrent la moitié de leur temps de travail à la table de parage (postes 13, 14 et 15). Le poste de dépeçage des poitrines occupe ensuite plus du quart de la journée alors que le dernier quart est passé aux quatre autres postes. Aux postes des hommes, le temps passé à chacun des postes est réparti de façon plus équitable: on n'occupe jamais le même poste plus de 20 p. 100 du temps sur une période de deux jours. On peut aussi visualiser par ces figures la succession des postes au cours de la rotation. Les travailleuses prennent quatre heures pour faire le tour de leurs postes avant de recommencer leur cycle de rotation. Les travailleurs, après avoir fait une heure d'accrochage au cours de la journée (poste 1), feront environ trois fois leur cycle de rotation des postes sur la plate-forme (poste 2 à 7) en prenant deux heures et demie chaque fois.

Comparaison des types d'opérations et des exigences des postes d'hommes et de femmes

Tous les postes de travail nécessitent le maintien statique de la position debout. Cependant, le statisme de la posture est plus important aux postes de parage (postes 13, 14 et 15) puisque les travailleuses demeurent debout face à leur table alors que l'avancement de la chaîne aux postes situés sur la plate-forme (postes 2 à 12), amènent les gens à piétiner sur place ou au moins à déplacer leur poids de gauche à droite. En effet, à ces postes, les travailleuses ont tendance à commencer leurs opérations sur la dinde un peu en amont de la chaîne (à gauche), elles continuent leur travail en suivant le mouvement de la chaîne et terminent leur cycle de travail un peu en aval de la chaîne (à droite). Les personnes travaillant sur la chaîne doivent maintenir les bras à la hauteur de la dinde suspendue ce qui entraîne le maintien ou la répétition d'abduction/flexion/rotation interne des épaules. Sauf au poste de l'accrochage (poste 1), tous les autres postes nécessitent l'usage d'un couteau qu'il faut régulièrement affiler sur un fusil si l'on veut entretenir le tranchant de la lame. Lors des entrevues, plus de la moitié des travailleuses et des travailleurs ont dit rencontrer des difficultés lors de l'affilage des couteaux.

D'après nos observations, on peut distinguer cinq types de postes dont les exigences et les contraintes sont différentes: les postes de préparation à la coupe, de coupe d'articulations, de dépeçage ou coupe de la chair, de finition et de nettoyage. Les postes sont classés au tableau 3. Trois postes appartiennent à deux catégories puisqu'on y exécute deux types d'opérations[3].

Pour chacun des postes de travail occupé de façon régulière, chaque personne répondant au questionnaire devait indiquer, selon une série de conditions de travail (force, cadence, précision, posture, température, couteau, gants), si elle n'avait aucune difficulté ou si elle trouvait le poste un peu difficile, pas mal difficile ou très difficile. Les réponses à ces questions seront en même temps présentées ainsi que certains éléments tirés des rencontres collectives.

Tableau 3 Caractéristiques des postes de la chaîne de découpe de dinde

	Préparation à la coupe	Coupe des articulation	Dépeçage	Finition	Nettoyage
Postes occupés par les hommes					
1. Accrochage	X				
2. Coupe des ailes		X	X		
3. Coupe des pilons et de la falle		X			
4. Enlèvement de la peau des hanches	X				
5. Renversement des cuisses	X	X			
6. Dépeçage des cuisses		X	X		
7. Enlèvement de la peau de poitrine	X				
Postes occupés par les femmes					
8. Dépeçage des poitrines			X		
9. Couteau rot./parure br.				X	
10. Couteau rég./parure br.				X	
11. Séparation des carcasses	X	X			
12. Couteau rot./parure bl.				X	
13. Parage des ailes					X
14. Parage des cuisses					X
15. Parage des poitrines					X

Les postes de préparation à la coupe: application de la force

On note d'abord au tableau 3 que les *postes de préparation* à la coupe sont presque essentiellement des postes d'hommes. Il s'agit de postes qui, selon nos observations, nécessitent peu ou pas l'usage du couteau et seraient moins exigeants du point de vue précision et qualité du travail, mais plus exigeants physiquement. Au poste de l'accrochage cinq hommes sur neuf rapportent souffrir de refroidissement aux mains puisque la dinde est saisie dans un contenant de glace. Les postes où on enlève la peau sont ceux où les répondants masculins rapportent le plus de difficulté en ce qui concerne l'application de la force (3 hommes sur 9). On se plaint aussi de difficulté avec les gants qui deviennent graisseux et très glissants. Au renversement des cuisses, la force représente également une difficulté à cause du geste de renversement de la hanche qui suit la coupe du tendon. La rotation des hommes les amène à passer le plus grand pourcentage de temps sur ces postes, soit 42 p.100.

La séparation des carcasses est le seul poste des femmes que l'on retrouve en partie dans cette catégorie. Cette opération ne représente que trois p.100 de leur temps de travail. Les travailleuses, après avoir coupé la carcasse, doivent en effet appuyer avec force sur celle-ci afin de la séparer. Ce poste est celui où le plus grand nombre de personnes a rapporté des difficultés au niveau de la cadence (huit personnes sur 17) et de la force (10 personnes sur 17). On mentionne également des difficultés avec le maniement du couteau (sept personnes sur 17). Il est cependant intéressant de noter que trois des quatre femmes qui vont régulièrement du côté des hommes vont également du côté des femmes; elles ont donc rapporté leurs difficultés pour l'ensemble des postes. Ces trois femmes n'ont signalé aucune difficulté avec l'application de la force au poste de la séparation des carcasses alors qu'elles en ont rapporté aux postes des hommes telles que l'enlèvement de la peau et le renversement des hauts de cuisse. Au moment de la rencontre avec les travailleurs, ceux-ci ont mentionné que souvent «les femmes ne sont pas assez grandes et elles doivent forcer de bas en haut pour renverser les hauts de cuisse ce qui peut décrocher la dinde». De plus, ces travailleuses ne peuvent pas bien voir l'endroit où il faut couper le tendon, ce qui peut augmenter ensuite leur difficulté à renverser la cuisse.

Coupe des articulations: du savoir-faire et un couteau bien affilé

Plusieurs postes masculins sont de ceux *où on coupe les articulations*. Le couteau doit être très bien affilé et les personnes doivent acquérir un savoir-faire qui leur permette de placer le couteau à un endroit bien précis afin de diminuer l'effort de coupe. Aux postes des hommes, on cherche l'endroit au niveau de l'articulation où on pourra couper les tendons des ailes et des cuisses. On y rapporte surtout des difficultés avec l'entretien du tranchant du couteau. Les hommes passent plus du tiers de leur temps à effectuer ce type d'opérations (39 p.100). Au poste de séparation des carcasses, les femmes au cours des premières opérations doivent aussi repérer la ligne de cartilage où elles devront effectuer la coupe. Cette opération ne représente cependant que trois p.100 de leur temps de travail.

Dépeçage: de la précision, de la qualité et un couteau bien affilé

Lorsque l'on doit *dépecer*, la chair doit être détachée de l'os. Ce travail demande un bon couteau et de la précision afin de ne pas laisser trop de chair sur l'os ni d'os dans la chair. Les hommes dépècent les ailes et les cuisses ce qui occupe 18 p.100 de leur temps alors que les femmes désossent les poitrines pendant 27 p.100 du temps. Les hommes éprouvent peu de difficulté sur ces postes, sauf avec le couteau au poste de coupe des ailes. Les femmes, par contre, rapportent des difficultés au niveau de la précision (cinq personnes sur 17), mais aussi avec le couteau que l'on n'a pas le temps d'affiler et les mains qui refroidissent à force de tenir la poitrine glacée. Il y a beaucoup d'incisions à pratiquer pour détacher correctement les poitrines. Les poitrines gauches sont plus difficiles à enlever, car le bras s'élève à plus de 90° C afin de contourner les os.

L'enjeu de ces postes est de récupérer le plus de chair possible. Au moment des rencontres, il a été plusieurs fois mentionné que le contrôle de qualité se faisait de façon plus insistante au poste de dépeçage de poitrine puisqu'il s'agit du morceau de volaille vendu le plus cher. La qualité du morceau dépecé dépend également de l'absence d'os dans la chair. En essayant d'obtenir le plus de chair possible, on peut en effet couper des parcelles d'os si les gestes ne sont pas suffisamment précis. Mais cette responsabilité appartient davantage aux travailleuses des postes de parage qui ont à enlever les os et les cartilages des morceaux dépecés. Le fait que les travailleuses aux postes de dépeçage de poitrine soient en rotation avec celles qui font le parage prend ici toute son importance. En effet, les travailleuses au dépeçage savent le travail qu'elles imposent à leurs compagnes du parage lorsqu'elles ne font pas le travail avec précision. Les travailleuses au dépeçage de poitrine ont intérêt à bien faire leur travail si elles veulent qu'on leur rende la pareille quand elles seront au parage. Mis à part le travailleur régulier aux postes des femmes, les hommes ne vont jamais au parage et n'en connaissent pas les contraintes. Certaines personnes, lors des rencontres ont mentionné qu'il serait important que les hommes aillent au parage afin d'acquérir cette conscience de l'impact de leur travail. D'autres ont suggéré que le parage soit fait au même poste que le dépeçage.

Finition: souci du travail bien fait

Aux *postes de finition*, toute la chair blanche et brune restant sur la carcasse doit être enlevée. On utilise soit un couteau ordinaire soit un couteau rotatif afin de récupérer le plus de chair possible. Seules des femmes sont assignées à ce poste et elles y passent 18 p.100 de leur temps. Très peu de difficulté y ont été mentionnées. Il faut que chaque personne ait la motivation de faire du bon travail pour que la carcasse soit bien nettoyée. Le contrôle de la qualité n'est cependant pas très important à ces postes comparés aux postes de parage.

Nettoyage ou parage: qualité, vitesse, résistance au froid et statisme postural

Les *postes de nettoyage* correspondent aux postes de parage: il faut nettoyer les morceaux coupés sur la chaîne des os, cartilages, etc. Il s'agit d'un travail minutieux où on contrôle la qualité des morceaux en coupant les parties indésirables. Encore une fois, seules les femmes occupent ces postes pendant la grosse partie de leur temps de travail (50 p.100). C'est aux postes de parage que l'on supporte la responsabilité de la qualité des morceaux. Si les personnes aux postes de dépeçage laissent des os dans la chair, ce sont les femmes aux postes de parage qui seront interpellées par le contremaître au moment du contrôle de la qualité.

On parle de difficulté au niveau de la cadence (sept sur 17) et du couteau (huit sur 17) surtout au poste de parage des ailes où une seule personne doit faire toutes les ailes. Ce sont aussi les postes où on relèvera le plus de problèmes reliés à la posture (six sur 17) et au refroidissement (sept sur 17). Il s'agit en effet d'un poste très stationnaire où la tête est toujours penchée vers le morceau à inspecter. Le dos peut également être courbé si la table est trop basse pour la personne.

Commentaires généraux comparant les postes des femmes et les postes des hommes

Aux postes des hommes, il est intéressant de noter que seules les travailleuses qui sont régulières à ces postes ont rapporté la mention «très difficile» en ce qui a trait à la force appliquée. Par ailleurs, seul l'unique travailleur du côté des femmes a mentionné des conditions «très difficiles» pour la précision et la posture.

On remarque que seul le dépeçage constitue l'une des cinq catégories où les hommes comme les femmes passent une proportion de temps significative (18 p.100 et 26 p.100). Les autres catégories regroupent soit des postes d'hommes, soit des postes de femmes. Les postes des hommes et les postes des femmes ont, d'un côté comme de l'autre, une catégorie qui domine: la catégorie où on doit appliquer la force chez les hommes (42 p.100 du temps) et la catégorie du parage chez les femmes (50 p.100) où on inspecte et nettoie avec minutie chaque morceau de dinde. Si l'on se rapporte aux figures 3 et 4, rappelons que les postes des différentes catégories alternent davantage du côté des hommes que du côté des femmes.

L'opinion des contremaîtres, des travailleurs et des travailleuses sur les exigences physiques des postes et les difficultés d'apprentissage

Selon les informations tirées des rencontres de discussion avec les deux contremaîtres, voici leur classification des postes en ce qui concerne les exigences physiques et les difficultés d'apprentissage.

Les exigences physiques seraient les plus importantes dans la catégorie des postes de préparation à la coupe (catégorie 1), viendraient ensuite, entremêlés, des postes appartenant à la catégorie de coupe des articulations et à celle du dépeçage (catégories 2 et 3) dans l'ordre suivant: coupe du pilon, dépeçage des poitrines, dépeçage des hauts de cuisse et coupe et dépeçage des ailes. La catégorie des postes de parage (catégorie 5) et la catégorie des postes de finition (catégorie 4) terminent la liste.

On considère généralement que l'apprentissage à un poste est difficile si les personnes prennent plus de temps à acquérir de la vitesse et à être suffisamment à l'aise pour avoir le temps d'affiler leur couteau, ou encore s'il y a une technique particulière à acquérir pour être en mesure de répondre aux exigences de qualité ou pour être capable d'exécuter les opérations sans trop d'efforts. Si l'on classe maintenant les postes par ordre de difficulté d'apprentissage, les contremaîtres proposent d'abord, encore une fois entremêlés, les postes des catégories 2 et 3 dans cet ordre: coupe des pilons, dépeçage des poitrines, coupe du tendon au renversement des hauts de cuisse, dépeçage des ailes, coupe du cartilage au poste de séparation des carcasses, dépeçage des cuisses. Viennent ensuite les postes de parage (catégorie 5), les postes de finition (catégorie 4) et les postes de préparation à la coupe (catégorie 1).

Les travailleurs et les travailleuses, lors des rencontres de discussion, rapportent à peu près les mêmes ordres de classification, mais il est intéressant de mentionner certains commentaires. Par exemple, une travailleuse qui connaissait tous les postes de la chaîne, rapportait qu'il était plus long d'apprendre à dépecer une poitrine qu'à couper un pilon. «Quand tu coupes le pilon, précise-t-elle, ce n'est pas nécessaire d'être aussi minutieuse, on ne te demande pas de faire une aussi belle «job», mais si tu ne coupes pas à la bonne place, par exemple, c'est là que tu te fatigues les bras». Quand on demande aux travailleuses quel est le temps nécessaire pour apprendre les opérations des postes, elles diront trois à quatre semaines au dépeçage des poitrines (catégorie 3), deux semaines à la séparation des carcasses (catégories 1 et 2) et deux ou trois jours au parage (catégorie 5). Cependant, le temps nécessaire pour être à l'aise serait de deux ou trois mois au dépeçage des poitrines, un mois à la séparation des carcasses et un mois aussi au parage. L'apprentissage aux postes de parage ne serait donc pas long; mais avant d'avoir la vitesse requise et répondre aux exigences de qualité, on a besoin de plusieurs semaines.

Un travailleur, de son côté, rapporte: «Les postes des hommes sont plus durs physiquement, mais on travaille de partout. C'est plus dur pour les femmes au dépeçage de poitrine parce qu'elles passent une heure à dépecer et c'est un poste dur pour les mains». Lors de la rencontre de discussion avec les travailleurs, ceux-ci ont insisté sur l'importance de la technique à leurs postes de travail et de l'affilage du couteau.

Sites de fatigue et de douleur et niveau de gravité

La différence entre les hommes et les femmes ressort tout spécialement lorsque l'on compare le nombre de personnes rapportant de la douleur et le niveau de gravité des problèmes. Le tableau 4 est très éloquent à ce sujet. En effet, alors que 70 p. 100 des hommes ne rapportent aucun site de fatigue ou de douleur, 41 p. 100 des femmes ont des douleurs qui les ont amenées, soit à s'absenter, soit à prendre des médicaments, ou à consulter un médecin. Notons que plus des trois quarts des femmes ont rapporté au moins un site de douleur ressentie pendant l'accomplissement du travail au cours de la dernière semaine de travail. Si l'on enlève du groupe des femmes celles qui vont aussi du côté des postes des hommes, ce pourcentage demeure le même. Du côté des travailleurs, les seuls trois hommes qui rapportent de la douleur ont atteint un seuil de gravité plus élevé que celui de ressentir de la douleur pendant le travail. Le travailleur du côté des femmes fait partie de ceux-ci.

Tableau 4   Pourcentage des hommes et des femmes rapportant au moins un site de fatigue ou de douleur selon le degré de gravité

	% Femmes N= 17	% Hommes N= 10
Aucun site rapporté	12	70
Fatigue	88	20
Douleur pendant le travail	76	30
Douleur après le travail	65	30
Consultation médicale ou médicament ou absence	41	10

La région du corps principalement affectée est la région cervico-brachiale comprenant le cou, le haut du dos et les épaules: plus de 55 p. 100 des personnes avaient ressenti de la douleur à cette région au cours de la dernière semaine. Il s'agit surtout de douleurs à l'épaule droite. Viennent ensuite les membres supérieurs, dont le poignet, et aussi les jambes.

Certaines douleurs sont ressenties au cours de l'exécution de certaines opérations. Sur le tableau 5, on retrouve le nombre de personnes qui ont associé leurs douleurs à des postes en particulier. Du côté des hommes, les postes où on enlève la peau et le poste où on renverse les cuisses (poste de catégorie 1 et 2) sont mentionnés mais presque uniquement par les quelques femmes qui occupent régulièrement ces postes. Du côté des postes des femmes, on note tout spécialement le dépeçage des poitrines (catégorie 3) et les postes de parage (catégorie 5). L'unique travailleur masculin de ce côté de la chaîne associe ses douleurs à l'exécution des tâches liées à ces mêmes postes.

Tableau 5 Nombre de personnes associant leur douleur à un poste et nombre d'accidents déclarés à chaque poste

	Nombre de personnes associant ses douleurs à un poste	Nombre d'accidents déclarés à un poste
1. Accrochage	0	3
2. Coupe des ailes	1	1
3. Coupe des pilons et de la falle	3	1
4. Enlèvement de la peau des hanches	5	7
5. Renversement des cuisses	4	7
6. Dépeçage des cuisses	2	0
7. Enlèvement de la peau de poitrine	3	0
8. Dépeçage des poitrines	10	3
9. Couteau rot./parure br.	2	0
10. Couteau rég./parure br.	1	0
11. Séparation des carcasses	4	10
12. Couteau rot./parure bl.	3	1
13. Parage des ailes	7	1
14. Parage des cuisses	7	2
15. Parage des poitrines	7	2

postes 1 à 7 : n=13 (9 hommes et 4 femmes)
postes 8 à 15 : n=17 (16 femmes et 1 homme)

Accidents

Entre janvier 1986 et décembre 1992, 26 des 27 travailleurs et travailleuses de la chaîne de découpe de dinde ont cumulé 102 accidents dont 86 depuis que chacun et chacune est assigné à la chaîne de découpe de dinde. La plupart de ces accidents, soit 50 sur 86, ont eu lieu alors qu'ils étaient en train de travailler sur les postes de la chaîne de découpe de dinde. Une proportion importante des accidents (36 sur 86) a donc été déclarée au moment où les travailleurs et les travailleuses de la chaîne de découpe de dinde étaient envoyés temporairement dans un autre département, à des postes inhabituels afin de remplacer des absents, par exemple. Nous ne connaissons pas la fréquence de ces remplacements pour chacun des travailleurs et des travailleuses. Sur les 50 accidents survenus sur la chaîne de découpe de dinde, 86 p.100 sont des problèmes musculo-squelettiques dont 88 p.100 concernent les membres supérieurs et la région cervico-brachiale. La fréquence moyenne d'accidents pour les personnes qui sont actuellement régulières à la chaîne de découpe de dinde — en ne considérant que les accidents qui ont eu lieu sur la chaîne de dinde entre janvier 1986 et décembre 1992 — est de 0,43 chez les femmes et de 0,41 chez les hommes.

Pour 38 des 50 accidents survenus à la chaîne, on a noté le poste sur lequel la personne travaillait au moment de la déclaration d'accident. Ces accidents peuvent donc se distribuer selon les postes. Les postes de la peau des hanches (sept accidents) et du renversement des hauts de cuisses (sept accidents) ressortent du côté des hommes ainsi que le poste de l'accrochage (trois accidents) (tableau 5). Ces postes appartiennent à la première catégorie de postes («préparation à la coupe») et sont considérés difficiles à cause de la force physique à appliquer. Il est intéressant de noter que les femmes ont déclaré huit des 19 accidents associés à un poste masculin. Ces huit accidents ne sont pas attribuables aux travailleuses qui sont régulières du côté des hommes. Il s'agit plutôt de travailleuses qui y travaillent parfois (cinq accidents) ou même rarement (trois accidents).

Le poste de séparation des carcasses, lui aussi de la catégorie 1 de «préparation à la coupe», domine du côté des femmes (10 des 19 accidents rapportés sur les postes des femmes). On rapporte également trois accidents au dépeçage de poitrine et cinq accidents aux postes de parage. Il est intéressant de noter l'importance que prend le poste de séparation des carcasses en ce qui concerne les accidents alors que ce poste occupe un faible pourcentage du temps des travailleuses comparé aux postes de parage, par exemple. Par ailleurs, contrairement au poste de dépeçage des poitrines, la séparation des carcasses n'est pas un poste où les travailleuses rapportent ressentir le plus de douleur, mais c'est bien celui où elles rapportent éprouver le plus de difficulté avec l'application de la force.

Préférence d'assignation

Les questions concernant les postes que les personnes préfèrent et ceux qu'elles n'aiment pas apportent un autre type de données qui va au-delà des contraintes physiques. Il est intéressant de comparer les raisons pour lesquelles les hommes et les femmes aiment ou détestent un poste de travail. Bien que la principale raison invoquée pour l'appréciation d'un poste soit qu'il est facile à faire ou relaxant, la seconde raison est la satisfaction du travail bien fait. Pour cette raison, cinq femmes auront comme premier choix le dépeçage de poitrine, malgré le fait que ce soit un poste où l'on rapporte souvent de la douleur. Les femmes mentionnent qu'à ce poste, elles ont un certain défi à relever, un savoir-faire à acquérir. Au total, 10 femmes vont donner leur préférence à ce poste. Du côté des hommes, les postes de dépeçage comptent aussi parmi les préférés.

En revanche, les postes de parage sont plus souvent mentionnés parmi les postes détestés à cause de la monotonie, de la précision et de la cadence. Le parage des ailes, en particulier, est rapporté par six personnes, dont le travailleur masculin. Le plus souvent, on n'aime pas un poste parce qu'il est physiquement trop exigeant. C'est le cas de trois postes de la catégorie de «préparation à la coupe», soit les postes d'enlèvement de la peau et de renversement des cuisses ainsi que celui de la séparation des carcasses qui est le poste le plus souvent mentionné par les femmes (huit personnes) comme étant celui qu'elles aiment le moins.

DISCUSSION

La fréquence des lésions musculo-squelettiques indemnisées est très élevée chez les travailleurs et les travailleuses de la chaîne de découpe de dinde étudiée. La description des contraintes aux postes de travail de ce département met en évidence des facteurs de risque reconnus pour favoriser le développement de ce type de lésions (Armstrong et al., 1987; Silverstein et al., 1986). Le travail est très répétitif. Les cycles de travail sont très courts: de 6 à 24 secondes. Il n'y a pas de possibilité de régulation de son rythme de travail puisqu'il faut suivre la cadence de la chaîne. Les membres supérieurs sont très sollicités, tous les postes exigeant des mouvements répétés de différentes articulations. Pour tous les postes se situant sur la plate-forme, on peut souligner le maintien des bras en hauteur pour avoir accès à la dinde. La température de la salle de travail est basse et les mains manipulent de la dinde glacée. Tout le monde travaille debout, de façon statique. Il s'agit ici de caractéristiques appartenant autant aux postes occupés en rotation par les femmes qu'aux postes assignés en rotation aux hommes.

Qu'est-ce qui explique que davantage de femmes rapportent des symptômes de douleur et à un niveau de gravité plus important que les hommes? En effet, 77 p.100 des femmes aux postes des femmes ressentent de la douleur en travaillant comparativement à 22 p.100 des hommes sur les postes des hommes. On peut se demander si les hommes ont été moins enclins que les femmes à rapporter leurs douleurs (Gervais, 1992). Pourtant d'autres études ont été menées par notre équipe dans le même secteur d'activité, mais où les emplois étaient occupés exclusivement par des hommes (abattoirs de porcs) et les travailleurs ont rapporté une fréquence de douleur élevée (Toulouse et al., 1992; Chatigny et Vézina, 1994). Dans ce milieu mixte que constitue la chaîne de découpe de dinde, peut-être devons-nous envisager la possibilité que d'un point de vue simplement culturel, les hommes n'aient pas rapporté leurs symptômes de la même manière que les femmes. Mais cette possibilité explique-t-elle entièrement la différence observée? D'autres questions nous ont semblé importantes à poser: Au-delà des ressemblances énumérées précédemment, est-ce que les différences entre les postes n'exposeraient pas les travailleurs et les travailleuses à des contraintes différentes? Ces contraintes diverses ne peuvent-elles pas avoir un impact différent sur le développement des problèmes musculo-squelettiques et dans leurs manifestations?

Mais on peut aussi poser le problème autrement. Puisque les taux annuels d'accidents à la chaîne de découpe de dinde chez le groupe de travailleurs et chez le groupe de travailleuses sont semblables, ce sont peut-être les hommes, au contraire, qui sont plus enclins à déclarer un accident plutôt que d'endurer de la douleur au travail. Mais d'une façon comme d'une autre, il importe de s'attarder sur l'exposition des deux groupes à des contraintes différentes. En effet, il est possible que les caractéristiques des postes des hommes obligent à une déclaration plus rapide des problèmes musculo-squelettiques.

Les hommes et les femmes travaillant à la chaîne de découpe étudiée sont exposés à des contraintes différentes

En effet, même dans les ressemblances qui ont été énumérées au début de cette section, des différences peuvent être notées. Tout le monde travaille au *froid*, mais les femmes souffrent davantage de refroidissement ce qui peut s'expliquer par le fait qu'elles passent la moitié de leur temps aux postes de parage où elles sont plus statiques et ont moins la possibilité de se réchauffer par l'intensité de l'activité musculaire. Par ailleurs, bien que tous soient *debout*, l'inconfort de la position debout est davantage ressentie, encore une fois, aux postes de parage à cause du caractère quasi statique de la posture et de la dureté du sol de ciment. La *hauteur de la chaîne* est la même pour tout le monde mais les femmes étant plus petites en moyenne de 10 centimètres, voilà autant de centimètres qu'elles doivent récupérer en soulevant les bras. La charge au niveau des épaules peut donc être plus importante pour plusieurs femmes. Les problèmes reliés à la *posture* sont aussi davantage rapportés au poste de parage à cause de la hauteur de la table et de la minutie des mouvements qui obligent à une flexion continuelle du cou pour diriger le regard vers les morceaux à parer (Charpentier et Gandon, 1989).

Aux postes des femmes, on rapporte plus souvent des difficultés au niveau de la *cadence*. La cadence est davantage ressentie au poste de séparation des carcasses car il y a beaucoup d'opérations à faire et une seule personne occupe ce poste. Aux postes de parage, la cadence est considérée comme difficile par plusieurs. En effet, il faut faire le parage de tous les morceaux désossés à la chaîne tout en respectant les consignes relatives à la qualité des morceaux. Par contre, ce qui caractérise le plus le travail des hommes, est sûrement l'application de la *force* aux postes de préparation à la coupe. Il s'agit de la catégorie d'opérations la plus importante chez les hommes (42 p.100 du temps). On applique une force importante soit pour accrocher les dindes aux crochets de la chaîne, soit pour arracher la peau, ou pour désarticuler les hauts de cuisse en les renversant. La force exigée est d'autant plus contraignante que les gants deviennent glissants et qu'il faut maintenir la cadence. Aux postes des femmes, on passe très peu de temps à ce type d'opérations qui ne se retrouvent qu'à la séparation des carcasses et 63 p.100 des femmes rapportent avoir de la difficulté à ce poste à cause de la force physique à appliquer.

L'ampleur des contraintes est aussi reliée aux différences dans l'organisation du travail

Si nous nous attardons sur ce qui différencie le travail des hommes de celui des femmes, soulignons aussi la différence dans l'ensemble de la journée de travail qui dépend de l'organisation des rotations. En comparaison de la rotation effectuée aux postes des femmes, la rotation entre les postes des hommes leur permet d'une part, de passer au cours d'une journée de travail des pourcentages de temps mieux partagés entre les différentes catégories de postes, et d'autre part, de rester moins de temps en continu sur des postes appartenant à la même catégorie et comportant le même type de contraintes. Durant une journée de travail, les hommes auront le temps de faire trois fois le tour de chacun de leurs postes de travail alors que les femmes n'auront pas le temps de faire deux fois le tour complet de leurs postes, ce qui diminue la variation des contraintes au cours de la journée de travail.

La précision des gestes: une contrainte liée aux exigences de qualité, à la cadence, à la force appliquée, aux difficultés d'apprentissage

La précision des gestes est un point intéressant à discuter, car la précision est présente à chaque poste de travail, mais avec une acuité différente et peut-être, surtout, pour des raisons différentes. On considérera qu'un poste demande beaucoup de précision si les coups de couteau doivent être donnés à des endroits précis. Ces postes exigent aussi que le couteau soit toujours très bien affilé. Il s'agit surtout des postes où on coupe les articulations (2ᵉ catégorie), ce qui occupe 39 p. 100 du temps des hommes et trois p. 100 du temps des femmes, et des postes où on fait du dépeçage (3ᵉ catégorie) occupant 18 p. 100 du temps chez les hommes et 27 p. 100 chez les femmes. Ces deux catégories occupent donc 57 p. 100 du temps chez les hommes et 30 p. 100 du temps chez les femmes. Les hommes ont donc souvent un travail très précis à effectuer. On distinguera cependant les postes de la deuxième catégorie, où on doit couper les articulations, des postes où on doit dépecer (3ᵉ catégorie), car les raisons qui expliquent l'importance de la précision sont différentes. Quand on coupe une articulation, la précision du geste influera sur la force qui sera nécessaire pour couper ainsi que sur le nombre de coups de couteau requis. si l'on réussit à trouver l'endroit où on peut couper le tendon, on facilite son travail. De là l'importance de l'apprentissage pour avoir la possibilité d'acquérir ce savoir-faire. Mais on n'exigera pas ce savoir-faire des travailleurs et des travailleuses dans la mesure où ils réussissent à suivre la cadence.

Par contre, quand on fait du dépeçage, la précision est nécessaire pour répondre aux exigences de qualité. Il faut couper au bon endroit car on ne peut pas recommencer la coupe du morceau ou essayer de continuer à enlever de la chair sur les os. Il faut faire en sorte que le ou les coups de couteau permettent d'obtenir un morceau le plus charnu possible, mais ceci est surtout contrôlé au dépeçage des poitrines coûteuses . Par ailleurs, le geste sera d'autant plus précis qu'on tentera de récupérer le plus de chair possible mais sans couper une partie d'os ou de cartilage; cela dépend alors de la volonté de chacun et de chacune de laisser moins de travail aux travailleuses de la table du parage qui, elles, ont la responsabilité de nettoyer les morceaux de ces particules indésirables. Cette conscience est plus facile à avoir quand on connaît le travail aux postes de parage.

Les postes de parage et de finition: de la précision ou de la minutie?

Sur les postes de parage et de finition, on préférera parler de minutie plutôt que de précision. Non que le travail ne demande pas de précision, puisqu'il faut réussir à récupérer le plus de chair possible; mais en comparaison des postes où on coupe les articulations et des postes de dépeçage, l'endroit exact où devra se placer le couteau est moins capital. On peut redonner un coup de couteau pour enlever un morceau de cartilage, par exemple. Par contre, la qualité du travail dépendra, en ce qui a trait au parage, de la minutie avec laquelle la personne inspectera chaque côté du morceau à nettoyer afin de repérer et de couper ce qui en diminue la qualité. Chaque fois il faudra être en mesure de juger à quel point on doit nettoyer un morceau. À l'étape de la finition, on jugera si l'on a suffisamment récupéré toute la chair sur la carcasse. Ce sont donc des postes où la qualité du travail et le nombre de coups de couteau donnés dépendent du souci de la personne à bien faire son travail, de sa minutie. Au parage ce travail de minutie est plus exigeant à cause de l'importance de la qualité des morceaux à nettoyer.

Pourquoi les femmes ne veulent-elles pas aller du côté des hommes et pourquoi les hommes ne veulent-ils pas aller du côté des femmes?

Si l'on résume les différences entre les postes des hommes et ceux des femmes, on pourrait dire qu'aux postes des hommes, les personnes sont beaucoup plus souvent appelées à fournir un effort important en appliquant de la force. Quand les femmes ont indiqué lesquels de leurs postes de travail elles aimaient le moins, la plupart ont indiqué le poste de séparation des carcasses où elles ont à appliquer de la force, même si ce poste occupe peu de temps dans leur journée de travail. On comprend donc que, de façon unanime, elles ont invoqué cette raison pour ne pas aller du côté des hommes. On peut penser que la force physique nécessaire pour occuper les postes des hommes représente le principal obstacle à la polyvalence des femmes. La force physique de la moyenne des femmes est moins importante que celle de la moyenne des hommes, surtout au niveau des membres supérieurs où elle représenterait moins des deux tiers de celle de la moyenne des hommes (Celentano et al., 1984; Pheasant, 1983). Les femmes pourraient donc être plus à risque que les hommes sur ce type de poste. Cela est confirmé par le nombre d'accidents subis par les femmes alors qu'elles occupaient un poste masculin.

Sur les quatre femmes qui se retrouvent régulièrement du côté des hommes, aucune n'a eu d'accident sur ces postes, mais trois ont rapporté des symptômes de douleur y compris la seule travailleuse non régulière sur les postes des femmes. Il est difficile de conclure quoi que ce soit à partir de ce groupe de travailleuses puisque trois d'entre elles sont aussi régulières du côté des femmes; cependant, ces femmes ont surtout associé leurs douleurs au travail sur les postes des hommes.

Couper les tendons lors de la coupe des articulations aux postes des hommes (2e catégorie) demande aussi un savoir-faire important et suppose un temps d'apprentissage assez long pour pouvoir, notamment, diminuer la force pour couper les morceaux. Si une femme décide d'aller du côté des hommes, qu'est-ce qui se passe? La période d'apprentissage peut être trop pénible, si en plus de faire les postes de la première catégorie (postes qui exigent de la force), elle doit aussi exercer de la force physique aux postes de la deuxième catégorie (coupe des articulations) parce qu'elle n'a pas encore intégré la gestuelle qui permet de couper au bon endroit. Elle peut aussi avoir à forcer davantage que la plupart des hommes parce que sa taille plus petite l'empêche de bien voir les tendons ou de placer son bras.

On se souvient des raisons pour lesquelles les hommes ne veulent pas aller du côté des femmes: routine ennuyeuse, trop vite, maux de dos, trop de précision, trop de minutie («zigonnage»). En effet, on ne dira pas des postes des femmes qu'ils sont trop éreintants; par contre, les travailleuses sont appelées à rester pendant de longues périodes sur le même type de postes, donc à conserver pendant longtemps des postures qui sont également plus statiques. Les exigences de qualité et de cadence apparaissent plus importantes et supposent davantage de tension et moins de temps de récupération.

Si le portrait des femmes est équivalent à celui des hommes en ce qui concerne le taux de lésions déclarées, il est plus inquiétant en ce qui a trait à l'état de santé comme le laisse supposer la fréquence et la gravité des symptômes musculo-squelettiques rapportés. Cette situation contribue peut-être aussi à la réticence des hommes à aller aux postes féminins, par crainte de développer les symptômes des femmes, et à la réticence des femmes à aller aux postes masculins, par crainte d'augmenter les symptômes qu'elles ont déjà. Cela nous amène donc à poser une dernière série de questions.

Les postes des hommes seraient-ils plus «limitants» et les postes des femmes plus «usants»?

Les hommes comme les femmes rapportent plus souvent leurs accidents aux postes où la force est nécessaire. Aux postes des hommes, presque tous les accidents sont déclarés soit à l'enlèvement de la peau, soit au renversement des cuisses, ou à l'accrochage des dindes. Du côté des postes féminins, il est surprenant de constater que plus de la moitié des accidents sont déclarés à la séparation des carcasses alors qu'une faible proportion du temps travaillé y est passé. Cette situation peut certainement s'expliquer, en partie, par le fait que lorsque l'on a à exercer une force soit pour tirer, soit pour pousser, comme c'est le cas aux postes de la catégorie 1, il est possible de donner un mauvais coup et d'avoir une lésion musculo-squelettique plutôt de type accidentel: «… en tirant, j'ai ressenti une douleur», ou bien «la dinde était dure et j'ai trop forcé», etc.

Il est possible également de développer une lésion du type «traumatismes répétés» (*cumulative trauma disorder*) et, au cours d'une journée de travail, ressentir une douleur qui sera impossible à supporter aux postes où on doit exercer une force. C'est alors que l'on arrête de travailler pour déclarer une lésion professionnelle. En effet, comment peut-on arracher de la peau lorsque l'on éprouve une douleur? Alors qu'il est peut être encore possible de continuer à travailler dans la douleur si l'on coupe de façon répétitive de petits morceaux dans un effort moindre, mais continu, comme aux postes de parage ou de finition.

Cette constatation peut nous aider à comprendre pourquoi les accidents sont déclarés au poste «forçants» alors que la douleur peut être ressentie et associée à d'autres postes, comme c'est le cas des travailleuses qui associent surtout leurs douleurs au poste de dépeçage de poitrine et aux postes de parage, alors que leurs accidents sont surtout déclarés à la séparation des carcasses. On peut alors considérer que le travail des hommes est plus «limitant», puisque l'importance des postes «forçants» peut représenter une limite, une barrière qui entraîne l'arrêt de travail. De même on peut comprendre la réticence des femmes qui rapportent de la douleur à se retrouver du côté des hommes.

Nous croyons qu'il est possible que l'état de santé du système musculo-squelettique des femmes soit plus endommagé et se manifeste par une fréquence et une gravité accentuées des symptômes. Les femmes pourraient avoir développé davantage que les hommes de chronicité dans la douleur parce qu'elles peuvent continuer à exécuter leur travail malgré l'inconfort ressenti, parce qu'elles peuvent retourner au travail alors que la douleur persiste. Le travail des femmes est moins dur physiquement? Peut-être parce qu'il ne demande pas de déployer un effort dynamique instantané aussi important, mais qu'en est-il du travail statique, qu'en est-il de l'endurance? Et surtout, combien de temps ces femmes peuvent-elles travailler dans la douleur avant de déclarer une lésion profession-nelle?

Est-il possible que les femmes continuent à travailler et à user leur système musculo-squelettique jusqu'à ce qu'elles ne peuvent plus du tout faire ce type de travail? Comment se fait-il qu'on ne retrouve aucune femme avec plus de six ans d'ancienneté alors que celle des hommes va jusqu'à 12 ans? Par contre, peut-être l'effet de sélection des plus résistants joue-t-il davantage chez les hommes, puisqu'on trouve soit des anciens (six ans et plus), soit des nouveaux (trois ans et moins).

Dans cette même entreprise, Lemay (1995) a tenté de suivre le cheminement de chacune des personnes qui avaient souffert d'une ten-dinite aux membres supérieurs en 1988. Le nombre de sujets était de 14 hommes et 24 femmes. Il s'agissait surtout de personnes provenant des départements de découpe de la dinde et de découpe du poulet. Ces personnes devaient être rencontrées en entrevue en 1993, mais 11 person-nes avaient quitté l'entreprise. Il s'agissait de sept hommes et de quatre femmes, ce qui représente 50 p. 100 du groupe des hommes et 17 p. 100 du groupe des femmes. Dans la région où se trouve l'entreprise étudiée, il est probablement plus facile pour un homme de se trouver un autre emploi. Il est possible que les hommes qui éprouvent des difficultés physiques quittent ce type d'emploi, alors que les femmes le conservent tant qu'elles sont capables d'accomplir leur travail[4]. C'est aussi ce que semble confir-mer la répartition de l'ancienneté: chez les hommes, on retrouve des employés soit de trois ans et moins, soit de six à 12 ans; alors que chez les femmes, plus de 80 p. 100 ont entre quatre et six ans d'ancienneté et aucune n'en plus de six ans.

CONCLUSION

Notre réflexion demeure suspendue à plusieurs questions concernant les caractéristiques du travail des hommes, les caractéristiques du travail des femmes et les situations de travail qui peuvent favoriser le développement des problèmes musculo-squelettiques. Est-ce que les postes des femmes «usent» différemment de ceux des hommes? Il est possible que les contraintes décrites aux postes des femmes soient plus dommageables, compte tenu, en particulier, de la difficulté de varier le travail et de récupérer.

Par ailleurs, est-ce que les postes des femmes leur permettent de tolérer plus longtemps leur douleur sans déclarer d'accident et d'atteindre ainsi un niveau d'usure plus important? Si l'on se rappelle que 41 p.100 des femmes ont consulté un professionnel de la santé ou prennent des médicaments pour leurs douleurs musculo-squelettiques, on peut en conclure que le système de santé publique pourrait donc être celui qui paie la note de l'état de santé des femmes plutôt que la Commission de la santé et de la sécurité au travail (CSST) financée par les entreprises.

Est-ce que la plupart des femmes auraient plus d'accidents si elles se retrouvaient régulièrement du côté des hommes? Est-ce que les hommes auraient plus de douleur s'ils se retrouvaient régulièrement du côté des femmes? Des questions pertinentes, certes, mais que peu de recherches peuvent envisager d'étudier faute d'un marché de travail vraiment «désexisé» où ces questions pourraient être examinées adéquatement (Messing et al., 1994).

NOTES

1. Au Québec, LATR: lésion attribuable au travail répétitif; au Canada anglais, RSI: *repetitive strain injury*, ou CTD: *cumulative trauma disorder*.

2. Certains postes sont en effet occupés par les travailleurs accidentés lors de leur retour au travail. Il s'agit alors d'une assignation temporaire.

3. Le temps passé à ces postes de travail sera partagé entre les deux catégories lors du calcul du temps passé par les travailleurs et les travailleuses dans chacune des catégories.

4. C'est ce que Neis conclut aussi dans son étude des travailleuses du crabe à Terre-Neuve. Voir article dans ce volume.

BIBLIOGRAPHIE

Armstrong, T.J., J.A. Foulke, B.S. Joseph et S.A. Goldstein. "Investigation of Cumulative Trauma Disorders in a Poultry Processing Plant." *American Industrial Hygiene Association Journal* 43, 2 (1982). pp. 103-16.

Armstrong, T.J., et B.A. Silverstein. "Upper-extremity Pain in the Workplace — Role of Usage in Causality," dans *Clinical Concepts in Regional Musculoskeletal Illness*. M. Nortin, et M. Hadler (éds.). Toronto: NC Press, 1987. pp. 333-54.

Celentano, E.J., J.W. Nottrodt et P.L. Saunders. "The Relationship Between Size, Strength and Task Demands." *Ergonomics* 27, 5 (1984). pp. 481-8.

Charpentier, P., et M. Gandon. «Organisation et conditions de travail dans les abattoirs de volailles». *La lettre d'informationde l'Agence Nationale pour l'Amélioration des Conditions de travail* 137 (janvier 1989). pp. 4-11.

Chatigny, C., et N. Vézina. «Conditions d'apprentissage du métier dans un abattoir: Un handicap pour les travailleurs qui utilisent un couteau». *Performances Humaines et Techniques* 71 (juillet-août 1994). pp. 29-38.

Courville, J., L. Dumais et N. Vézina. «Conditions de travail de femmes et d'hommes sur une chaîne de découpe de volaille et développement d'atteintes musculo-squelettiques». *Travail et santé* 10, 3 (septembre 1994). pp. S17-23.

Gervais, M. *Interprétation des enquêtes de santé.* Montréal: IRSST, janvier 1992.

Hinnen, U., T. Laübli, U. Guggenbülh et H. Krueger. "Design of Check-out Systems Including Laser Scanners for Sitting Work Posture." *Scandinavian Journal of Environmental Health* 18 (1992). pp. 186-94.

Hünting, W., T. Laübli et E. Grandjean. "Postural and Visual Load at VDT Workplaces: 1. Constrained Postures." *Ergonomics* 24 (1981). pp. 917-31.

Kilbom, A., J. Persson et B.G. Jonsson. "Disorders of the Cervicobrachial Region Among Female Workers in the Electronic Industry." *International Journal of Industrial Ergonomics* 1 (1986). pp. 37-47.

Laville, A. "Postural Stress in High Speed Precision Work." *Ergonomics* 28 (1985). pp. 229-36.

Lemay, N. «La récidive de la tendinite au membre supérieur au sein d'une industrie de transformation de la volaille», dans *Mémoire de Maîtrise en Sciences Biologiques.* Non publié. Montréal: UQAM, 1995.

Mergler, D., C. Brabant, N. Vézina et K. Messing. "The Weaker Sex? Men in Women's Working Conditions Report Similar Health Symptoms." *Journal of Occupational Medicine* 29 (1987). pp. 417-21.

Messing, K., et J.P. Reveret. "Are Women in Female Jobs for their Health? A Study of Working Conditions and Health Effects in the Fish-processing Industry in Quebec." *International Journal of Health Services* 13, 4 (1983). pp. 635-47.

Messing, K., J. Courville, M. Boucher, L. Dumais et A-M Seifert. "Can Safety Risk of Blue-collar Jobs be Compared by Gender?" *Safety Science* 18 (1994). pp. 95-112.

Patry, L., D. Laliberté, J. Pelletier, L. Gilbert, M.A. Telle et J.G. Richard. «Problèmes musculo-squelettiques et mouvements répétitifs dans les abattoirs de volailles». *Compte rendus du 3e colloque annuel de l'Association des médecins du réseau public en santé au travail du Québec* (1993). pp. 56-72.

Pheasant, S.T. "Sex Differences in Strength, Some Observations on Their Variability." *Applied Ergonomics* 14, 3 (1983). pp. 205-11.

Ryan, G.A. "The Prevalence of Musculo-skeletal Symptoms in Supermarket Workers." *Ergonomics* 32, 4 (1989). pp. 359-71.

Silverstein, B.A., L.J. Fine et T.J. Armstrong. "Hand Wrist Cumulative Trauma Disorders in Industry." *British Journal of Occupational Medicine.* 43 (1986). pp. 779-84.

Toulouse, G., N. Vézina, L. Geoffrion, C. Lapointe, C. Larue et C. Chatigny. «Application de l'ergonomie à la prévention des LATR dans les abattoirs de porcs». *Rapport IRSST* (1992).

Viikari-Juntura, E. "Neck and Upper Limb Disorders Among Slaughterhouse Workers: An Epidemiologic and Clinical Study." *Scandinavian Journal of Work, Environment and Health* 9 (1983). pp. 283-90.

Susan R. Stock

A Study of Musculoskeletal Symptoms in Daycare Workers

Cet article décrit un projet de «recherche-action» chez un groupe d'éducatrices de garderie. Le projet avait comme objectif d'aider les éducatrices et la direction de la garderie à déterminer l'ampleur des problèmes musculo-squelettiques chez les éducatrices, à déterminer les facteurs qui y auraient contribué et à élaborer des solutions pour réduire ces problèmes.

Le projet consistait en une étude épidémiologique descriptive utilisant des questionnaires administrés à chacune des travailleuses pour déterminer la prévalences des symptômes musculo-squelettiques, l'inconfort associé aux tâches profesionnelles, la perception des difficultés reliées aux facteurs environnementaux et organisationnels et aux autres facteurs contribuant au stress. Les résultats du questionnaire ont démontré une prévalence très élevée des maux de dos et une prévalence moins élevée des douleurs au cou et à l'épaule. Les éducatrices ont déterminé les facteurs suivants comme étant pénibles: la manutention fréquente de charges encombrantes, les charges physiques et psychologiques de travail très élevées, une latitude décisionnelle plutôt limitée et l'exposition au bruit.

Les résultats ont été restitués à toutes les travailleuses et à la direction. L'équipe de projet a organisé des sessions de résolution de problèmes avec des groupes de cinq à huit personnes, lors desquelles les travailleuses ont participé à l'élaboration des solutions et à l'établissement des priorités.

Le projet nous a amené à discuter de la nature de la «recherche-action» et de l'utilité d'une meilleure collaboration entre les épidémiologistes, les ergonomes et les chercheurs des sciences sociales pour comprendre et prévenir les problèmes musculo-squelettiques reliés au travail.

This paper describes an "action research" project addressing musculoskeletal symptoms in 21 female daycare workers. The project's objectives were to assist the daycare workers and the administrators of a particular centre to assess the extent of work-related musculoskeletal symptoms among these workers, identify potential contributing factors, find solutions to reduce the number of symptoms and prevent development of new symptoms.

The project included a descriptive epidemiologic study with structured interview of all workers to identify the prevalence of musculoskeletal symptoms, perceived discomfort associated with work tasks, environmental and organizational difficulties, and factors perceived as work stressors. Results of the questionnaire revealed that this group of daycare workers experienced very high rates of back pain and moderately high rates of neck and shoulder pain. The results of the study generated several hypotheses about the occupational health preoccupations among these daycare workers. These preoccupations included frequent and awkward lifting and carrying, high physical work loads, high psychological work loads, moderate to low control over decisions affecting working conditions and noise exposure.

Findings were reported to all members of the staff of the daycare centre. The action-research project team then facilitated small group problem-solving sessions, in which all members of the staff participated, to identify solutions and set priorities.

This study is a point of departure for a discussion of the nature of action research and the need for greater collaboration among epidemiologists, ergonomists and social scientists in order to understand and address the problems of workers at risk for work-related musculoskeletal disorders.

INTRODUCTION

This paper offers some personal reflections on "action research" in occupational health in the context of providing public health services in an occupational health clinic for the prevention and management of work-related musculoskeletal problems. It describes an action research project, addressing musculoskeletal symptoms in 21 female daycare workers, which highlights some of the questions currently facing public health professionals and researchers. The objective is to stimulate discussion on how, as occupational health professionals and researchers, we can improve how we carry out this type of research: what methods are best for obtaining accurate measures of what we wish to study?; how do we ensure rigor while providing for genuine participation of workers?; how do we ensure that the focus on "action" — not just "research" — is maintained? Often, in public health and in universities, we tend to carry out "Health Hazard Evaluation" studies whose goal is to demonstrate the presence or absence of specific health problems or exposures, or the association between exposures and health problems. Once such associations are identified, it may be possible to use these research findings to facilitate a process in which the workplace parties identify workable solutions taking into account and addressing the organizational barriers.

In this paper, "action research" refers to the application of research methods to identify occupational health problems and the factors that may be causing them, the identification of potential solutions and the application of research methods to evaluate the implementation or effectiveness of those solutions in eliminating or reducing the health problems or the causal factors. The collaborative nature of this type of research has been well described by Barbara Israel et al. (1989): "an action research approach in a work setting involves researchers and organization members in a joint process aimed at meeting both research and intervention objectives. [It] involves a cyclical problem-solving process with five phases: diagnosing, action planning, action taking, evaluating, and specifying learning. Organization members and the research team collaboratively carry out the process."

The quality of action research depends on the active participation of worker and employer representatives from the study workplace in each of the steps. Participation of workers is necessary for truly good science to take place, because actively listening to workers' experience is essential to understanding the problem and asking the right questions. If we don't ask the right questions our research may be quite irrelevant no matter how elegant our methods. Moreover, appropriate, feasible and effective solutions to problems are more likely to be identified if we seek the participation of those who will implement the changes and experience their effects. This perspective, while widely accepted in some disciplines and settings, is far from the dominant view in epidemiology and occupational medicine.

The project to be described grew out of patient care management of a 45-year-old daycare worker with back pain who presented herself at the author's office in a Hamilton occupational health clinic. In order to advise her about continuing or stopping work, it was necessary to see her workplace and assess whether the work could be modified. Her other two co-workers had been advised by their doctors to restrict lifting tasks, which suggested that the problem might not be just this patient's but one affecting several workers. The employer and employees readily agreed to a workplace visit by an occupational health physician. Numerous ergonomic hazards were identified during the site visit and a short epidemiologic study was proposed and accepted by the workplace.

PROJECT AND STUDY OBJECTIVES

It may be useful to distinguish between the objectives of the overall action research project and the objectives of the epidemiologic study conducted within the project. The project's objectives were to assist the 21 daycare workers and the two administrators of a particular daycare centre to assess the extent of work-related musculoskeletal symptoms among these workers, to identify potential contributing factors, and to find solutions to reduce the number of symptoms among them and prevent development of new symptoms. The goal of the epidemiologic study was more narrow — i.e., to identify the prevalence of musculoskeletal symptoms, perceived discomfort associated with work tasks, perceived environmental and organizational difficulties, and factors perceived as work stressors.

METHODS
Study Population/Setting

The daycare centre was a large private, non-profit church-run centre in Hamilton, Ontario. It was non-unionized. Administration of the centre was carried out by two individuals, a director and assistant director, who were accountable to a church Board of Directors. The decision-making process was hierarchical. There was an active health and safety committee and regular staff meetings were held to discuss administrative and programme issues. Provincial regulations concerning child/daycare worker ratios were respected. The centre had a strong early childhood education orientation and had regular, frequent student placements from a local community college and a local high school. Children cared for ranged from young infants to four year olds. The centre employed 21 daycare workers: 36 percent of the staff cared for infants; 40 percent for toddlers; 12 percent for junior pre-school; and 12 percent for senior pre-school. Mean age of the daycare workers was 35.2 years (standard deviation 9.7; range 23-52). The mean years of seniority was 3.0 (standard deviation 2.1; range 1 month to 6.3 years).

Project Design

The project included the following steps:
1. an initial worksite evaluation;
2. questionnaire development and pre-testing;
3. a descriptive epidemiologic study (structured interview of all workers);

4. reporting of findings to all members of the staff of the daycare centre;

5. staff education on the nature of work-related musculoskeletal disorders and the factors that may contribute to them;

6. the facilitation of priority setting and solution identification by all workplace parties through small group problem-solving sessions.

The project was also intended to include the implementation of solutions and an evaluation of the intervention but these were not carried out as discussed below.

The initial worksite evaluation included an ergonomically oriented "walk through" visit of the daycare centre and unstructured interviews with staff and administrators to observe the work process and organization of work, identify tasks and collect perceptions of workplace conditions.

On the basis of the initial work site evaluation a four-page questionnaire was developed which was an adaptation of the Nordic musculoskeletal symptom questionnaire (Kuorinka et al., 1987) with additional questions relevant to this workplace. Health outcomes measured included pain for each musculoskeletal body site in the past 12 months, disabling pain in the past 12 months and pain in each body site in the past seven days. The musculoskeletal body sites surveyed and grouped together included neck, shoulders and upper back; hands, wrists and forearms; elbows; low back; hips and thighs; knees; and ankles and feet.

Perceptions of the difficulty of carrying out 20 work tasks were measured on a discomfort scale with four choices: not a part of my job; not a problem; leads to minor discomfort; leads to major discomfort. The work tasks measured were as follows:
- lifting children
- feeding infants
- lifting objects less than 10 pounds (4 kilograms)
- lifting objects 10 to 25 pounds (4 to 10 kilograms)
- lifting objects greater than 25 pounds (10 kilograms)
- moving furniture
- setting up beds/cots
- serving meals
- sitting on a child's chair
- pulling children on a rope
- picking up toys etc. from floor
- sweeping/mopping
- cleaning counters/tables
- playground duties (specify)

- carrying objects up/down stairs
- carrying children
- carrying other objects
- dressing children

Perceptions of the presence of the following 13 environmental and organizational factors were also measured:
- high level of noise
- poor level of lighting
- hot temperature in summer
- cold temperature in winter
- difficulty communicating with co-workers
- difficulty communicating with supervisor(s)
- too much work
- too many children to look after
- looking after children with behaviour problems
- not enough staff to do the job
- not enough influence in decisions that affect work
- not enough training
- not enough breaks

Open-ended questions were included about the five most difficult physical tasks and the five most stressful factors.

The questionnaire was administered to all 21 workers by two nurse interviewers.

ANALYSIS

Descriptive statistics were calculated. Correlation coefficients were calculated to correlate age and seniority with musculoskeletal symptoms, and Chi square or Fisher's exact tests (with Yates correction where appropriate) were carried out for relationships between frequencies of symptoms and frequencies of work task and work organizational variables.

Following completion of the study and preliminary analysis of results, two of the researchers presented the initial results of the study and an educational session on basic ergonomic principles during a staff meeting devoted to this topic. Following these presentations, the 21 staff were divided into small groups according to the age group of the children they worked with and asked to identify the five most important ergonomic or other organizational problems they believed contributed to musculoskeletal symptoms and to propose solutions. They were asked to identify potential barriers to implementation and to propose methods of overcoming them. The staff and administrators planned to continue the problem solving and solution-implementation process. The daycare staff and researchers agreed to meet three months later to evaluate the project.

RESULTS OF THE STUDY

Results of the questionnaire revealed that 81 percent of the 21 daycare workers had reported low back pain and 57 percent had reported pain in the neck, shoulders or upper back during the previous 12 months; 62 percent had reported back pain interfering with work or home activities (thus "disabling") in the previous 12 months; 24 percent had disabling neck or shoulder pain; 19 percent disabling hand, wrist or forearm pain; and 10 percent disabling lower limb pain. Fifty-two percent had reported low back pain and 48 percent had reported neck, shoulder or upper back pain during the previous seven days (see Figure 1).

Figure 1   Disabling Pain in Past 12 Months

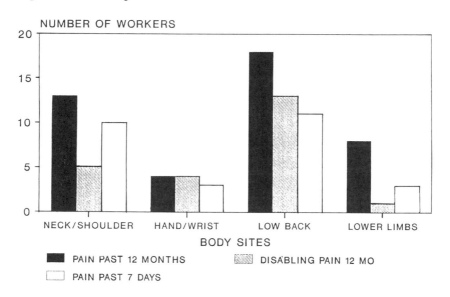

Tasks perceived to be associated with discomfort by more than 50 percent of workers included: lifting objects greater than four kilograms; lifting and carrying children; moving furniture; playground related activities (such as lifting children onto swings, leading 10 to 15 children on walks while holding onto a rope, carrying and storing bicycles, etc.); carrying and storing beds for naps; sitting in child-sized chairs; and carrying children and furniture up or down stairs. Environmental or organizational problems identified by 50 percent or more of the daycare workers included too heavy a workload; caring for children with behavioral problems; and high noise level.

The tasks rated most physically difficult included lifting and carrying children (for activities such as diapering, putting them into cribs, strollers, or swings, or carrying them up and down stairs); lifting and carrying heavy objects (such as furniture, food trays, "sensory bins" [very large bins filled with water or sand which are emptied after each use], laundry or other equipment); and bending or leaning over cribs or low tables and counters. The five most frequently mentioned perceived stressful working conditions included lack of pay for time spent on tasks such as employer-initiated professional development, staff meetings and administrative paper work (mentioned by 43 percent); not enough time allocated for scheduling and "transition" at start and end of shift (43 percent); lifting and carrying children repetitively (29 percent); dealing with children with behaviour problems (29 percent); and lifting and carrying equipment and furniture (24 percent).

Statistically significant correlations were observed between low back pain in the past seven days and the following factors: years of seniority (but not age); perception that the daycare staff-to-toddler ratio was too high; and difficulty lifting and carrying children and objects over 10 pounds (four kilograms). The details of these analyses are not reported here because our confidence in the larger relevance of these results is low. There were few subjects upon which these observations are based. The apparent statistically significant relationships may actually be due to chance because of multiple comparisons. Moreover, the design of this study cannot indicate the temporal relationship between the back pain and the explanatory variables.

Despite initial marked enthusiasm by staff and administrators at the time of the problem-solving session, labour relations between staff and administrators deteriorated significantly. The administrators decided unilaterally not to continue with the project or implement the solutions generated, and it was no longer possible for the investigators to conduct any follow-up. Follow-up with the initial patient revealed that most of the cohorts studied left this daycare centre over the course of the following year.

Discussion

The scope of this study was quite limited and we are limited in our conclusions about causal relationships because of the small numbers and the lack of a control group. But we have been able to generate relevant hypotheses about the main occupational health preoccupations among these daycare workers — frequent and awkward lifting and carrying; high physical work loads; high psychological work loads; moderate to low control over decisions affecting working conditions; and noise exposure — as well as demonstrate that this group experienced extremely high rates of back pain and moderately high rates of neck and shoulder pain. These results corroborate observations of daycare workers reported by other research groups (Markon and LeBeau, 1993; Morisette, 1993; Proteau, 1990; Tessier et al.; Tougas, 1988).

Perhaps more importantly, it allowed the women in this workplace the opportunity to explore in depth amongst themselves the nature of these problems and how they might resolve them. The research group was very struck by how highly motivated these workers were to participate in the small group problem solving exercise and how each group came up with very specific priority problems and solutions. Several factors aside from their obvious interest in the topic and its relevance to their experience probably contributed. Communication among co-workers was good. Their education level was relatively high and they were used to regular meetings as a method of discussing issues of concern to them. There was considerable similarity among their jobs and each person belonged to a group of women who did the exact same job.

Although our experience with the group problem-solving session persuaded us that this approach has merit, the project did not succeed in implementing solutions. We believe there are important lessons to be learned from this experience and have hypothesized some possible explanations for the lack of success in implementing solutions. The severity of the labour relations problems were not apparent in the initial interviews with daycare educators and administrators. The project may have been carried out far too quickly. For a number of external reasons this project had to be carried out extremely quickly (eight weeks from contact with the initial patient to presentation of results and problem-solving session), and some of the steps we believe to be important were omitted. Although worker and employer participation was sought, a formal joint worker-management committee to collaborate with the research team was never set up and the health and safety committee did not act in this capacity. The project was discussed with members of the health and safety committee and permission to carry out the project was given by the Director. It was initiated by individual workers of the centre and their enthusiasm for and participation in the project was high. Although both administrators participated in the initial worksite assessment and the session in which results and educational ideas were presented and small group problem-solving exercises carried out, they likely were never fully committed to the project. This workplace was not unionized and there were no workers who were mandated to represent the others. A formal joint worker-management committee to collaborate with the research project could have been mandated to review the study protocol, participate in discussions of the questionnaire, review results of the pre-test, participate in planning the presentation of results and the education and problem-solving session, oversee implementation of solutions and participate in an evaluation process. Because of the small number of workers, their strong support for the project and extraneous timetable pressures on the researchers, the process was speeded along and many of the above steps were not formally discussed. Although a joint committee process would have taken much longer, it might have allowed the workplace parties to take greater ownership of the project, explore advantages and disadvantages and identify and express possible reservations towards carrying out such a process. Such concerns might have been addressed through a process of consensus building and might have prevented the administrators from unilaterally terminating the project prematurely despite apparent endorsement at the time of the study and problem-solving session. Refusal by the administrators to accept a bi-partite project committee or failure to reach consensus would have indicated the depth of labour relations problems earlier and the potential difficulties implementing solutions.

This project's outcome points out our need to articulate the most efficient and effective ways of collaborating with workplace parties willing to engage in action-oriented research. Effective methods for participation are needed in all phases of the research, including the design of the study, design of research tools, implementation of the study and the generation of the potential solutions — particularly in complex settings or ones with difficult labour-management relationships.

There are also other methodologic concerns, which can influence the quality of results of such research, that warrant mention. To improve the ability of such studies to accurately identify health problems and exposures, we need rigorous measurement methods. This includes the development of valid and reliable measures of health effects (e.g. questionnaires for assessment of musculoskeletal symptoms and disorders), workplace biomechanical and work organizational exposure factors, and important non-work confounders (i.e. variables that can cause or prevent a health outcome of interest and are not associated with the exposures under investigation, and which must be measured and controlled in order to obtain an accurate estimate of the effect of the exposures under investigation). Few existing questionnaires have been adequately tested for reliability, sensitivity, specificity and other measures of validity. Such studies are currently being carried out and more standardized instruments with known measurement properties are currently under development (Baron, 1994; Armstrong, 1994). Such standardized measures allow comparison of high and low risk workplaces, and are particularly useful when studying small workplaces without potential control groups as the rate of the health effects in such a workplace population can be compared to a known low risk standard rate which can serve as a control. The Nordic questionnaire used in this study has been tested for reliability in Scandinavian populations. It is a limited questionnaire and requires additional questions.

Adequate and systematic pre-testing is also needed to ensure the applicability and appropriateness of given standardized measures to the specific study population. This is particularly true when such tools are translated or were developed in another culture or are used in a multi-ethnic population different from the one in which reliability and validity were demonstrated. While there are obvious advantages to using standardized tools, they must be pertinent to the study population and questions relevant to a specific setting frequently must be added. Not only does pre-testing allow one to identify questions that may be ambiguous, inappropriate or disconcerting to members of the study population, it also allows interviewers to become more familiar with the questionnaire and anticipate potential problems in administration or interpretation. This was one of the steps which was not fully carried out in this study and is therefore another limitation.

This study relied on epidemiologic methods and general workplace observations and did not include systematic ergonomic measures. An ergonomist was not included in the research team because of a lack of resources. But the need was recognized for more interdisciplinary collaboration in order to better understand the complex biomechanical and organizational interactions associated with musculoskeletal and mental health symptoms in the workplace. In general, many such studies can benefit from collaborations among those with expertise in epidemiology, occupational medicine, ergonomics, sociology, psychology, workplace anthropology, health economics and other disciplines dealing with work organization and organizational change. Multidisciplinary methods for the evaluation of workplace interventions to prevent musculoskeletal disorders are also needed. Such evaluations pose enormous methodologic challenges. While epidemiologic methods may allow for improved generalizability, such methods have inherent limitations when studying complex and dynamic systems. A more complete understanding of complex interrelationships may be found with detailed observational methods. The hypotheses generated through detailed observations may be more amenable to epidemiologic study. Different research strategies can complement each other and lead to a more complete understanding of workers' and workplace experience and the process of change leading to improved health outcomes.

Epidemiologists, ergonomists and social scientists have much to learn from each other and our methods can complement each other. The collaborative nature of action research, the increased levels of trust between the workplace parties and researchers frequently associated with this approach and the detailed observational methods in ergonomics and some of the social sciences can provide insights unavailable through traditional epidemiologic methods. Conversely, the concern with rigor and the reduction of potential sources of bias in epidemiology can greatly enhance an understanding of what is truly being observed and its potential for generalizability. The focus on intervention inherent in action research is consistent with a public health mandate and thus offers epidemiologically oriented public health departments alternative strategies for fulfilling the mandate to improve the health of our communities.

REFERENCES

Armstrong, T., et al., and ANSI Committee for the Prevention of CTDs. *Draft CTD Prevention Standards, July 1994.* Presented at International Conference on Work-related Musculoskeletal Disorders of the Upper Extremity, San Francisco, CA, December 1994.

Baron, S. *NIOSH Musculoskeletal Questionnaire.* Presented at University of Massachusetts, Worcester and NIOSH Conference on Outcome Measures, Denver, CO, November 1994.

Israel, B.A., S.J. Schurman and J.S. House. "Action Research on Occupational Stress: Involving Workers as Researchers." *International Journal of Health Services* 19 (1989). pp. 135-55.

Kuorinka, I., B. Jonsson, A. Kilbom, et al. "Standardised Nordic Questionnaires for the Analysis of Musculoskeletal Symptoms." *Applied Ergonomics* 18 (1987). pp. 233-7.

Markon, P., and D. Le Beau. *La santé et la sécurité au travail pour les éducatrices en garderie.* Chicoutimi, QC: Laboratoire d'ergonomie, Université du Québec à Chicoutimi, Bibliothèque nationale du Québec, 1993. p. 223.

Morisette, L. "La problématique des lésions professionnelles en garderie." *Objectif Prévention* (automne 1993). pp. 14-25.

Proteau, R-A. "Garderies: une approche globale." *Objectif Prévention* (printemps 1990). pp. 20-6.

Tessier, R., M.C. Blais and G. Dion. *Stress et santé au travail dans les garderies au Québec.* Research Report. Montreal: Groupe interdisciplinaire de recherche sur l'organisation, la santé et la sécurité du travail (GIROSST) de l'Université Laval. p. 133.

Tougas, G. "Le travail de l'educateur(trice) en garderie: les activités de travail en relation avec les maux de dos." Presented at the 10th Congress of L'association pour l'hygiène industrielle au Québec, June 1988.

Ellen Balka

Technology as a Factor in Women's Occupational Stress
The Case of Telephone Operators

Le stress au travail a été étable comme étant un problème de santé prioritaire pour les femmes (Lowe, 1989). Malgré l'augmentation des recherches depuis 10 ans dans le double domaine de la santé des femmes au travail et des effets de la technologie sur les travailleuses, l'intersection entre ces deux préoccupations n'a pas été beaucoup explorée. Cet article fait le lien entre les recherches sur le stress au travail et celles qui portent sur les femmes et les changements technologiques, dans le but d'élargir notre analyse théorique des rapports entre la complexité technologique et les déterminants psychosociaux du stress professionnel. Ces rapports sont analysés en observant le travail d'opératrices de téléphone à la lumière du modèle de Feldberg et Glenn (1983) sur les changements technologiques dans le travail des femmes (modèle qui met l'accent sur les changements occupationnels, les changements organisationnels, et sur la transformation des procédés de travail) ainsi que le modèle de Karasek (1979) sur le stress au travail (qui met l'accent sur la marge de manoeuvre dans les décisions et sur les exigences de la tâche). À travers une discussion sur l'impact des techniques de pointe implantées chez Newfoundland Telephone en termes de changements occupationnels, organisationnels et dans les procédés de travail, je démontre que ces transformations ont contribué à diminuer la marge de manoeuvre des opératrices et à accroître les exigences de leur tâche. Je suggère que certains problèmes de stress au travail pourraient être diminués si l'on sollicitait la participation des travailleuses lors de la conception et de l'implantation de ces techniques de pointe.

Occupational stress has been identified as one of the leading health problems for women (Lowe, 1989). Although, in the last decade, there has been an increase in research concerned with both women's occupational health and safety and the effects of technology on women workers, the intersectionofthesetwotopicshasbeenleftlargelyunexplored.Thispaper links research into occupational stress with research about women and technological change, in an effort to extend our theoretical understanding of the connections between complex technologies and psychosocial determinants of occupational stress. These linkages are discussed by examining the work of telephone operators in relation to Feldberg and Glenn's (1983) model of technological change in women's work (which focuses on occupational change, organizational change and changes in work processes), and Karasek's (1979) model of occupational stress (which focuses on decision latitude and job demands). Through a discussion of how technological change at Newfoundland Telephone has contributed to occupational change, organizational change and changes in work processes, I demonstrate how technological change has contributed to a decline in decision latitude and an increase in demands on telephone operators. I suggest that some occupational stress problems can be alleviated by engaging in a more participatory design and implementation process with workplace technology.

INTRODUCTION

In the last decade there has been an increase in research concerned with both women's occupational health and safety, and the effects of technology on women workers, but the intersection of these two topics has been left largely unexplored.[1] For example, in collections about women and technological change such as *Machina Ex Dea* (Rothschild, 1983) and *Women, Work, and Technology* (Wright, 1987), health in general and stress in particular are virtually unmentioned. Similarly, in texts on occupational health and safety, such as that of Reasons, Ross and Paterson (1981), technology is neglected. Although technology is often a focal point in ergonomic literature (for example, in portions of Galitz, 1984), the complex nature of processes surrounding the social relations of technology and related health impacts are often obscured by comments, such as the following, which fail to address the social relations and gendered nature of the labour process, as well as work speed and physical stress:

> Research also indicates that the kind of job being performed correlates with reported physical ailments associated with video display terminal (VDT) use. Professional users report fewer discomforts than do their clerical counterparts. *Evidently one's job significantly colors one's attitudes about automation* (Galitz, 1984:59; emphasis added).

Although Galitz points out that professional users of computers reported fewer discomforts than their clerical counterparts, he fails to recognize that there is a correlation between professional jobs and high decision latitude, and clerical jobs and low decision latitude.

Alcalay and Pasick (1983), writing about psychosocial factors and technologies of work, made an observation similar to Galitz' but also concluded that, in general, among blue collar and clerical workers, technology is often a controlling element, to the detriment of health. In contrast, among professionals and managers technology can be an aid to work and may facilitate positive health. As Amick, Weisman and Smith (1984) point out, in one of the rare articles that specifically addresses technology and occupational stress, the focus on individuals in research (rather than the relationship between the organization and the individual), has resulted in stress management programmes becoming the primary intervention available to management. Amick et.al. explored the effects of technology on job attitudes and workers' health. They found it was not technology *per se* that affected job satisfaction, but the constellation of job characteristics associated with a particular technology. Although advances in occupational health research have broadened the scope of interventions available since Amick, Weisman and Smith's article, their conclusion — that "it may be a more effective strategy to propose organizational changes which affect jobs (481-2)" — remains relevant.

With the growth of women's employment outside of the home in recent years, occupational stress has become an increasingly important issue for women. It has been identified as one of the leading health problems for women (Lowe, 1989), incurring heavy personal and social costs. For example, Karasek, Gardell and Lindell (1987) found that, for full-time Swedish white collar workers (male and female), the psychosocial situation at work appears to have a greater impact on psychological well-being than do family situations. Although there has been a proliferation of literature concerned with occupational stress in recent years (e.g., Karasek and Theorell, 1990), women have often been excluded as subjects of study.

Although many theories of occupational stress exist (see for example Mawson's 1993 work that outlines four explanations of women's occupational stress based on social inequality), the dominant perspective on job stress is the "demand-control model" (Lowe and Northcott, 1994) developed by Karasek (1979), and subsequently expanded by Karasek and Theorell (1990). The demand-control model suggests that most adverse reactions to psychological strain (such as fatigue, anxiety, depression and physical illness) occur where the psychological demands of the job are high and the worker's decision latitude in the task is low.

Karasek (1979) suggested that psychological strain is not the result of a single aspect of the work environment, but rather results from the joint effects of the demands of a work situation and the range of decision making freedom (or discretion) available to a worker in facing those demands. It is the combination of low decision latitude combined with high job demands (or workload demands) that results in strain. Intellectual responsibility is treated as a measure of decision latitude, and time pressure is treated as a measure of job demands related to workload (Karasek, 1979). Karasek and Theorell (1990) suggest that social support at work (overall levels of helpful social interaction available on the job from co-workers and supervisors) can act as a buffer to psychological strain. They suggest that the three dimensions of work — demand, control and social support — are capable of predicting a wide range of depression symptoms.

Alcalay and Pasick (1983) argue that there are several psychosocial pathways through which workplace technology can affect health. They also point out that these are for the most part left uncharted, and that an inclusive, theoretical framework that links the use of complex technologies with psychosocial determinants of health must be developed.

My aim here is to contribute to the development of such a framework through a focus on technology as a factor in women's occupational stress. I will introduce readers to the literature on women and technological change, as well as women's occupational stress, through a case study of telephone operators. Howard (1985) suggests that the work of telephone operators respects Karasek's (1979) definition of a high-strain job since it combines high levels of psychological demand with little ability to control and shape work. Thus, a focus on telephone operators is a good starting point for the investigation of how technology contributes to occupational stress through simultaneously increasing psychological demands while lowering decision latitude. My hope is to provide some conceptual tools that will help practitioners understand the complex web of relationships surrounding technology, gender, work and stress.

I will begin my analysis by reviewing literature concerned with women and technological change — a review that ends with a discussion of Feldberg and Glenn's (1983) framework for analyzing the effects of technology on women workers. That framework is particularly useful in considering technological change as a source of occupational stress. In the second section, I will review previous studies concerned with telephone operators' occupational health issues in general and stress in particular. In the third section I will provide an overview of technological change at Newfoundland Telephone between 1988 and 1993, following Feldberg and Glenn's framework.[2] In the fourth section, I will consider technological change at Newfoundland Telephone in relation to Karasek's (1979) model of occupational stress. By discussing how technological change at Newfoundland Telephone has contributed to occupational change, organizational change and change in the work process, I will demonstrate how technology can lead to a decline in decision latitude and increasing psychological demands, which in turn leads to increased occupational stress. Finally, in my conclusion, I will suggest that occupational stress problems can be reduced through a reconceptualization of technological change, and a more participatory process in technological design and implementation.

This research is based on interviews with selected informants, employment data provided by the personnel department at Newfoundland Telephone, and information contained in Newfoundland Telephone's corporate reports.

WOMEN AND TECHNOLOGICAL CHANGE: A REVIEW OF THE LITERATURE

In the early 1980s, as personal computers were becoming more widespread in workplaces, articles began appearing about the effects of technology on women workers. Initially, there were few studies that addressed technology and women's work. There were numerous articles that addressed the potential of technology to create new jobs and eliminate jobs that involved drudgery. However, many scholars and trade unionists read Braverman's (1974) *Labour and Monopoly Capital*, and, inspired by his analysis, began doing research that derived from his work. Braverman's analysis suggested that technology is designed to increase managerial control of the labour force and reduce it in size, which is accomplished through embedding skill in technology and thus deskilling workers. Although Braverman looked at clerical work in his book, most of his analysis involved work environments typically populated by men. Braverman himself was a machinist, and he tended to view work through the eyes of a male shop floor labourer. In simplistic terms, Braverman's analysis has been deemed by some (for example Linn, 1987) as deterministic, placing too much emphasis on how technology acts on workers, and not enough emphasis on how workers can determine the shape of technological change (see also Noble, 1982).[3]

Once women were considered the subjects of study in research concerned with technological change in the workplace, the limitations of Braverman's (1974) analysis became clear. Feldberg and Glenn (1983) pointed out that Braverman assumed that work changes related to new technology were experienced by workers who ended up in subdivided and standardized jobs, and that this resulted in a focus on the divisions between capital and labour, while neglecting the divisions within each. Workers were viewed as a uniform group with identical relationships to work, who were similarly affected by technology. Challenging Braverman's analysis, Feldberg and Glenn argued that, historically, labour has been divided into many segments, each representing different pools of workers with access to different kinds of work and with interests that may be contradictory. Thus, Feldberg and Glenn argued that "an accurate assessment of the effects of technology requires identifying the social divisions within the labor force, describing the impacts for each group, and analyzing the connections and differences between what happens to one group and what happens to another group."[2]

Working with a model of technology similar to that of Noble (1979 and 1984), Feldberg and Glenn (1983) emphasize the way social relations affect the development and use of technology. They investigate technological changes in relation to change at each of three levels: the occupational structure, the organizational structure and the work process. Occupational level changes are reflected in the content and/or scope of activities which constitute a job, the number and types of jobs, and the ratio of one job category to another. Among the characteristics which Feldberg and Glenn (1983) cite as indicative of change on the occupational level are greater job specialization and standardization (which result from a reorganization of the work), shifts in the number and type of jobs, and elimination of some occupations through labour savings.

Changes at the organizational level refer to changes in the ratio of workers in different job categories within a workplace or organization. An organization's workforce often becomes increasingly gender stratified with technological change, and opportunities for upward mobility are reduced through compression of the occupational hierarchy. When jobs are reorganized, deskilling may result (Feldberg and Glenn, 1983) although the trend is not uniform (Cohen and White, 1987). Cockburn (1983) points out that it is important to distinguish loss of skill from degradation of work, and we should not assume that deskilling for one group implies deskilling throughout an organization or occupation.

Changes in the work process refer to changes in the content and organization of jobs. Among the characteristics which reflect changes in the work process are the level of autonomy associated with a job; the extent to which jobs are specialized, varied or routine; and the amount and type of skill associated with a job (Feldberg and Glenn, 1983).

Work by Feldberg and Glenn (1983) and Hacker (1979) suggested that, with the implementation of new technology in different sectors of the labour force, layoffs related to the new technology were often masked behind an implementation and adjustment period. During the adjustment period, the size of the workforce often increased, as workers completed one-time-only tasks (such as converting paper records to electronic records). At the same time, new technology often resulted in changes in the tasks associated with a job. For example, many typists and secretaries became responsible for document layout when they discarded manual typewriters in favour of word processors and computers. Finally, the introduction of new technologies often resulted in changes in the occupational structure, evidenced by the disappearance of some job categories (such as teletypists) and the emergence of new job categories (such as word processing operators). Cockburn (1985) found that in some industries, as new technology was introduced and the nature of jobs changed, so too did the gender of workers completing certain tasks, and that the introduction of new technology served to increase the distance between men's jobs and women's jobs in terms of skill and wages.

Feldberg and Glenn's (1983) framework is particularly useful in terms of understanding the interaction of technology, gender and occupational stress issues, as it encourages analysts to look not only at how the content of a specific job may have changed with the introduction of new technology, but also at how the relations of one group of workers to another may change with the introduction of new technology.

Before I provide an overview of technological change in the telephone industry along the lines suggested by Feldberg and Glenn, I feel it is important to consider some of the different groups of workers who utilize telecommunications technologies in their employment.

One of the things that has happened in the last decade is that many more of us have become users of telecommunication services. My colleagues and I at the university increasingly use electronic mail and fax machines as a viable means of communication. We work with telecommunications technology, but we are not telecommunications workers — we rely on, but do not produce, telecommunication services.

I've raised this last point because it is important to realize that one of the major differences between my consumption of telecommunication services and the use of similar technology by the people producing those services for the rest of us to consume has to do with how the work is organized. As a professional, I am able to exercise a high degree of decision latitude in my use of telecommunications services. In contrast, telephone operators producing those services have little scope for exercising decision latitude in their work. It is important to remember that the use of telecommunication services (by those of us in the university and government) differs dramatically from that of women in the clerical workforce and women who produce some of the services that we take for granted — such as a functional long distance telephone system.

In this paper I will be focusing mostly on telephone operators, though some of my comments will be pertinent for clerical workers as well. It is important that the reader bear in mind the intensity of supervision experienced by these workers.

A REVIEW OF HEALTH ISSUES FOR TELEPHONE OPERATORS

Although my focus in this paper is on occupational stress rather than all occupational health issues telephone operators may face, it is important to note that telephone operators are often exposed to numerous other occupational health risks. Because of the computer-intensive nature of their work, telephone operators are exposed to stressors associated with computer use. These include repetitive movements, postural constraints and eye problems. In addition, telephone operators may be exposed to common environmental stressors such as indoor air problems and noise.

Some research into occupational health issues faced by workers in the telecommunications industry may be relevant to telephone operators, although telephone operators were not subjects of those studies. For example, Phillips (1983) considers occupationally induced hearing loss in the telecommunications industry. Reid, Ewan and Lowy (1991) discuss repetitive strain injuries in two groups of women, one of which is comprised of telecommunications workers. Similarly, some general work (such as Bradley's 1988 article on women, work and computers) as well as some research concerned with aspects of jobs that constitute a portion of telephone operators' jobs (eg. Teiger and Bernier's 1992 article about data entry clerks in the computerized service sector) suggest that telephone operators are exposed to some occupational stressors that are not unique to their occupation.

Few studies have addressed health and safety concerns of telephone operators. The studies that have been conducted, discussed briefly below, outline a range of health problems. Unfortunately, most of them fall short of making recommendations to ameliorate health problems. Even in the limited literature available on the health of telephone operators, it is clear that stress is a major issue for these workers. Although technology may contribute significantly to the work stress experienced by telephone operators, it is rarely identified as a factor worthy of attention (Yassi, Weeks, Samson and Raber, 1989 are the exception).

Starr, Thompson and Shute (1982) considered the effects of video display terminals on telephone operators. They compared directory assistance operators using computers to directory assistance operators using the older, manual paper-based system. They found very few significant differences between the two groups, although other researchers (DeMatteo, 1985) have suggested that a wide range of health problems are related to extensive use of video display terminals. Ivanovich, Kolarova, Enev, Tzenova and Topalova (1994) investigated the health effects of noise loading on telephone operators in Bulgaria. The annoying effects of the noise were subjectively evaluated as "very high" or "high" by most of the operators in all three departments studied. The authors advocated redesign of the workplace as a preventative health measure.

Electronic performance monitoring, defined as "computerized collection, storage, analysis and reporting of information about employees' productive activities on a continuous basis" (OTA, 1987, quoted in Carayon, 1993:385), has been the subject of some investigations of telephone operators' work. Ditteco (1987) considered the effects of machine pacing and electronic monitoring on telephone operators. Writing for the popular media, Coutts (1989) also considered this topic. Monitoring has also been addressed by scholars concerned with technological change (Zureik, Mosco, and Lochhead, 1989) and work and stress (Yassi et al., 1989). Although monitoring the pace of telephone operators' work is a common practice (see Howard, 1985), Zuriek et al. argue that it may decrease overall job satisfaction. They also suggest that the more satisfied the worker is with management strategy regarding the new technology and the impact of technology on management/worker relations, the less likely it is that monitoring will be perceived as a problem. Bell Canada ended electronic monitoring in some areas after a joint union-management study (in cooperation with the Health and Safety Institute of Quebec) showed surveillance to be one of the biggest causes of stress for workers (Coutts, 1989).

Kamphuis and DeGroot (1993) investigated the mental task load of international telephone operators in the Netherlands. Their task analysis of operators' work determined that 85 percent of time spent on the task was effectively used, compared to a norm of 65 to 75 percent of time effectively used in other occupations. They also found that there was a fair amount of multiple task performance (performing a task either concurrently or alternatively with one or more other tasks) and a frequent blockage of the work in progress resulting from a sluggish computer system. Gaillard (1993) suggests that multiple task performance requires continuous attention because task demands change quickly. The higher the demands, the more sensitive the task is to changes in a worker's energy state.

Gaillard (1993) makes a distinction between mental load and stress. He points out that mental load has to do with the limits of a worker's capacity to process information, whereas stress has to do with the factors in a work environment (such as decision latitude, control and social support associated with a particular job) that produce cognitive strain and increased health risks. Kamphuis and DeGroot (1993) found that, compared to their clerical counterparts, operators in general, and older operators in particular, reported more feelings of tension, mental effort and load. The researchers concluded that "a conflict exists between the demands of the operator task and the conditions under which it must be performed" (p. 130), which they speculate may be the cause of the high rates of health complaints and absenteeism of telephone operators. They recommended to the phone company that they provide for more variation in the operators and tasks, and more frequent pauses during work.

Perhaps the most striking aspect of previous research concerned with the health and safety of telephone operators is that, despite a general dearth of research in this area, three studies have addressed psychogenic epidemics.

Boulougouris, Rabavilas, Stefanis, Vaidakis and Tabouratzis (1981) investigated fainting episodes of 250 (of 990) women telephone operators in Athens in 1975. Their research argued that the fainting, which generally occurred during the earliest (and busiest) hours of the day, was a form of transitory anxiety attack in response to environmental or situational stress, and was related to neither hysteria nor an anxiety state. Alexander and Fedoruk (1986) investigated what they concluded was an epidemic psychogenic illness or mass hysteria in a telephone operators' building. Their case began when a male employee stated that he had smelled a strange odor in one of two sections of the telephone operator's building in a California community. Over the next few days, 81 of 153 employees (all but three of whom were women) at the telephone operator's building were treated at area hospitals for symptoms which included headaches, dizziness, nausea and upper respiratory distress. After an exhaustive environmental assessment by a private industrial hygienist failed to demonstrate evidence of toxins, the researchers concluded that "all elements required for the diagnosis of epidemic psychogenic illness

... were present in the affected group" (p. 44). Alexander and Fedoruk noted that the telephone operators' work was highly routine unskilled or semiskilled work performed for an hourly wage, and that the age, sex ratio and type of work the operators performed conformed to other reports of psychogenic illness.

In 1986, after two brief power failures affected the operation of computers in a section of the Manitoba telephone company, three telephone operators reported tingling sensations in their arms and one side of their bodies, which they referred to as "shocks." In the two weeks following the power outages, 92 similar incidents were reported by 55 telephone operators. Extensive investigations were carried out and an independent medical panel assessing the results concluded that there was no immediate hazard to life or health. After reports of the shock incidents persisted, a multidisciplinary committee, convened for further investigation, ruled out all known hazards other than electrostatic shock and occupational stress. Nearly two years after the initial reports of "shocks," it had become obvious that the main problem was a collective stress reaction.

In all three studies, steps were taken to identify and reduce sources of stress in the workplace. Few incidents of shocks were subsequently reported. In their article about the events at Manitoba telephone, Yassi, Weeks, Samson and Raber (1989) argue that the costly and lengthy investigation at Manitoba Telephone underlined "the desirability of considering the psychosocial effects of technology and regimented tasks" (p. 816).

Yassi et al.'s (1989) analysis of psychogenic illness amongst telephone operators differs significantly from other reported cases by Boulougouris et al. (1981) and Alexander and Fedoruk (1986). First, Yassi and her colleagues make the point that the use of the diagnostic label of psychogenic illness or mass anxiety is precarious, as the symptoms are perceived by affected populations as real, rather than viewed as stress-induced. Yassi et al. argue that Boxer's (1985) diagnostic term "collective stress reaction" is a better term as it does not negate other causative factors and is less suggestive of victim blaming than the more commonly used terms. Finally, Yassi et al. suggest that in order for collective stress reaction to become an accepted diagnosis by the affected population, an understanding of the underlying stressors must be reached and steps must be taken to reduce workplace stress.

Although Yassi et al. (1989) identified a number of factors related to technology (such as machine pacing, electronic monitoring and task fragmentation) as stressors at Manitoba telephone, and recognized that collective stress reactions are found in computer driven populations (as opposed to those who "use computers as tools" [p. 819]), their work was not intended as an analysis of technology in the workplace, aimed at ameliorating health risks. Similarly, Statham and Bravo (1990) make a convincing argument for considering the introduction of new technology in the context of workplace health issues, but they provide only a limited analytic view of technology. In the next section, I provide an overview of technological changes at Newfoundland Telephone, following Feldberg and Glenn's (1983) model. This provides the context for a more detailed discussion of technology and occupational stress.

TECHNOLOGICAL CHANGE AT NEWFOUNDLAND TELEPHONE
Methodology

Material in this section is derived from corporate documents, articles from newspapers, business and academic publications, interviews with selected informants, and employment data provided by an employee in the personnel department at Newfoundland Telephone. Corporate documents used were Newfoundland Telephone and NewTel (Newfoundland Telephone's holding company) Annual reports. Only two in-depth interviews were conducted, a circumstance that reflects the preliminary nature of the study and difficulties in gaining access to informants. Access posed a problem for several reasons. First, telephone operators work in a secured building, and come on and off shifts at staggered times. Second, because operators typically receive their schedules one week in advance of working, it is often difficult for them to incorporate additional activities into their lives. As well, many of the telephone operators have heavy family responsibilities, one result of which is little discretionary time.

One of the operators interviewed was active in the union; the other was a shop floor supervisor.

Overview of Technological Changes

In local 410 of the Communications, Electrical and Paper Workers (formerly the Communications Workers of Canada) in Newfoundland, there are three separate groups of workers. Two groups are composed largely of women (clerical workers and staff in operator services) while the third group (craft workers who do installation, repair and line work) are all men. Not surprisingly, craft workers are better paid than staff in either the clerical or operator groups.

Newfoundland Telephone provides all local residential telephone service in Newfoundland and Labrador. Recently, the Canadian Radio-television and Telecommunications Commission (CRTC) ruled against Newfoundland Telephone in allowing competition in the long distance calling market. Losing its status as the sole provider of telephone service (and many additional telecommunications services) in the province during a general economic decline has fueled the pace of technological change at Newfoundland Telephone.

Efforts to upgrade the telecommunications infrastructure have been underway in Newfoundland for a number of years. They have included replacing old switching equipment with digital switching equipment and replacing old lines with fiber optic cable, which allows both faster communication and the potential for the exchange of more information. These capabilities, along with the introduction of touch tone telephones, have provided the basis for massive changes in the services Newfoundland Telephone offers customers.

In 1988, two technological changes had a large impact on administrative and clerical staff: a computerized system for handling customer trouble reports was introduced; and the computerized payroll and personnel systems within the company were integrated. Also during 1988, a major new billing and cost reporting system was developed.

In December of 1988, Newfoundland Telephone purchased Terra Nova Telephone, the only other telephone service provider in the province. In 1989, federal regulation was extended to all members of Telcom Canada, which included Newfoundland Telephone. This decision removed Newfoundland Telephone from provincial jurisdiction and brought it under the federal jurisdiction of the CRTC. This may have signaled industry-wide deregulation, and contributed to the escalation of technological change.

During 1990, the computerization of manual record-keeping systems (e.g., for processing service orders) began. In 1991, a corporate reorganization occurred, along with a number of technological changes to service functions. Newfoundland Telephone was realigned into five departments. Among the five, the new technology department was given a mandate to continue the company's efforts to mechanize service functions.

Also in 1991, the directory assistance services were automated. A computer-generated voice was used to provide customers with the telephone number they requested, and the new system automatically recorded the telephone numbers of customers calling directory assistance, for billing purposes. Also, an interactive voice system was introduced, and there was a general equipment upgrading of operator services which included the introduction of new "multipurpose"' work positions for operators in the St. John's office.

In 1991, as part of a large-scale reorganization which included shutting down several phone company offices and reducing the hours of service in others, Newfoundland Telephone created the Provincial Network Operations Centre (PNOC). The PNOC became the sole facility for monitoring the status of the company's communication network, consolidating services that had been provided by operators elsewhere on the island as well as in Labrador.

In 1992, Newfoundland Telephone continued to make progress with the development of an online service order system and the capability to activate a customer's service from a computer terminal, without a field visit. The company also developed an active partnership with the Atlantic Provinces Telecommunications Council (APTC) and began planning to provide network surveillance and management for all Atlantic provinces. The end of the year brought yet another company reorganization, which the technology department survived. In 1993, an automated billing system was introduced, which allowed customers to place and bill long distance and collect calls without interacting with an operator.

For the telephone operators affected by the above changes, new technologies have a potential effect on occupational stress. In the rest of this section I will examine the relationship between technological changes and occupational stress, using Feldberg and Glenn's (1983) framework of occupational change, organizational change and change in the work process.

Changes in Occupational Structure

Changes in the occupational structure are difficult to monitor in the best of circumstances. Inadequate attention to gender during data collection often makes it difficult to track the gendered nature of occupational change. (See Armstrong and Armstrong, 1990, who discuss problems in the use of quantitative data concerned with women in the economy.) Such an examination is particularly difficult in the context of telephone operators because of the inability to distinguish clerical workers in telecommunications from those in other sectors, and the general invisibility of women within the category of "telecommunications worker."

For example, women were virtually absent from a discussion of telecommunications work in the 1983 edition of the International Labour

Organization's (ILO) Encyclopedia of Occupational Health and Safety. Although the description of work was generally accurate, operators were only mentioned in relation to older switchboard systems. In descriptions of internal work (installation and maintenance) and external work (line and cable work) there was no mention of any of the clerical functions required for these operations. Similarly, telephone operators were neglected in Phillips' (1983) study of occupationally induced hearing loss amongst employees in the telecommunications industry, as well as Clark, McLoughlin, Rose and King's (1988) study of technological change in the modernization of telephone exchanges in Britain.

Changes in Organizational Structure

Changes in an organizational structure because of technological change are reflected in changes in the ratio of workers in different categories in the organization's workplace. As Figure 1 indicates, unionized employees have constituted about 65 percent of the Newfoundland Telephone Company's labour force in recent years, with the exception of 1988, when unionized employees made up less than half of the total workforce. (This reflected the company's acquisition of Terra Nova Telephone.) With the exception of 1988, the ratio of unionized to non-unionized employees has remained remarkably stable. However, as Figure 2 indicates, the ratio of one group of workers to another within Newfoundland Telephone has changed dramatically. Since 1987, telephone operators have held a declining share of jobs within their bargaining unit. Having left the Communications Workers of Canada (CWC), Newfoundland Telephone Operators are currently represented by Local 410 of the Communications, Electrical and Paper Workers union, which some claim is more male-dominated than the CWC.

Another component of change within the organizational structure is found in reorganized jobs. These changes are perhaps best understood through a discussion of the work process, which includes changes to both the organization of work and the content of jobs.

Changes in Work Process

Telephone operators at Newfoundland Telephone perform three general functions. They handle toll calls (long distance), directory assistance, and special services which include ship to shore communication, radio calls from areas of Labrador not serviced by phone, conference calls and TTY calls (for hearing and vocally impaired persons).

Prior to 1991, there were telephone company offices all over the province which offered a mix of operator services, and there were two types of operators. Toll operators handled long distance calls. In addition, they had a headset on their desk for Special Operator Services Traffic (SOST), which allowed them to handle special services calls. Directory assistance operators handled directory assistance calls only.

Figure 1   Total Number of Employees and Number of Unionized Employees, Newfoundland Telephone

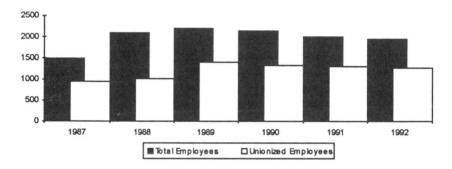

Figure 2   Number of Employees in Each Bargaining Group, Newfoundland Telephone

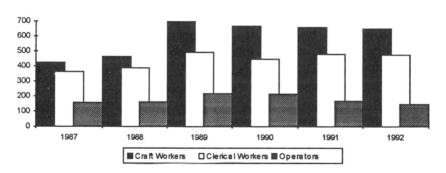

In 1991, the office in Goose Bay (Labrador) was closed down, and toll/special service and directory assistance calls were rerouted. Around the same time, the automated directory assistance service was introduced and multipurpose positions were introduced in the St. John's office. Directory assistance operators went from a completely manual system, where operators looked up phone numbers and then recorded the caller's number on slips of paper, to a system that required them to type information into a computer to obtain a number for a caller. The computer based billing portion of the system automatically traced the caller's number, which eliminated a component of the directory assistance job (asking for and recording the caller's number).

The "multipurpose" work stations introduced in 1991 are actually computers that can handle both directory assistance and toll calls through one computer. Although they were first used exclusively by directory operators, by April 1992 all toll operators had been trained to use the multipurpose work stations as well. With the introduction of the multipurpose system, both directory and toll operators are using the same computer system. When they come into work they log onto the computer as either a directory, toll, or multipurpose operator (handling both types of calls). "Cross-training" (teaching directory assistance operators how to handle toll calls and vice versa) has all but eliminated the distinction between directory assistance and toll operators. Current cross-training efforts are underway to ensure that all operators are also proficient in handling special services calls.

The combination of digital communications switching equipment and computers has made it easy to reroute telephone traffic from one location to another. As a result, the phone company was able to shut down an office in Labrador and change the mix of services handled in other locations. By March of 1993, all operators in St. John's were using multipurpose work stations, and two offices that had operated twenty-four hours a day in Gander and Corner Brook were closed at night. When the smaller offices closed down at night, the toll traffic was routed to St. John's, where it was handled through the multipurpose work stations. One phone company employee described this as three toll offices "homing" off of one switch, and proudly pointed out that this technology allowed the St. John's office to pick up long distance calls during busy daytime periods, reducing the need for additional staff in smaller offices. Directory assistance jobs were eliminated in all areas of the province except for St. John's, and all operators in St. John's now handle a broader mix of services.

Prior to the massive reorganization and automation that occurred in 1991, the special services calls required a dedicated piece of equipment, but each location handled a different mix of services (e.g., one office handled ship to shore, another "fringe radio" etc.). With automation, the phone company was able to reduce the number of offices handling Special Operator Services Traffic (SOST) from four to one (located in St. John's). Currently, SOST has a separate group of operators, who also provide after-hours telemarketing. Now an effort is underway to have all operators in St. John's handle marine calls, which were historically handled through the toll/SOST operators, and subsequently through the SOST group.

In July 1993, an automated billing system was introduced for toll calls. It eliminates the live operator interface, and allows customers to make collect and third party calls with no operator intervention. One operator viewed this as a threat to jobs, and also noted that many customers (especially seniors) found the new automated billing system difficult to use. A supervisor countered this by suggesting that customers could choose to bypass portions of the automated billing system when placing long distance calls. An advertisement placed in a local St. John's newspaper (*Express*, October 20, 1993, B3) by Local 410 of the Communication, Electrical and Paper Workers (which represents the telephone operators) provided instructions towards this end. The advertisement began with the heading "YOU HAVE A CHOICE!" and included the following text: "When placing third party, collect and credit card calls, dialing '0' when the recording begins will get you an operator. Insist on an operator. It's your right. It's your choice!"

Referring to a similar system developed by Northern Telecom, a Northern employee indicated that more than 95 percent of calls are completed or ended on the first or second try (Canadian Press, 1991), while another source (Surtees, 1991:B5) indicated that "more than 80 percent of calls using the system are completed without an operator." Again, Northern's Moris Simson (Canadian Press, 1991:B11) pointed out that "neither we nor the phone companies view this system as a replacement for operators ... rather than replace them, it displaces them to do other things for telephone users" such as act as service agents, set up conference calls, handle emergencies and so on. This phenomenon is occurring at Newfoundland Telephone, where the separate group of SOST operators provides after-hours telemarketing services for the company.

Not surprisingly, extensive use of new technology at Newfoundland Telephone has led to massive service increases, with no corresponding increase in staff (see Figure 3).

DISCUSSION AND ANALYSIS OF OCCUPATIONAL STRESS AT NEWFOUNDLAND TELEPHONE

Some of the health risks telephone operators may be exposed to are inherent in the technology, and will occur to a degree that reflects the extent of use and other factors (such as how work is organized). For example, Amick and Celentano (1991) argue that machine-paced

Figure 3 Service Statistics and Employment Levels, Newfoundland Telephone

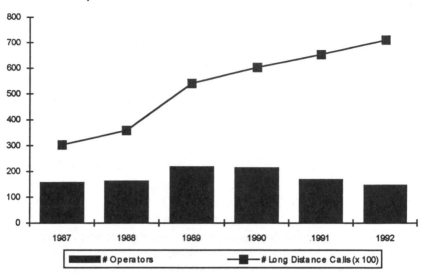

technology produces higher levels of job demand and lower levels of autonomy and co-worker support when compared with self-paced technologies. Thus, a computer-driven system that places calls in a queue and automatically delivers them to an operator as soon as she has completed her previous call will increase demands and reduce autonomy and control to a greater extent than a system that allows the operator to accept a call at her own discretion. The diminished autonomy that results from such an automatic call-queuing system is also likely to have an indirect effect on social support in the workplace, as it prohibits operators from chatting with their co-workers between calls.

Some of the health hazards telephone operators face are the result of employer practices, which result in the use of technologies in ways that reduce telephone operators' control on the job. One example of this, reported by an operator at Newfoundland Telephone, is the practice of electronically monitoring the length of an employee's absence from her terminal when she goes to the bathroom. (Howard, 1985, found this practice common in New York as well.) One union official in Ontario referred to this as "the culture of the company." Operators are clearly suspected of stealing from the company at each turn, and there is no tolerance. For example, workers are called at home when they take a sick day, to check that they are not simply taking the day off, and they can be fired for making an outgoing call during work time.

Several researchers have considered the health impacts of the threat of unemployment. For example, Brenner and Levi (1988) suggest that the threat of becoming unemployed may in itself lead to psychiatric problems. Brenner and Mooney (1983) point out that the threat of unemployment creates problems for those who remain employed, and Karasek and Theorell (1990) note that both skill obsolesence and fear of losing a job are stressors that are components of psychological job demands, and may also be a source of job-related stress. Kerkhoff and Beck (1968) found that when workers under heavy stress were unable to take coping actions because of the threat of layoffs, the most severe behavioral symptoms of strain occurred.

In the case of telephone operators at Newfoundland Telephone, the threat of occupational change (represented in the movement of jobs from smaller communities to St. John's, as well as the elimination of positions altogether) as a result of technological change is tremendous. For example, when several technological changes made it possible to shut down the Goose Bay telephone office in 1991, the 23 operators who worked there at the time were given an opportunity to transfer. Not surprisingly, because of family committments, very few were able to relocate.

For those operators who maintained their jobs outside of St. John's, the threat of job loss resulting from the movement of jobs out of their communities became very real. With recent speculation that the Atlantic Provinces Telecommunications Council has made decisions about further reorganizing work (e.g., moving all directory services to New Brunswick where the database is maintained, moving all billing to another Atlantic location and so on), and eliminating some tasks in some provinces, the threat of job loss continues to be very real for all telephone operators at Newfoundland Telephone. Ironically, the threat of lost work is, for telephone operators, made possible as a result of the telecommunications services that they are helping to provide.

For those operators who have kept their jobs, new technology has resulted in reduced decision latitude in both their professional and personal lives, and increased psychological demands. For example, the new multipurpose positions and automated call-queing system used by both directory assistance and toll operators in St. John's diminish operators' ability to pace work. At the same time, supervisors can monitor how long operators spend on each call. Operators are supposed to spend only 23 seconds on each call (Howard, 1985, found that the desired average call time for New York City telephone operators was 30 seconds per call). Operators with slow averages (28 seconds per call) at Newfoundland Telephone report being thwarted in their efforts to move within the company, although the ability to handle calls at this rate was not a performance requirement of jobs elsewhere in the company.

The new system also tracks call volume, which has made it possible to more accurately schedule operators' shifts to coincide with high call volumes. Where, in the past, an operator's shift might have included some busy and some slow times, "traffic monitoring" has enhanced the company's ability to schedule operators to handle higher call volumes throughout their shifts. Thus, the technical capability to monitor call volume has facilitated an increase in the mental load handled by operators, while the same technology allows electronic performance monitoring, which poses a constraint to exercising decision latitude and control.

Finally, labour savings related to the automated directory assistance and toll systems have resulted in layoffs and significant scheduling changes for those operators who remain. (The 1993 advertisement placed in the *Express* by the union representing telephone operators indicated that 15 operators had been laid off). Both labour savings and the redistribution of work (e.g., moving all night shifts to St. John's), have necessitated that operators with extensive seniority have had to return to night and weekend shifts in order to retain their jobs. The relationship between shift work, erratic scheduling and stress are well documented (see, for example, Sprout and Yassi, this volume). In addition, if the high demand/low control model is applied to the work of reconciling home and paid work demands, then schedule changes are likely to increase the demands of this work.

It is clear that mental load and psychological demand have increased because of changes in the work process as a result of technological change. Both learning how to use the new computer-based system, and the nature of the steps the automated system requires of operators to perform tasks, has contributed to mental load and psychological demand. For example, with the ABS, there are now four different "screens" an operator must rapidly distinguish amongst in order to complete a long distance call for a customer. And, given that generally operators only intervene with a toll call when the ABS has failed (for example, because a customer responded to a computer generated question with something other than a yes or no response allowed by the ABS), the majority of the calls now handled by toll operators are "trouble" calls, often involving a frustrated ABS user.

Finally, efforts to cross-train telephone operators has required the assimilation of not just a new computer system, but, additionally, an entire new set of work tasks and procedures. Coutts (1989) reports that a study (that led to a reduction in monitoring of operators' average work times in some parts of the Bell system) found that 70 percent of operators reported that the conflict between providing good service and the pressure to work quickly was the most stressful aspect of their jobs. For operators at Newfoundland Telephone, a similar conflict exists. Random quality monitoring (listening in on calls) makes it difficult for operators to advise callers who are having difficulty about how to bypass the ABS.

The ability to monitor individual operators and the length of time operators spend on a call has been designed into the software. Similarly, some sort of social vision (although it is perhaps not recognized as such) has informed the system design that resulted in a telephone system that allows work to be easily moved from one geographic location to another. The work practices in Newfoundland Telephone's Operator Services division represent social decisions that reflect attitudes about management practices and groups of workers. However, the social nature of these technological decisions is often hidden. Also, each of a society's needs do not receive equal treatment. For example, as Rothwell (1984: 122-3) points out, "when asked about how employees' needs affected their work, most system designers admitted 'little or none.'" Similarly, managers who were questioned about job design and work satisfaction admitted that they did not really think in those terms, and that such factors would hardly be seen as criteria for implementing new technology (Rothwell).

Other problems that have arisen for telephone operators at Newfoundland Telephone are related to a failure to understand technology as more than hardware, and a failure to understand the context into which technology is introduced. For example, a common problem in operator services is that many of the workers were never taught how to adjust the workstations (positions), or the screens on the machines (for contrast). As a consequence, the technology is not being utilized as it was intended to be, and operators are not accruing the benefits it offers. A failure to recognize that human beings interact with technology to perform a task (which results in no provision for training and unrealistic expectations about what can be accomplished as a result of the introduction of new technology) can lead to injury, such as eyestrain, and musculoskeletal disorders. These problems can easily be corrected with a shift in how we view technology, along the lines of Linn (1987), who suggests we must also consider how workers interact with and shape technological systems.

CONCLUSION

Previous research suggests that a number of variables bear upon how workers view — and experience — technological change. For example, in their research about the effects of video display terminals on telephone operators, Starr, Thompson and Shute (1982) suggested that some aspects of work other than the use of VDTs (such as task design, office and workstation design, and organizational factors) may affect the subjective experiences of telephone operators.

Consistent with Yassi et al.'s (1989) review of the literature (which indicated that the degree of job involvement or participation and organizational support were significant in terms of stress reduction related to technology), Zureik et al. (1989) found that the quality of management/worker interaction and the method of introducing technology is what counted most in the minds of their respondents.[4] They also found that the more satisfied a worker was with management's methods of introducing new technology, and the positive impact of technology on management/worker relations, the greater the level of job commitment and sense of control over the work environment.

Turner and Karasek (1984) suggest that despite unequivocal evidence for musculoskeletal and eye strain problems, that it is not the physical characteristics of technology (such as screen glare) that have the most profound impacts on workers' health. They argue that it is the manner in which control over computer software and hardware is related to workers' control over their jobs that makes the biggest difference. Stratham and Bravo (1989) suggest that providing workers with opportunities for input into job redesign related to new technology would lower the incidence of health problems related to loss of control. Their research found that the most commonly reported health problems in their sample increased in frequency as problems resulting from the implementation of new technology increased.

Zuriek et al. found that the majority of workers in their sample felt that not much could be done about the march of technology. These findings are consistent with Balka's (1986) findings that, among two groups of workers (airline workers and university clerical workers), there was an overwhelming sentiment that technological change would occur whether workers wanted it to or not (92 percent of airline workers and 89 percent of clerical workers agreed with this statement). This suggests that a workplace-based educational programme that challenges the ideology of technology as fixed and inevitable might have positive health outcomes (see Balka, 1986, for elaboration).

In her review of microlevel and macrolevel strategies for reducing stress at work, Mawson (1993) suggests that stress management interventions or policies can target stress at several levels. These include the individual level, the work-group unit, the organizational level (system or structural changes) and the interaction between the organization and the individual. Mawson points out that there are fewer interventions available at the macrolevel than at the microlevel, because macrolevel interventions are more difficult to implement and require more management involvement. Often macrolevel interventions require large scale structural changes, and pose a threat to management styles and existing power structures.

Mawson cautions her readers that it is important to ensure that diagnoses of stress are made at the right level, because placing the burden on individual workers is not likely to result in change if the stressor occurs at the organizational level. Unfortunately, although technology is a regular feature of most of our lives, it is infrequently examined from a social perspective and it is poorly understood as a variable in organizational structure. Thus, technology has often been neglected as a variable in stress intervention strategies. Nonetheless, the relationship between technological change and changes in work provides an excellent opportunity to identify (and subsequently target) stress at all levels of work.

Although several strategies can be identified to help ameliorate the effects of technological change on workers' health (such as developing technology clauses that require worker input in collective agreements, strengthening health and safety monitoring practices, and negotiating social solutions such as the elimination of monitoring) real change will require nothing short of a reconceptualization of technology and work. This process will entail a more sophisticated understanding of the technological change process (see, for example, Bush's 1983 definition of technology, or Franklin's 1990 characterization of technology). Such a reconceptualization of the technological change process should be based on an expanded notion of profit which gives weight to social costs and personal costs as well as business profitability. This, combined with the idea that technological change can take more than one form and is not inevitable, might lead to participatory job redesign strategies, which have improved working conditions in numerous workplaces (see, for example, Green, Owen and Pain, 1993; Greenbaum and Kyng, 1991; Schuler and Namioka, 1993; Trigg, Anderson and Dykstra-Erickson, 1994).

Namioka and Schuler (1990:ii) point out that "despite a proliferation of methodologies for designing computer systems, we commonly end up with systems that are difficult for workers to master, poorly suited for their tasks, and perceived by them as job-threatening or job-degrading." They argue that participatory design represents an approach that differs from traditional design processes in many respects. For example, it rejects the assumption that the goal of computerization is to automate the skills of human workers, and instead sees automation as an attempt to give workers better tools for doing their jobs. Participatory design also assumes that users of technology are in the best position to determine how to improve their work and work lives, and, in incorporating users into the design process, that the traditional designer/user relationship must undergo significant change. Concern for social as well as technical aspects of new technology is central to participatory design strategies. Such an approach at Newfoundland Telephone might lead to innovations such as computer-based phonetic spellers (that do not dramatically reduce average work time as the current phonetic spellers in use at Newfoundland Telephone do) for directory assistance operators.

Suchman (1993) asserts that what distinguishes participatory design from other approaches to system development is the "central and abiding concern for direct and continuous interaction with those who are the ultimate arbiters of system adequacy; namely, those who will use the technology in their everyday lives and work (vii)." Participatory design offers the possibility of placing concerns about occupational stress and technology high on the occupational health agenda. It offers the possibility of reducing occupational stress by encouraging workers and employers to simultaneously consider social and technical aspects of technological change. In short, participatory design should be a process through which workers can investigate (and ideally change) the levels of decision latitude, control and social support associated with technology at work.

NOTES

1. For exceptions, see: Marshall and Gregory, *Office Automation: Jekyll or Hyde?* Cleveland: Working Women Education Fund, 1983; Statham and Bravo (1990); Cohen and White (1986); Alcalay and Pasick (1983); Amick, Weisman and Smith (1984) and Amick and Celentano (1991).

2. Although I find Feldberg and Glenn's (1983) model works well, other frameworks exist for tracking the effects of technology on groups of workers. Of particular note are Karasek and Theorell's (1990) model and DiCindio and Simone's (1993) universes of discourse.

3. Linn (1987) offers a critique of Braverman's thesis in terms of its neglect of what Linn refers to as "human capital" — the workers ability to intervene in the technological change process.

4. Items reflecting this sentiment: satisfaction with management's methods of producing technological change; management's recognition of workers' performance; and the extent to which technological change has affected the relationship between management and workers.

REFERENCES

Alcalay, R., and R. J. Pasick. "Psycho-social Factors and the Technologies of Work." *Social Science and Medicine* 17, 16 (1983). pp. 1075-84.

Alexander, R. W., and M. J. Fedoruk. "Epidemic Psychogenic Illness in a Telephone Operators' Building." *Journal of Occupational Medicine* 28, 1 (January 1986). pp. 42-5.

Amick, B. C., and D. D. Celentano. "Structural Determinants of the Psychosocial Work Environment: Introducing Technology in the Work Stress Framework." *Ergonomics* 34 (1991). pp. 625-46.

Amick, B.C., C.S. Weisman and M.J. Smith. "The Implications of Technological Change for Worker Health: The Role of the Job Redesign Model in Public Health," in *Human Factors in Organizational Design and Management.* H. W. Hendrick and O. Jr Brown (eds.). Amsterdam: North-Holland, 1984. pp. 481-7.

Armstrong, P., and H. Armstrong. "Beyond Numbers: Problems with Quantitative Data" in *Women and Men: Interdisciplinary Readings on Gender.* Greta Hoffman Nemiroff (ed.). Toronto: Fitzhenry & Whiteside, 1990. pp. 54-79.

Balka, E. *Women and Workplace Technology: Educational Strategies for Change.* Master's Thesis. Burnaby, B.C.: Simon Fraser University, 1986.

Boulougouris, J. C., et al. "Epidemic Faintness: A Psychophysiological Investigation." *Psychiatria-Clinica* 14, 4 (1981). pp. 215-25.

Boxer, P. A. "Occupational Mass Psychogenic Illness: History, Prevention, and Management." *Journal of Occupational Medicine* 27 (1985). pp. 867-72.

Bradley, G. "Women, Work and Computers." *Women and Health* 13, 4 (1988). pp. 117-32.

Braverman, H. *Labor and Monopoly Capital.* New York: Monthly Review, 1974.

Brenner, M. H., and A. Mooney. "Unemployment and Health in the Context of Economic Change." *Social Science and Medicine* 17 (1983). pp. 1125-38.

Brenner, S. O., and L. Levi. "Long Term Unemployment Among Women in Sweden." *Social Science and Medicine* 25 (1987). pp. 153-61.

Bush, C. G. "Women and the Assessment of Technology: To Think, To Be; To Unthink, To Free," in *Machina Ex Dea: Feminist Perspectives on Technology.* Joan Rothschild (ed.). New York: Pergamon, 1983. pp. 150-71.

Canadina Press. "Anglo-phones, Franco-phones." *Vancouver Sun* (6 March, 1991). p. B11.

Carayon, P. "Effect of Electronic Performance Monitoring on Job Design and Worker Stress: Review of the Literature and Conceptual Model." *Human Factors* 35, 3 (1993). pp. 385-95.

Clark, J., et al. *The Process of Technological Change: New Technology and Social Choice in the Workplace.* Cambridge: Cambridge University Press, 1988.

Cockburn, C. *Brothers: Male Dominance and Technological Change.* London: Pluto Press, 1983.

— *Machinery of Dominance: Women, Men and Technical Know-how.* London: Pluto Press, 1985.

Cohen, M., and M. White. *Playing with our Health: Hazards in the Automated Office.*

Vancouver: Press Gang, 1986.

Cooper, C. L., and J. Marshall. "Occupational Sources of Stress: A Review of the Literature Relating to Coronary Heart Disease and Mental Ill Health." *Journal of Occupational Psychology* 49 (1976). pp. 11-28.

Coutts, J. "Bell Stops Snooping on its Operators." *The Globe and Mail* (14 September, 1989). p. A16.

deCindio, F., and Carla S. "The Universes of Discourse for Education and Action/Research," in *Gendered by Design? Information Technology and Office Systems*. Eileen Green, Jenny Owen and Den Pain (eds.). London: Taylor and Francis, 1993. pp. 173-93.

DeMatteo, B. *Terminal Shock: The Health Hazards of Video Display Terminals*. Toronto: NC Press, 1985.

Ditecco, D., and M. Andre. *Report to the Health and Safety Sub-committee on Machine Pacing and Remote Electronic Monitoring* (March edition). Montreal: Communications and Electrical Workers/Bell Canada, 1987.

Edwards, R.C. *Contested Terrain: The Transformation of the Workplace in the Twentieth Century*. London: Heineman, 1979.

Feldberg, R.L., and E.N. Glenn. "Technology and Work Degradation: Effects of Office Automation on Women Clerical Workers," in *Machina Ex Dea: Feminist Perspectives on Technology*. Joan Rothschild (ed.). New York: Pergamon, 1983. pp. 59-78.

Franklin, U. *The Real World of Technology*. CBC Massey Lecture. Toronto: CBC Enterprises, 1990.

Gaillard, A.W. K. "Comparing the Concepts of Mental Load and Stress." *Ergonomics* 36, 9 (1993). pp. 991-1005.

Galitz, W.O. *Humanizing Office Automation: The Impact of Ergonomics on Productivity*. Wellesley: QED Information Sciences, 1984.

Green, E., J. Owen, and D. Pain (eds.). *Gendered by Design? Information Technology and Office Systems*. London: Taylor and Francis, 1993.

Greenbaum, J., and M. Kyng (eds.). *Design at Work: Cooperative Design of Computer Systems*. Hillsdale, NJ: Lawrence Erlbaum Associates, 1991.

Hall, E.M. "Gender, Work Control and Stress: A Theoretical Discussion and an Empirical Test." *International Journal of Health Services* 19, 4 (1989). pp. 725-45.

Howard, R. *Brave New Workplace*. New York: Viking, 1985.

Ivanovich, E., et al. "Noise Evaluation and Elimination of Some Specific and Non-specific Health Indicators in Telephone Operators." *Review of Environmental Health* 10, 1 (January-March 1994). pp. 39-46.

Kamphuis, A., and J. P. deGroot. "Mental Task Load of International Telephone Operators: Assessment by Task Analysis, Physiological Measures, Reaction Times and Questionaires." *International Journal of Psychophysiology: Official Journal* 14, 7 (1993). pp. 130-1.

Karasek, R. A. Jr. "Job Demands, Job Decision Latitude, and Mental Strain: Implications for Job Redesign." *Administrative Science Quarterly* 24 (1979). pp. 285-307.

Karasek, R. A., B. Gardell and J. Lindell. "Work and Non-work Correlates of Illness and Behaviour in Male and Female Swedish White-collar Workers." *Journal of*

Occupational Behaviour 8 (1987). pp. 187-207.

Karasek, R.A., and T. Theorell. *Healthy Work: Stress, Productivity, and the Reconstruction of Working Life*. New York: Basic Books, 1990.

Linn, P. "Gender Stereotypes, Technology Stereotypes," in *Gender and Expertise [Special Issue] Radical Science Journal 19*. London: Free Association Books, 1987. pp. 127-51.

Long, B.C., and S.E. Kahn. "A Theoretical Integration of Women, Work and Coping," in *Women, Work and Coping*. Bonita C. Long and Sharon E. Kahn (eds.). Montreal and Kingston: McGill-Queen's, 1993. pp. 296-311.

Lowe, G.S. *Women, Paid/Unpaid Work and Stress*. Ottawa: Canadian Advisory Council on the Status of Women, 1989.

Lowe, G.S., and H.C. Northcott. *Queen's Papers in Industrial Relations: Stressful Working Conditions and Union Dissatisfaction*. Kingston, Ontario: School of Industrial Relations, Queen's University, 1994.

Mawson, D.L. "Implications for Employment Intervention and Policy," in *Women, Work and Coping*. Bonita C. Long and Sharon E. Kahn (eds.). Montreal and Kingston: McGill-Queen's, 1993. pp. 51-69.

Namioka, A., and D. Schuler (eds.). *PDC'90: Conference on Participatory Design, Seattle, WA*. Palo Alto, CA: Computer Professionals for Social Responsibility, 1990.

Newfoundland Telephone Company Limited. *Newfoundland Telephone Annual Report 1988*. St. John's: Newfoundland Telephone Company Limited, 1988.

— *Newfoundland Telephone Annual Report 1990*. St. John's: Newfoundland Telephone Company Limited, 1990.

— *Newfoundland Telephone Annual Report 1991*. St. John's: Newfoundland Telephone Company Limited, 1991.

Newtel Enterprises Limited. *Annual Report for 1989*. St. John's: Newtel Enterprises Limited, 1989.

— *Annual Report 1990*. St. John's: Newtel Enterprises Limited, 1990.

— *Annual Report 1991*. St. John's: Newtel Enterprises Limited, 1991.

— *Annual Report 1992*. St. John's: Newtel Enterprises Limited, 1992.

Noble, D.F. "Social Choice in Machine Design: The Case of Automatically Controlled Machine Tools," in *Case Studies on the Labour Process*. A. Zimbalist (ed.). New York: Monthly Review, 1979. pp. 18-50.

— *Forces of Production: A Social History of Industrial Automation*. New York: Knopf, 1984.

— "Present Tense Technology." *Democracy* 3 (1982). pp. 8-24.

Parmeggiani, I. (ed.). *Encyclopedia of Occupational Health and Safety*. Third Revised Edition, 2. Geneva: International Labour Office, 1983.

Phillips, F. N. "A Study of Occupationally Induced Hearing Loss with Associated Tinnitus Attributable to Acoustic Trauma Amongst Employees in the Telecommunications Industry," in *On the Prevention of Occupational Accidents and Diseases: Xth World Congress*. Canadian Centre for Occupational Health and Safety (ed.). Hamilton, Ontario: Canadian Centre for Occupational Health and Safety, 1983. pp. 119-20.

Reasons, C.E., L.L. Ross and C. Paterson. *Assault on the Worker: Occupational Health and Safety in Canada*. Toronto: Butterworths, 1981.

Reid, J., C. Ewan and E. Lowy. "Pilgramage of Pain: The Illness Experiences of Women with Repetition Strain Injury and the Search for Credibility." *Social Science and Medicine* 32, 5 (1991). pp. 601-12.

Rothschild, J. (ed.). *Machina Ex Dea: Feminist Perspectives on Technology*. New York: Pergamon, 1983.

Rothwell, S. G. "Company Employment Policies and New Technology in Manufacturing and Service Sectors," in *Microprocessors, Manpower and Society*. M. Warner (ed.). New York: St. Martin's, 1984.

Schuler, D., and A. Namioka (eds.). *Participatory Design: Principles and Practices*. Hillsdale, NJ: Lawrence Erlbaum Associates, 1993.

Starr, S.J., C.R. Thompson and S.J. Shute. "Effects of Video Display Terminals on Telephone Operators." *Human Factors* 24, 6 (1982). pp. 699-711.

Statham, A., and E. Bravo. "The Introduction of New Technology: Health Implications for Workers." *Women and Health* 16, 2 (1990). pp. 105-29.

Suchman, L. "Foreword," in *Participatory Design: Principles and Practices*. Douglas Schuler and Aki Namioka (eds.). London: Lawrence Erlbaum Associates, 1993. pp.vii-ix.

Surtees, L. "Bell Automates Collect Calling: Voice Recognition Key to New System." *The Globe and Mail* (4 March 1991). p. B5.

Teiger, C., and C. Bernier. "Ergonomic Analysis of Work Activity of Data Entry Clerks in the Computerized Service Sector Can Reveal Unrecognized Skills." *Women and Health* 18, 3 (1992). pp. 67-77.

The Express. *The Express* (October 20, 1993).

Trigg, R., S.I. Anderson and E. Dykstra-Erickson (eds.). *PDC '94: Proceedings of the Participatory Design Conference*. Palo Alto, CA: Computer Professionals for Social Responsibility, 1994.

Turner, J. A., and R. A. Karasek. "Software Ergonomics: Effects of Computer Application Design Parameters on Operator Task Performance and Health." *Ergonomics* 27 (1984). pp. 663-90.

United States Office of Technology Assessment. *The Electronic Supervisor*. OTA-CIT-333 (ed.). Washington D.C.: United States Government Prnting Office, 1987.

Wright, B.D. (ed.). *Women, Work, and Technology: Transformations*. Ann Arbor: University of Michigan, 1987.

Yassi, A., et al. "Epidemic of 'Shocks' in Telephone Operators: Lessons for the Medical Community." *Canadian Medical Association Journal* 140 (1 April 1989). pp. 816-20.

Zureik, E., V. Mosco and C. Lochhead. "Telephone Workers' Reaction to the New Technology." *Relations Industrielles* 44, 3 (1989). pp. 507-31.

Janet Sprout and
Annalee Yassi

Occupational Health Concerns of Women who Work with the Public

Les femmes qui travaillent auprès du public constituent une part de la main-d'oeuvre en forte croissance. Pourtant, les problèmes de santé et de sécurité des travailleuses de ces secteurs ont reçu peu d'attention. Les recherches montrent que ces femmes sont exposées à des risques psychosociaux, chimiques, biologiques, physiques ou ergonomiques. Cet article souligne en particulier les risques psychosociaux reliés au stress, à la violence et aux conflits entre le travail et la famille, et leur impact sur la santé des femmes travaillant auprès du public. On y présente différentes méthodes pour aborder ces problèmes, à partir d'une enquête pan-canadienne auprès des spécialistes du travail et de la gestion, et d'une étude documentée publiée ou à paraître. L'article souligne la nécessité de poursuivre la recherche sur les moyens de limiter les risques dans ces emplois traditionnellement féminins.

Women who work with the public constitute a rapidly increasing proportion of the labour force. However, the occupational health and safety concerns of women workers in these sectors have received little attention. Research is showing that women workers in these occupations are at risk for psychosocial, chemical, biological, physical and ergonomic hazards. This paper highlights the psychosocial hazards of stress, violence and work/family conflict and their impact on the health of women working with the public. Examples of methods to address these problems in the workplace are discussed, based on a cross-Canada survey of key inform-ants in labour and management, as well as a review of published and unpublished literature. Further research into measures to control hazards in women's traditional work is needed.

INTRODUCTION

Over the last 20 years, the increase in the number of women in the labour force has exceeded that of their number in the population. Most of this growth has occurred in the service industries, due to a general shift in Canada away from goods producing sectors, which have traditionally employed men, to the service sector, which employs predominantly women. Despite the growing importance of this sector, the occupational health and safety concerns of workers in this sector have been largely ignored by traditional health and safety professionals and researchers. The purpose of this paper is to discuss some of the occupational health issues facing women working with the public and some approaches taken in the workplace to address these problems.[1]

Table 1 Principal Occupations of Women in Canada who Work with the Public, 1986

Occupation	Major Group	Number (x1000)	% of Female Workers	% of Total Employed Women
Social work & related	Social sciences	11	72.4	1.7
Kindergarden, elementary & secondary teachers	Teaching & related	295	70.2	4.6
Cashiers & tellers	Clerical & related	297	88.2	4.7
Insurance banks & other finance clerks	Clerical & related	48	85.3	0.8
Stenographers & typing	Clerical & related	496	98.3	7.8
Receptionists & information clerks	Clerical & related	132	93.1	2.1
Telephone operators	Clerical & related	27	89.2	0.4
Sales clerks & sales persons	Sales	380	53.9	6.0
Food & beverage preparation service	Service	451	64.7	7.1
Occupations in lodging & other accommodation	Servicet	43	71.4	0.7
Barbers & hairdressers	Service	81	83.4	1.3
Childcare Workers	Service	127	96.7	2.0
Travel & related attendants	Service	9	77.9	0.1
Total in above occupations	Service	2497		39.3

Source: Statistics Canada, Census 1991 Catalogue No. 93-327

We will focus on the following major occupational groups: clerical, service, sales, teaching and social sciences. Specifically, the focus will be on salespeople/cashiers, flight attendants, restaurant and hospitality workers, hairdressers and cosmetologists, clerical workers, telephone operators, bank workers, daycare workers, teachers and social service agency workers (Table 1). Together these workers constitute nearly 40 percent of the female labour force in Canada. It is recognized that many groups of women who work with the public are not included in this discussion — for example, health care workers, women in the police force, prostitutes and women in the unpaid labour force were excluded. Each of these women have their own occupational health and safety concerns, some of which are similar to those addressed in this paper, and some of which go far beyond the areas discussed here. In addition, there

Table 2 Workplace Injuries by Occupation and Gender, Canada, 1991

Occupation	Total (X 1000)	% Injured In Last Year		Work Days Lost Due to Injury							
				0 days		1-3 days		4-5 days		6+ days	
Clerical: total	2122	96	4.5	*22	23	*23	24	*10	10	*42	44
Women	1720	*54	3.1	*18	33	*13	24	*3	6	*20	37
Men	403	*43	10.6	4	9	10	23	6	14	22	51
Service: total	2036	173	8.5	*49	28	*30	17	*26	15	68	39
Women	1159	78	6.8	*25	32	*14	18	*15	19	*24	31
Men	877	95	10.8	*24	15	*16	17	*11	12	*44	46
Sales: total	1381	96	9.5	*23	24	*32	33	*11	11	*29	30
Women	664	*41	10.2	*8	20	*15	37	*3	7	*15	37
Men	717	*55	6.5	*15	27	*17	31	*8	15	*15	27
Teaching: total	715	*43	6.1	*23	53	*9	21	-	-	*9	21
Women	425	*21	5.0	*5	24	*7	33	-	-	*7	33
Men	290	*22	7.6	*18	82	*3	14	-	-	*2	9
Social Sciences: Total	278	*10	3.7	*5	50	-	-	-	-	*6	60
Women	155	*7	4.4	*2	29	-	-	-	-	*5	71
Men	124	*4	2.9	*2	50	-	-	-	-	*1	25

Source: General Social Survey, 1991, unpublished data; Percentages were rounded and so may not add up to 100 percent.

*Estimated number based on a sample site of less than 30. Therefore numbers may not add up to total numbers

- Data not available

are numerous books, review articles, and collections of publications on
the hazards of health care work (eg. M. Hagberg et al., 1993), as well as
specific articles regarding psychosocial hazards in this field (eg. Yassi and
Miller, 1990; Yassi, 1994).

HAZARDS FACING WOMEN WORKING WITH THE PUBLIC

Historically, working with the public has been viewed as relatively safe.
It has been assumed that this type of women's traditional work is not
hazardous because it does not involve the obvious hazardous conditions
found in some male-dominated jobs such as construction, forestry or
mining. Therefore women's working conditions have not been well
studied (Mergler et al., 1987). Yet workers in these occupations are
indeed at risk. In 1991, 8.5 percent of service workers, 9.5 percent of sales
workers, 6.1 percent of teachers and 4.5 percent of clerical workers
reported experiencing a workplace injury in the previous year (Table 2).
The majority of these required time loss from work. Proportionally fewer
women workers reported experiencing an occupational injury in the
previous year than did men in the same sector, except in sales and social
sciences, which likely reflects differences in working conditions.

Table 3 outlines the type of accidents sustained by women that have
resulted in accepted time loss workers' compensation claims. Overexer-
tion injuries accounted for the largest percent of time loss claims for
women in each of the five major occupational groups that work with the
public. Table 4 outlines the accepted time loss workers' compensation
injury claims for women and again according to major occupational
group and this time focusing on the nature of the injury. Strains and
sprains accounted for by far the largest proportion of injuries, indicating
possible ergonomic hazards in these occupations. It is noteworthy that
infectious diseases, which generally account for a very tiny percent of
total injuries, accounted for 1.6 percent of injuries in female teachers.

In the 1991 General Social Survey conducted by Statistics Canada, a
substantial number of women in these occupations reported exposure to
perceived occupational health hazards (Table 5). Nearly 65 percent of women
in the clerical field reported occupational exposure to computer screens, 24
percent reported poor air quality and 22 percent noted dust in the air. Even
loud noises (8.7 percent) and chemicals (5.4 percent) were perceived as a
problem for some female clerical workers. Women in sales occupations
reported similar exposure to loud noises (16.2 percent) and chemicals (13.1
percent), in addition to poor air quality (12.1 percent) and dust (20.9 percent).
A large number of female teachers reported exposure to all these hazards.

Table 3   Accepted Time-loss Injury Claims for Canadian Women by Major Occupational Groups and Type of Accident

Type of Accident	% Clerical	% Service	% Sales	% Teaching	% Social Sciences
Struck against	5.8	7.3	9.5	3.8	3.8
Struck by	9.71	13.2	16.6	12.1	15.8
Fall from elevation	7.6	4.8	7.0	8.9	5.7
Fall on same level	16.7	16.1	11.8	24.0	14.9
Caught	3.5	3.9	4.0	1.7	1.8
Rubbed and abraded	0.9	2.3	1.8	0.5	0.5
Bodily reaction	17.7	14.1	13.2	18.9	12.0
Over exertion	31.5	25.6	30.7	21.5	32.2
Contact — extreme temperatures	1.4	8.1	1.4	0.4	0.9
Contact — toxic substances	1.4	2.2	0.7	2.0	1.4
Vehicle accident	0.9	0.5	1.4	0.9	3.6
Others	2.9	1.9	1.9	5.3	7.4
Total	13006	32169	8113	3441	2018

Source: Statistics Canada, National Work Injuries, Statistics Program, 1992.

Table 4   Accepted Time-loss Injury Claims for Canadian Women, by Major Occupational Group and Nature of Injury, 1990

Nature of Injury	% Clerical	% Service	% Sales	% Teaching	% Social Sciences
Burns	1.4	8.2	1.4	0.2	0.8
Contusions	18.1	16.7	16.7	19.5	17.3
Cuts/lacerations	4.7	11.7	14.6	3.0	3.5
Fractures	4.6	3.3	4.1	7.8	4.5
Dermatitis	0.3	0.9	0.3	-	-
Inflammations	6.5	4.3	3.7	2.3	1.9
Abrasions	1.5	1.7	2.0	1.6	1.5
Sprains/strains	51.5	44.4	47.3	50.0	59.0
Multiple injuries	1.4	1.0	1.4	1.2	1.9
Infectious diseases	0.2	0.3	-	1.6	0.6
Other occupational injuries	3.9	4.2	4.6	5.8	5.0
Other	5.9	3.3	3.9	7.0	4.0
Total	13006	32169	8113	3441	2018

Source: Statistics Canada, National Work Injuries, Statistics Program, 1992.

In addition to these perceived risks, there are the hidden hazards of working with the public, such as violence, stress, sexual harassment and work/family conflict. The focus of this paper will be on these occupational health hazards and some of the ways to address them.

Table 5 Exposure to Risks at Work by Occupation and Sex, Canada 1991

Occupation Groups	% Dust in Air	% Chemicals	% Loud Noise	% VDT Use	% Poor IAQ	% Other Dangers
Clerical: total	24.3	7.6	11.7	60.7	23.8	2.3
Women	122.1	5.4	8.7	64.7	24.2	1.8
Men	33.8	16.8	24.4	43.7	22.5	4.4
Service: total	26.5	19.3	22.5	8.9	16.2	6.5
Women	20.6	13.1	16.2	6.3	12.1	3.9
Men	34.3	27.6	31.0	12.4	21.7	10.0
Sales: total	21.7	10.9	9.7	28.2	12.8	2.3
Women	20.9	5.6	4.6	27.9	15.2	2.8
Men	22.5	16.0	14.5	28.4	10.5	1.9
Teaching: total	19.6	9.3	13.6	43.1	22.6	3.8
Women	20.2	7.1	13.8	34.2	18.2	3.6
Men	18.8	12.5	13.4	56.1	29.0	4.2
Social service: total	14.6	5.7	6.2	33.4	25.1	3.3
Women	18.9	5.8	10.0	38.9	29.9	2.8
Men	9.2	5.4	1.4	26.5	19.2	3.9

Source: General Social Survey, 1991; unpublished data.

STRESS

It is now widely recognized that health is not only the absence of disease, but a state of physical, mental and social well-being. Moreover, it is now known that psychological and social factors can play a major role in causing illness. There are many definitions of stress, but occupational stress can arise in a situation in which job related factors interact with individual characteristics of a worker to change her psychological or physiological well-being.

Stress is becoming an increasing occupational concern. The 1991 General Social Survey revealed that over three quarters of women working in the social sciences fields reported experiencing stress, as did a large number of women teachers (69.6 percent), women in sales occupations (58.7 percent), clerical workers (50.7 percent) and service workers (46.3

percent) (Table 6). The latter three categories were responsible for more than 44 percent of the total number of Canadian workers' compensation claims for work injuries of a psychological nature such as stress (Geran, 1992).

Table 6 Percent of Workers Reporting Stress by Sex and Occupation, Canada, 1991

Occupation	Very Stressful	Somewhat Stressful	Not Very Stressful	Not at all Stressful
Clerical: both sexes	8.3	43.1	35.5	13.1
Women	8.2	42.5	36.9	12.4
Men	8.8	45.7	29.5	16.0
Services: both sexes	8.6	37.9	38.2	15.3
Women	9.7	36.6	36.9	16.8
Men	7.3	39.5	39.8	13.4
Sales: both sexes	9.4	51.1	30.8	8.8
Women	7.0	51.7	33.4	8.0
Men	11.6	50.5	28.3	9.6
Teaching: both sexes	12.8	55.1	24.9	7.2
Women	13	56.6	26.2	4.1
Men	12.6	52.9	22.9	11.7
Social sciences: both sexes	13.5	55.3	21.8	9.5
Women	14.8	61.7	19.1	4.4
Men	11.9	47.3	25.0	15.8

Source: General Social Survey, 1991; unpublished data.

Prepared by Social Environment Information. Policy, Planning and Information Branch, Health and Welfare Canada, June 1991.

In fact, contrary to the belief that it is the chief executive officers and professionals who have the high-stress jobs, it is now recognized that the jobs most likely to involve stressors that impair health combine high levels of demand (the amount of work required) with little control over the work process (such as having the ability to decide how to do it, what skills to apply, whom to contact, etc.) (Karasek, 1984). Such jobs are typically low level and low paying. Although both men and women are employed in these types of jobs, women are more likely to find themselves restricted to these jobs by social factors such as sexist attitudes and discrimination (Baruch et al., 1987).

Several studies on stress have used the high demand/low control index as a measure of stress and have found that a high score not only increases the risk of spontaneous abortions and low birth weight infants (Brandt and Nielsen, 1992), but also the risk of depression (Braun and Hollander, 1988) and the rate of coronary heart disease (Karasek, 1984; Reed et al., 1989). Lowe (1989) also noted that the combination of constant work pressures and responsibility with little authority increased the likelihood of health problems such as eyestrain, headaches, nausea and depression.

In many jobs dealing with the public (waitress, cashier, social worker), the worker does not have much control over how to relate to the client but the client has considerable needs or demands. Many of these jobs are in large organizations with restrictive work rules that may prevent the workers from responding to the clients' needs in the way that they would like.

Machine-paced jobs offering little opportunity for decision making also fall into this category. Telephone operators, airline reservation agents, bank credit card centre clerks and those who are constantly working with computers while being monitored experience how automation, while improving some working conditions, has exposed women to major new stressors. Research at the University of Stockholm on computerization and the psychosocial work environment showed that women employees are consistently less satisfied with various aspects of the psychosocial work environment than are men. These differences appear to reflect the actual circumstances of working women: women have less varied work tasks, less independence in their jobs, fewer opportunities for promotion and lower prestige — all factors known to be related to dissatisfaction at work (Bradley, 1988).

Another common occupational stressor for many women working with the public is work overload. Several studies revealed that women who had to perform fast-paced work — a form of overload — complained more of fatigue, insomnia, aches and pains, and digestive problems than women who did not report performing fast-paced work (Messing and Reveret, 1983; Tierney et al., 1990). The hard economic times presently being experienced in Canada have resulted in an increasing requirement for government social services at the same time that government is undergoing cutbacks, often resulting in less staff to service the increasing demand. For government workers, this has led to a form of work overload and job burnout, as shown for example by Lowe's study (1991) of job stress among 537 employees (76 percent female) at Newfoundland's Department of Social Services (DOSS). The survey revealed that too heavy a workload was the major cause of stress among Newfoundland's DOSS workers, who include social workers, clerical workers, financial assistant officers, employment opportunity workers, homemakers and child management specialists. Heavy workload was also a major predictor of job dissatisfaction and fear of job loss.

Shift and night work is another major occupational stressor for women working with the public. Some studies have shown that people who work shifts more often experience tiredness, gastrointestinal disorders, sleep disorders and irritability than do day workers (Sutherland and Cooper, 1988; Seward, 1990). Of special concern for pregnant women are several studies suggesting that shift work increases the risk of miscarriages (Goulet and Theriault, 1987), although not all studies have supported this finding. Not only can shift work disrupt the normal sleep/wake cycle, temperature pattern and adrenaline rhythm in the body, it can affect family and social life. Shift workers will often have difficulty maintaining normal social contact and community involvement. It is difficult to arrange childcare outside of normal working hours, so spouses may have to work staggered shifts. This factor, plus altered sleep patterns, may limit interaction with children and spouses (Volger, 1988).

The hospitality industry provides an excellent example of this problem, hotels and many restaurants are 24-hour-a-day businesses. The hours of work are unpredictable and in some cases the workers only have a few days' notice of their next week's work schedule. Bell Telephone in Quebec and Ontario also post schedules with only five days' notice and schedules change radically for each operator from week to week. Interviews with factory workers, waitresses and telephone operators revealed that most feel that they do not sleep enough, that they are always tired and that they experience frequent headaches (Vandelac and Methot, 1993; Messing, in press). These symptoms, in turn, may affect their relationships with family and friends. For example, Vandelac and Methot described the situation of one single mother who started work at 6:30 am in a factory. In order for her child to get to the daytime caregiver, the child had to wake up at 4:30 am. The child thus had to be awake for four hours before school started. At the time when most children do their homework, this child was too tired to work and the mother was also too tired to help. The mother felt guilty when the child failed his school year.

Controlling Occupational Stress

The approach to controlling stress at the workplace should resemble that for any occupational hazard. The hazard should be controlled at the source by eliminating job components which produce stress. Some solutions include increasing staff, providing automatic pay increases, abolishing rotating shifts, stopping machine monitoring practices, changing the organizational structure or management style, providing daycare services at the worksite and altering work roles or functions.

The second choice among approaches to hazard control is to modify the hazard between the source and the worker, in this case by increasing worker participation. Generally, studies have shown that participation in decision making is crucial to reducing stress and increasing job satisfaction (Cherniss, 1985; Miller et al., 1990; Israel et al., 1989; McLaney and Hurell, 1988). New management initiatives, termed "industrial democracy," "quality circles" and "total quality management" are being implemented in the workplace, with the idea of procuring greater worker input into decision making. However, there is considerable controversy as to the effectiveness of these management initiatives in reducing stress or in effecting other positive outcomes (Buch, 1991; Bushe, 1988; Jennings, 1988; Peterson and Tracy, 1992; Johnson, 1992). Moreover, unions are sceptical of this initiative, claiming that this is just another management tool to reduce jobs while increasing the workload, and that management does not want true worker participation, accepting only those ideas which support management's plans. For example, Hydro-Quebec introduced its total quality participation programme just before unilaterally cutting thousands of jobs in 1993.

The last and generally least effective method of hazard control, and yet the most common approach used for stress reduction, is to reduce the impact of the hazard on the worker by introducing employee assistance programmes (EAP) and stress management courses to improve the individuals' "coping styles." An analysis of the literature associated with stress management programmes revealed that positive benefits, such as a reduction in anxiety or depression, diminish over time and that programmes do not produce impressive changes in productivity or absenteeism (Murphy, 1985). Only one out of nine studies reported objective evidence of improved stress management by employees (Pelletier and Lutz, 1989).

Another approach to preventing occupational stress is to pass occupational health and safety laws addressing issues such as working in isolation, barriers to advancement, monetary concerns and lack of control over work planning and pacing (Geran, 1992). Similarly, clauses can be introduced into collective bargaining agreements to provide for worker participation in decisions affecting job process, the formation of workplace stress committees, or the consideration of the social effects on workers prior to the introduction of new technology (Arndt, 1981; Lowe, 1991; Bradley, 1988; O'Mara, 1986).

Bell Canada and its union, the Communication, Energy and Paper Workers Union of Canada, have developed several mechanisms to reduce the stressors on telephone operators, who were under considerable stress due to the routine nature of their work, fast work speed, monitoring practices, the demand for a low expected average of time spent per call, and having to constantly remain at their work stations. As a result of a survey and discussion with the union, Bell Canada abolished the average time per call for individuals and instead set an office productivity objective. As long as the office is meeting its objective, its productivity is considered acceptable. The operators have also been given increased autonomy and skill variety. For example, some operators have the opportunity to do telemarketing for half of their shift. As well, operators have had an "on-off" mute switch installed on their headsets so that customers are not able to hear when an operator wishes to talk to another operator, and operators in some offices are now allowed to leave their work station to take a short "stress" break to talk to another person. Although this does not make the handling of calls any easier it affords operators more control in their job and, for difficult calls, it does allow the operator an outlet for emotions. Other telephone companies, in conjunction with their unions, have implemented similar programs.

VIOLENCE

Women who work directly with the public may face contemptuous, aggressive or violent behaviour. The awareness of this problem is growing, and there is the shocking recognition that this occupational hazard is all too prevalent. However, it is important to recognize that violent actions are not random unforeseeable acts. Workers in certain industries and occupations are known to be at greater risk for violence than are other workers. Table 7 summarizes some of the occupations and factors identified as increasing the risk of experiencing violence in the workplace.

For example, a survey of 1,111 social service and institutional workers conducted by the Alberta Union of Public Employees in 1985 found that 29.5 percent had been physically assaulted and approximately 5 percent had lost time from work due to physical assault, 19 percent had personal property damaged due to a physical assault, 41.5 percent had been physically threatened and 61.3 percent verbally threatened (Darcy, 1991). A survey of Manitoba teachers from grades K-12 revealed that 39 percent of teachers experienced some form of abuse within a 15 month period (Manitoba Teachers' Society, 1990). Of those who experienced abuse, 88 percent reported emotional abuse, 28 percent damage to personal property, and 17 percent physical abuse. A small number of teachers encountered attacks on their family. Female teachers were more likely to suffer abuse in the form of physical assault or harassment than male teachers.

Rape and murder are the most extreme forms of violence against women. Women employed in convenience food stores have the greatest risk of being raped — 20 times that of women employed in other workplaces (Seligman et al., 1987). Other occupations at risk for rape are hotel chamber maids and residence managers (ibid.).

Homicide is the leading cause of traumatic workplace deaths among women in the United States (Bell, 1991). Although Canada does not have as many occupationally related homicides as does the United States, women who work with the public are still at risk. An Ontario study revealed that a quarter of all occupational fatalities in women in Ontario over a 10 year period were attributable to workplace violence (Liss and Craig, 1990). Women employed in the retail trade and service industries have the highest risk of being murdered at work, with robbery being the most common motive (Liss and Craig, 1990; Levin et al., 1992). The workplaces at greatest risk are food/convenience stores, eating and drinking establishments, and gasoline service stations. The occupations at highest risk are sales personnel, service employees such as waitresses and grocery baggers, managers and clerical workers. The risk of homicide is closely related to extensive exposure to the public, the exchange of money, and evening employment (Bell, 1991).

Sexual harassment, another form of violence, can have a profound impact on women's physical and mental health and job performance (Shrier, 1990; Kasinsky, 1992; Crull, 1982). Studies have shown that victims of sexual harassment reported physical symptoms such as nausea, headache and chronic fatigue; reactions such as general tension or nervousness, persistent anger, fear and helplessness have also been reported (Shrier, 1990). Other common symptoms attributed to sexual harassment are depression, embarrassment, sleeplessness, and guilt (Kasinsky, 1992). All the studies have examined sexual harassment from co-workers or superiors; none specifically looked at the extent of sexual harassment from the public or client, although this is known anecdotally to be quite common. This area begs further research.

In fact, employer requirements in some jobs for women working with the public may actually encourage sexual harassment. Women may be encouraged to make themselves "sexually appealing," particularly in the hospitality/restaurant industry. Some women have found that their tips improved when they wore sexier clothing. In the past, women in other public service occupations were forced to attire themselves in ways which some women found objectionable; for example, it was not too long ago that a flight attendant was disciplined for refusing to wear make-up.

Table 7   Occupations at High Risk of Work-related Violence

Type of Activity	Occupations at Risk
Handling money or valuables	Cashiers Bank workers Retail clerks Convenience store clerks Supermarket cashiers
Providing care, advice, or dealing with complaints	Social service workers Teachers Daycare workers Residential centre workers Receptionists Library staff
Working with drunk, drugged, or mentally disturbed people	Food and bar waitresses Flight attendants Social workers Hotel staff
Working alone	Hotel housekeepers Convenience store clerks
Inspecting and enforcing legislation and policies	Social workers Inspectors Welfare agency workers U.I.C. workers and Workers' compensation employees

Adapted from: NALGO Safety Representative, September 1985, and other sources cited in the text.

Controlling Occupational Violence

Because violence towards public and service sector workers has only recently been recognized as an occupational health hazard, there is a paucity of research into prevention strategies. Nevertheless, the traditional occupational health hazard prevention approach can be applied, beginning with the reduction of job components which increase the risk of violence. Some examples of the changes that can be made are: increasing staffing ratios; making changes in the way money is handled (such as issuing chits instead of money, maintaining only a minimum of cash on hand); making administrative making changes (such as altering hours of operation, reviewing client files before start of shift); and altering the design of the workplace (such as ensuring that the cash register and personnel are visible to the outside, and providing well-lit parking lots, alarm devices and procedures).

Experience with workplace violence in England has shown that changing work practices is more effective than using security devices such as alarms (Poyner, 1989). Staff can be trained to spot and diffuse potentially violent situations.

Other approaches to prevention of workplace violence can include incorporating a workplace violence clause in the collective agreement (for an example of contract language, see Table 8) and legislation such as Manitoba's Working Alone Regulation or Saskatchewan's requirement for a workplace policy on violence, including sexual or racial harassment.[2]

Table 8 Example of Contract Wording Regarding Workplace Violence

Definition of Violence Violence shall be defined as any incident in which an employee is abused, threatened or assaulted during the course of employment. This includes the application of force, threats with or without weapons, severe verbal abuse and persistent sexual or racial harassment.
Violence Policies and Procedures The employer agrees to develop explicit policies and procedures to deal with violence. The policy will address the prevention of violence, the management of violent situations and the provision of legal counsel and support to employees who have faced violence. The policies and procedures shall be part of the employer's health and safety policy and written copies shall be provided to each employee. **The policies and procedures will include but not be limited to:** **a.** provision of adequate information about the previous actual or potential violent behaviour of a patient, resident or client towards employees; **b.** adequate arrangements to investigate cases where violence and assaults against employees have occurred; and **c.** provision for a Joint Union/Employer Health and Safety Committee to review the effectiveness of antiviolence policies.
Violence Prevention The employer agrees that in all cases where employees or the union identify a risk of violence to staff, the employer shall establish and maintain measures and procedures to reduce the likelihood of incidents to the lowest possible level. It is understood that the measures and procedures are in addition to and not a replacement for a training programme about dealing with violence.
Training The employer agrees to provide training and information on the prevention of violence to staff to all employees who come into contact with potentially aggressive persons. The training programme will include adequate opportunities for participation by union instructors. All employees working areas where there is a risk of violence shall be trained with a course including but not limited to: causes of violence; factors that precipitate violence; recognition of warning signs; prevention of escalation; controlling and defusing aggressive situations.

Source: CUPE Local 3499 and Central Interior Family Foundation Collective Agreement April 1, 1992-March 31, 1993.

Winnipeg's Welfare Office, for example, instituted physical and administrative changes in response to staff experiencing some problems with violent clients. The department erected shield barriers between waiting areas and receptionists; cashiers were provided with barriers; and locks were installed on the doors and a security system established to enter the welfare offices in which clients had to be "buzzed in." The office established a "Care and Caution" Committee with two management and two staff representatives. The intent of the Care and Caution Committee is to review clients placed on the department's "care and caution" list (and hence deemed to be violent or potentially violent) in order to determine the method of service delivery for the client. Employees can place a client on this list if they have reason to believe that the client is potentially violent. The normal procedures of seeing and interviewing the client are replaced by alternate procedures.

WORK/FAMILY CONFLICT

Women's work with the public, which requires responding to the needs of others, has some similarities to work required at home. A stressful job compounds the impact of domestic pressures and vice versa. Grahame Lowe's study (1991) of job stress at Newfoundland's Department of Social Service found that those with excessive job demands and other stressful working conditions experienced greater work/personal life conflict. Multiple demands and expectations at home, in the community and at work often result in women suffering from the stress associated with having two jobs at once — one at their workplace and one in their home. This stress results from two factors — role conflict and work overload (Lowe, 1989).

Several studies have shown that working women still perform the vast majority of household and childbearing tasks. This double workload, by itself, can be a source of tension, fatigue, and stress (Meleis and Stevens, 1992; Tierney et al., 1990; De Koninck, 1984; Le Bourdais et al., 1987) which can also make women sick. Several investigations have found higher levels of illness, such as coronary heart disease, respiratory illness, exhaustion, depression and poor mental health, among employed women whose spouses do not share the household and childrearing tasks (Meleis and Stevens, 1992; Baruch et al., 1987; Karasek et al., 1987).

It is not just caring for husband and/or children that is creating role conflicts and work overload for working women. Many elders with disabilities are requiring care from their extended family, usually women (McGovern and Matter, 1992). Some women are both raising children and taking care of elderly family members. Caregiving to the elderly is associated with exhaustion and physical, emotional, and financial strain (ibid.).

This double workload affects women's paid employment. Women are too tired or simply not available to work overtime, travel or participate in extra work activities and this affects women's job advancement opportunities and earnings. As well, women experience more work absences than men (Akyeampong, 1992a; 1992b). This difference is almost entirely family related. Statistics Canada's 1990 Labour Force Survey showed that the presence of children living at home, particularly pre-school children, dramatically influences the number of days women are absent from work for personal reasons. Women with children missed an average of 7.9 days due to family obligations, especially if they had at least one pre-school child (25.1 days). This compares to 1 day missed by men with children and 2.3 days by women without children at home (ibid.).

Reducing Work/Family Conflict

There is now increasing recognition of the need to balance work and family responsibilities. Paid leave for family responsibilities is becoming more common. Unions and employers have negotiated family leave provisions which allow days to be taken without loss of pay to attend to the health needs of family members. These policies help women caring for elderly parents or young children to take time from work without having to use their own sick days, vacation days or leave without pay. Quebec is the only province providing five unpaid days per year for parents to attend to children's health or educational needs.

A variety of options are being provided by some employers to assist their employees in reconciling the double workloads. Some of these work options are outlined in Table 9. Some Canadian banks have utilized flexible working options with good success. The Bank of Montreal, for example, has a programme which allows employees to alter their work schedule (flex-time) or place of work (flex-place). Joanna Totta, Vice President Workplace Equity for the Bank of Montreal, indicated that there were initial concerns that the programme would result in a scheduling nightmare, but this has not occurred and those who have opted into the programme have viewed it positively.

Many unions, however, are reticent about some of these work options, arguing that absence with pay for family responsibilities is preferable. Unions are concerned that flexible working options may pave the way towards permanent part-time work or permanent at-home work with fewer or no benefits. Unions also argue that many women do not fully understand the impact of the work options on their pensions, benefits and career advancement before they undertake the program. According to some union representatives, some of these flexible work options are promoted by some employers primarily as a means of reducing costs rather than from a genuine desire to accommodate workers. However, some unions have managed to negotiate provisions which protect benefits for those workers who choose the work options, and/or have set a minimum number of full-time jobs an employer must have.

Table 9   Some Work Options to Help Resolve Work/Family Conflicts

Job sharing:	Two or more people share the duties of a full-time position with pro-rated pay and benefits.
Flex-time:	Working a standard number of hours per week with flexible starting and quitting times.
V-time:	A voluntary time/income trade-off that allows people to reduce work hours by 5 to 40 percent for a specified period of time.
Flex-place:	People can choose to do some of their work at home, at a satellite office or anywhere that is most convenient and productive for them.
Modified work week:	The normal work day is extended to bank time towards days off.
Phased retirement:	An option of reducing work time in anticipation of full retirement without loss of eventual pension entitlement.
Banked overtime:	A form of voluntary compensatory time off in lieu of overtime pay.
Leaves of absence:	A broad range of both paid and unpaid leaves.
Permanent part-time:	A permanent reduction in working hours.

Source: Williams, 1990.

CONCLUSION

Historically, research on occupational health and safety hazards has focused on jobs with obvious physical and chemical hazards — jobs traditionally held by men — while addressing women's health concerns only with respect to women in nontraditional jobs.

Women who work with the public face real health and safety hazards; as such, there is certainly no justification for trivializing the occupational health concerns facing women in these jobs. The hazards identified in this paper focused entirely on the psychosocial hazards of stress, violence, and work/family conflict, although women in these jobs also face a variety of other hazards including chemical, biological, physical and ergonomic hazards.

This report indicates that women's health and safety is affected by these hazards, that control measures are possible and that attention is needed to ensure that these concerns are addressed.

While further research on hazard identification is clearly required, our findings suggest that the major research needed is on hazard control. Occupational health programmes are most important for women working in low paying, largely non-unionized yet highly hazardous jobs commonly found in the service sector, such as waitressing and retail sales. While some workplaces have initiated programmes to address these hazards, government initiatives to regulate and enforce compliance with measures to address these hazards lag far behind.

NOTES

1. This paper uses some of the data and information gathered for a study conducted under the direction of Dr. Annalee Yassi while under contract for Labour Canada. This is combined with information, observations and experience gathered during years of work in the field of occupational health. The report of the Labour Canada study is in the process of peer review.

2. In the time since this paper was presented, British Columbia promulgated a "Protection of workers from violence in the workplace" regulation.

REFERENCES

Akyeampong, E.B. "Absences from Work Revisited." *Perspectives, Statistics Canada* (Spring, 1992a). pp. 44-53.

— "Absenteeism at Work." *Canadian Social Trends* (Summer, 1992b). pp. 26-8.

Arndt, R. "Coping with Job Stress: The Role of the Union Safety and Health Committee." *Labour Studies Journal* 6, 1 (1981). pp. 53-61.

Baruch, G.K., L. Biener and R.C. Barnett. "Women and Gender in Research on Work and Family Stress." *American Psychologist* 42, 2 (1987). pp. 130-6.

Bell, C.A. "Female Homicides in United States Workplaces, 1980-1985." *American Journal of Public Health* 81, 6 (1991). pp. 729-32.

Bradley, G. "Women, Work and Computers." *Women and Health* 13, 3-4 (1988). p.117-32.

Brandt, L.P.A., and C.V. Nielson. "Job Stress and Adverse Outcome of Pregnancy: A Causal Link or Recall Bias?" *American Journal of Epidemiology* 135, 3 (1992). pp. 302-11.

Braun, S., and R.B. Hollander. "Work and Depression among Women in the Federal Republic of Germany." *Women and Health* 14, 2 (1988). pp. 3-26.

Buch, K. "Quality Circles in a Unionized Setting: Their Effect on Grievance Rates." *Journal of Business and Psychology* 6, 1 (1991). pp. 147-54.

Bushe, G.R. "Developing Cooperative Labor-management Relations in Unionized

Factories: A Multiple Case Study of Quality Circles and Parallel Organizations Within Joint Quality of Work Life Projects." *The Journal of Applied Behavioral Science* 24, 2 (1988). pp. 129-50.

Cherniss, C. "Stress, Burnout and the Special Services Provider." *Special Services in the Schools* 2, 1 (1985). pp. 45-61.

Crull, P. "Stress Effects of Sexual Harassment on the Job: Implications for Counselling." *American Journal of Orthopsychiatry* 52, 3 (1982). pp. 539-44.

Darcy, J. "Violence in the Workplace — It's Not Part of the Job." Keynote address to the CLC Health and Safety Conference. Health and Safety Department, Canadian Union of Public Employees, 1991.

De Koninck, M. "Double travail et santé des femmes." *Santé mentale au Canada* 32 (septembre, 1984). pp. 14-7.

Geran, L. "Occupational Stress." *Canadian Social Trends* (Autumn, 1992). pp. 14-7.

Goulet, L., and G. Theriault. "Association Between Spontaneous Abortion and Ergonomic Factors: A Literature Review of the Epidemiologic Evidence." *Scandinavian Journal of Work, Environment and Health* 13 (1987). pp. 399-403.

Hagbert M., F. Hofmann, U. Stobel and G. Westlander (eds.). "Occupational Health for Health Care Workers." Presented at International Congress on Occupational Health, 1993.

Israel, B.A., J.S. House, S.J. Schurman, C.A. Keany and R.P. Mero. "The Relation of Personal Resources, Participation, Influence, Interpersonal Relationships and Coping Strategies to Occupational Stress, Job Strains and Health: A Multivariate Analysis." *Work and Stress* 3, 2 (1989). pp. 163-94.

Jennings, K.R. "Testing a Model of Quality Circle Processes: Implications for Practice and Consultation." *Consultation: An International Journal* 7, 1 (1988) pp. 19-28.

Johnson, W.R. "The Impact of Quality Circle Participation on Job Satisfaction and Organizational Commitment." *Psychology, A Journal of Human Behavior* 29, 1 (1992).

Karasek, R.A. "Characteristics of Task Structure Associated with Physiological Stress and Cardiovascular Illness." *Annual American Conference on Industrial Hygiene* 8 (1984). pp. 27-32.

Karasek, R.A., B. Gardell and J. Lindell. "Work and Non-work Correlates of Illness and Behaviour in Male and Female Swedish White Collar Workers." *Journal of Occupational Behaviour* 8 (1987). pp. 187-207.

Kasinsky, R.G. "Sexual Harassment: A Health Hazard for Women Workers." *New Solutions* (1992). pp. 74-83.

LeBourdais C., P.J. Hamel and P. Bernard. "Le travail et l'ouvrage: Charge en partage des taches domestiques chez les couples québecois." *Sociologie et sociétés* XIX, 1 (1987). pp. 37-55.

Levin, P.F., J.B. Hewitt and S.T. Misner. "Female Workplace Homicides: An Integrative Research Review." *AAOHN*, 40, 5 (1992). pp. 229-36.

Liss, G.M., and C.A. Craig. "Homicide in the Workplace in Ontario: Occupations at Risk and Limitations of Existing Data Sources." *Canadian Journal of Public Health* 81 (1990). pp. 10-5.

Lowe, G.S. *Women, Paid/Unpaid Work, and Stress: New Directions for Research.* Background paper. Ottawa: Canadian Advisory Council on the Status of Women, 1989.

— "Workplace Stress in the Newfoundland Department of Social Services." Report prepared for the Newfoundland Association of Public Employees, 1991 (a).

Manitoba Teachers' Society. *Report of the Task Force on the Physical and Emotional Abuse of Teachers.* Winnipeg: Manitoba Teachers' Society, (1990).

McGovern, P., and D. Matter. "Work and Family, Competing Demands Affecting Worker Well Being." *AAOHN* 40, 1 (1992). pp. 24-35.

McLaney, M.A., and J.J. Hurrell. "Control, Stress and Job Satisfaction in Canadian Nurses." *Work and Stress* 2, 3 (1988). pp. 217-24.

Meleis, A.I., and P.E. Stevens. "Women in Clerical Jobs: Spousal Role Satisfaction, Stress, and Coping." *Women and Health* 18, 1 (1992). pp. 23-39.

Mergler, D., C. Brabant, N. Vézina and K. Messing. "The Weaker Sex? Men in Women's Working Conditions Report Similar Health Symptoms." *Journal of Occupational Medicine* 29, 5 (1987). pp. 417-21.

Messing K., and J.P. Reveret. "Are Women in Female Jobs for Their Health? A Study of Working Conditions and Health Effects in the Fish-processing Industry in Quebec. Health of Women in Employment Ghettos." *International Journal of Health Services* 13, 4 (1983). pp. 635-47.

Messing K. *Occupational Safety and Health Concerns of Canadian Women: A Background Paper.* Ottawa: Women's Bureau, Labour Canada, 1991.

Miller, K.I., B.H. Ellis, E.G. Zook and J.S. Lyles. "An Integrated Model of Communication, Stress and Burnout in the Workplace." *Communication Research* 17 (1990). pp. 300-26.

Murphy, L.R. *Industrial Coping Strategies Division of Biomedical and Behaviour Sciences.* Cincinnati, OH: NIOSH, 1985.

NALGO Safety Representative. "Violence — A Work hazard." Presented in London, England, September, 1985.

O'Mara, N. "Occupational Stress and VDU Usage," in *Trends in the Ergonomics of Work, Proceedings of the 23rd Annual Conference of the Ergonomics Society of Australia and New Zealand, 1986.* D. Morrison, L. Hartley, and D. Kemp (eds.). pp. 201-5.

Pelletier, K.R., and R. Lutz. "Mindbody Goes to Work: A Critical Review of Stress Management Programmes in the Workplace." *Advances* 6, 1 (1989). pp. 28-34.

Peterson, R.B., and L. Tracy. "Assessing Effectiveness of Joint Committees in a Labor-management Cooperation Program." *Human Relations* 45, 5 (1992). pp. 467-88.

Poyner, B. "Working Against Violence." *Occupational Health* 41, 8 (1989). pp. 209-11.

Reed, D.M., A.Z. LaCroix, R.A. Karasek, D. Miller and C.A. MacLean. "Occupational Strain and the Incidence of Coronary Heart Disease." *American Journal of Epidemiology* 129, 3 (1989). pp. 495-502.

Seligman, P.J., S.C. Newman, C.L. Timbrook and W.E. Halperin. "Sexual Assault of Women at Work." *American Journal of Industrial Medicine* 12 (1987). pp. 445-50.

Seward, J.P. "Occupational Stress," in *Occupational Medicine*. LaDou J. Norwalk (ed.). Connecticut: Appleton and Lange, 1990. Chapter 35, pp. 467-80.

Shrier, D.K. "Sexual Harassment and Discrimination: Impact on Physical and Mental Health." *New Jersey Medicine* 87, 2 (1990). pp. 105-7.

Statistics Canada. *Work injuries, 1989-1991*. Catalogue 72-208 Annual, 1992.

Sutherland, V.J., and C.L. Cooper. "Sources of Work Stress," in *Occupational Stress: Issues and Developments in Research*. Hurrell, Murphy and Sauter (eds.). New York: Taylor and Francis, 1988.

Tierney, D., P. Romito and K. Messing. "She Ate Not the Bread of Idleness: Exhaustion is Related to Domestic and Salaried Working Conditions among 539 Quebec Hospital Workers." *Women and Health* 16, 1 (1990). pp. 21-42.

Williams, G. "A Manager's Guide to: Evaluating Work Option Proposals," in *Work Well — Promoting Flexible Work Options*, 1990.

Yassi, A., and B. Miller. "Technological Change and the Medical Technologist: A Stress Survey of Four Biomedical Laboratories in a Large Tertiary Care Hospital." *Canadian Journal of Medical Technology* 52, 4 (1990).

Yassi, A. "Assault and Abuse of Health Care Workers in a Large Teaching Hospital." *Canadian Medical Association Journal* 151, 9 (1994).

Vivienne Walters, Barbara
Beardwood, John Eyles,
Susan French

Paid and Unpaid Work Roles of Male and Female Nurses

Cet article fait l'analyse préliminaire d'une enquête auprès de 2285 infirmières et infirmiers de l'Ontario. L'échantillon est composé de femmes et d'hommes infirmières(ers) licenciées(és) (Registered Nurses ou RN) ainsi que d'infirmières auxiliaires (Registered Nursing Assistants ou RNA). Nous examinons les inquiétudes et les gratifications, ainsi que le stress, l'autonomie et le soutien social relatifs au travail rémunéré et au travail non-rémunéré, en cherchant à identifier les ressemblances et les variations en fonction du sexe et du type d'emploi (RN/RNA). Nous visons à constituer une banque de données sur le travail des infirmières-ers et leurs responsabilités familiales aux fins de recherches futures sur les effets sur la santé du travail rémunéré et non-rémunéré, sujet qui a reçu peu d'attention dans les analyses sur la santé au travail des femmes. Plusieurs thèmes communs sont apparus chez les deux groupes d'emploi lors de l'analyse. On exprime de l'inquiétude par rapport à la surcharge de travail, aux dangers présents dans le milieu, aux horaires rotatifs, au manque de soutien de la part des superviseurs; ces facteurs étant souvent considérés comme sources de stress. En revanche, elles-ils se réjouissent des gratifications que leur apportent le soin aux patients et la latitude décisionnelle inhérente à la profession. Elles-ils considèrent aussi leurs responsabilités familiales comme étant gratifiantes. L'analyse a aussi montré des différences marquées selon l'emploi et le sexe. Par exemple, les RNA rapportent en moins grand nombre avoir de l'autonomie. Un plus grand nombre d'entre elles estiment que leur emploi est un cul-de-sac et subissent du stress lors de leur proximité avec la mort et les mourants, ou avec les patients et leurs familles. Bien que les femmes RN disent plus souvent avoir de l'autonomie, elles ont aussi identifié des sources de stress: surcharge de travail, doute quant aux traitements prodigués, peur d'être blâmées en cas d'erreur. Quant aux hommes RN, ils ont décrit leur travail comme étant un cul-de-sac et ils ne semblaient pas trouver de support social dans leur milieu de travail. Ils sont plus souvent préoccupés par la discrimination sexuelle, raciale ou ethnique. Jusqu'ici, l'analyse a montré que les différences les plus importantes étaient relatives à la division sexuelle des tâches domestiques: les femmes investissent beaucoup plus de leur temps à ces tâches et, devant faire face à une varité de demandes domestiques, elles disposent par conséquent peu de temps pour elles-mêmes.

In this article we report on the first stage of the data analysis for a study of 2,285 nurses in Ontario. The sample includes women and men who are Registered Nurses (RNs) and women who are Registered Nursing Assistants (RNAs). We focus on nurses' concerns, rewards, stress, control and social support with respect to paid and unpaid work, identifying common themes and variations with respect to sex and job (RN/RNA). In documenting features of nursing work and home responsibilities, we establish a basis for future analyses of the effects on health of paid and unpaid work — an issue that has received relatively little attention in research on women's occupational health. Several themes were common to RNs and RNAs. Both expressed concerns about overload, exposure to hazards in the workplace, rotating shifts and lack of support from supervisors. These were often seen as a source of stress. On the other hand, nurses acknowledged the rewards of helping others and of decision authority. Generally, they also considered their home responsibilities to be rewarding. There were some pronounced differences between RNs and RNAs. For example, RNAs were less likely to experience control in their work, more likely to view their job as "dead-end," and more likely to report stress from dealing with death and dying and from caring for patients and their families. Women RNs experienced greater control at work than RNAs, but they identified stress in heavy workloads, uncertainty concerning treatments and the fear of being blamed for mistakes. Male RNs described their jobs as "dead-end," felt their work environment was not supportive and were more likely to express concerns about sex, race and ethnic discrimination. It was striking that home responsibilities were very traditionally gendered. Women spent significantly more time on domestic tasks, did not have enough time for themselves and faced problems in meeting diverse demands on their time.

INTRODUCTION

In the past decade or so, women's ongoing participation in the labour force has been acknowledged and their experiences explored in increasing detail (Lowe, 1989; Messing, 1991). More attention is being paid to the effects on women's health of both paid and unpaid work, and apparently contradictory findings (that paid labour is both "good" and "bad" for women's health) have spurred researchers to consider the complex links between the public and private spheres (Barnett et al., 1991; Frankenhauser and Chesney, 1991; Hall, 1992; Lowe, 1989; Messing, 1991; Tierney et al., 1990). We are now attuned to variations among occupations as well as differences in family structures. Yet this growing body of research is still in its infancy.

Few studies compare women and men in the workplace because segmented labour markets have generally segregated them in the labour force; even when women and men are in the same occupations, they may do different work. Moreover, gendered notions of appropriate roles appear to have shaped the research agendas of both traditional scholars and feminists. While men's occupations have been a focus of attention, women's experiences in particular occupations have less often been the subject of research. On the other hand, the problems for men of combining work and family responsibilities have been neglected. This means that we run the risk of developing a "job" based understanding of men and a "gender" based understanding of women (Lowe, 1989).

In this paper, we report preliminary findings from a study of the combined effects of paid and unpaid work on nurses' health. We compare women doing different types of work within nursing, and women and men employed in similar nursing roles. We also explore their domestic responsibilities, being alert to how these might be shaped by gender and by occupational roles. Despite our comments about the lack of attention to women's experiences in the workplace, in the literature on nursing there has been a general neglect of men and few attempts to compare male with female nurses (but see: Egeland and Brown, 1988; Gans, 1987; Villeneuve, 1994; Williams, 1989). Differences between RNs and RNAs have also received relatively little attention.[1]

Our approach has been influenced by the work of Karasek and Theorell (1990) while incorporating concerns raised by Barnett et al. (1991) and Hall (1992). Karasek and Theorell have emphasized the importance of decision latitude and social support, as well as work demands, in understanding stress and heart disease. Both decision latitude and social support may mitigate the effects of a high demand job. One critical reaction to this model is that it has tended to focus on the more traditional high-strain jobs in the manufacturing sector in which men are employed. It may be less applicable to the service sector where other types of rewards are available, and it may be less applicable to women (Barnett et al., 1991). Moreover, the data on which the Karasek and Theorell thesis is based do not include important concerns of women in the workplace, such as sexual discrimination and harassment. Neither do they situate their findings in the context of domestic responsibilities.

Our aim in this paper is to identify the ways in which sex and job are predictors of nurses' concerns, rewards, stress, control and social support with respect to paid and unpaid work.[2] As our discussion below will indicate, it was sex that was most closely associated with many aspects of unpaid work — the type of homemaking responsibilities of the respondents, the hours they spent on homemaking, the degree of control they experienced in their home life and their main concerns about their home responsibilities. In this sense, the data fit with other studies that have focussed on gendered roles within the family — roles which are shaped by notions of what is "appropriate" work for women and men (Michaelson, 1985; Tierney et al., 1990).

With paid work roles, it is the job that stands out as an important predictor of nurses' reactions to their work environment. Though there were many common themes across the different work roles, female RNs and RNAs differed in their work-related concerns, rewards, sense of control and sources of job-related stress. However, sex was also associated with variations in nurses' experiences of their work. While many responses were common to female and male RNs, there were significant differences that may reflect the gendered aspects of the work setting. The work that women and men do may vary, though women and men may also experience different rewards and concerns when they do the same work.[3]

THE SAMPLE

At our request, the Ontario College of Nurses generated a random sample of women RNs and RNAs who were registered in 1992 in three regions in Ontario: the Northwest, Eastern and Central West regions. Also, we asked for the names and addresses of all male nurses registered in the province.[4] A questionnaire was mailed to 5,205 nurses in January 1993 and this was followed by a reminder letter in March 1993. Phone calls and returned questionnaires identified 90 nurses who were not eligible because they had died, moved from the province, retired, left nursing for other work, or were unemployed. In all, a total of 2,288 usable questionnaires were returned. These were distributed as follows: 1,188 female RNs; 646 female RNAs; 451 male RNs; and 3 male RNAs. The overall response rate was 44.7 percent: 48 percent for women and 34.9 percent for men. The comparisons reported here are between women who work as RNs and women who work as RNAs, and between female and male RNs.

Our questionnaire had four sections: the first collected information on features of the respondents' paid work; the second focussed on the domestic sphere; the third section included measures of health and well-being; and the final section collected data on where respondents worked, their qualifications and other demographic information. Here, we report results from the first two sections. In developing the questionnaire, we relied on existing research instruments, modified slightly on the basis of nurses' comments in focus groups and their responses to a pilot questionnaire. Our measure of job-related concerns and rewards closely followed the index of Barnett et al. (1991). With respect to sources of occupational stress, we used the nursing stress scale of Gray-Toft and Anderson (1981), adding many items. A question about the amount of control nurses exercised in the work setting was modelled on the work of Hall (1992). In the case of unpaid work we relied on the work of Michaelson (1985) to identify the distribution of tasks.

THE RESULTS

In analyzing the data we started with an interest in sex and job as predictors of nurses' experiences in their paid and unpaid work roles and so we explored differences between the female RNs and RNAs and between female and male RNs. Such an emphasis on statistically significant differences can obscure important commonalities, so we also wanted to identify salient features of paid and unpaid work roles that were shared by nurses. The data are presented in Tables 1 to 10. We look first at the domestic sphere, highlighting sources of difference and shared themes. Following this, we present the data with respect to paid work experiences. Because of the large sample size, we emphasize findings that were significant at the .001 level but we also report the more liberal .05.

The Home

Table 1 presents the mean ratings with respect to nurses' homemaking activities. They were asked to rate their contribution to these activities in an average week, using a scale of one (representing none/almost none) to five (representing all/almost all). The mean ratings are shown in the first two columns for female RNs and RNAs. The third column shows the t test for significant differences between these means. The fourth column shows the means for male RNs and the final column gives the t test value for differences between the means for female and male RNs. Most striking is the similarity in the domestic responsibilities of women, whether they are RNs or RNAs, and the pronounced differences in the responsibilities of female and male RNs. Even in this relatively highly educated sample there was little evidence of a redefinition of traditional gendered roles within the home.

Table 1   Homemaking Activities by Occupation and Sex

Homemaking Activities	Women			Men	
	RN	RNA	t sig	RN	t sig
Meal preparation	4.06	4.17	.055	2.69	.000
Dish washing	3.63	3.78	.015	2.80	.000
Laundry	4.25	4.23	.692	2.49	.000
Ironing	3.89	4.03	.064	2.61	.000
Indoor cleaning	3.89	4.09	.001	2.61	.000
Grocery shopping	4.12	4.15	.654	2.95	.000
Outdoor jobs	2.39	2.43	.499	4.04	.000
Maintaining/repairs to car	1.84	1.81	.718	4.02	.000
House/apartment repairs and maintenance	1.97	1.91	.389	4.03	.000
Home improvement	2.45	2.36	.208	3.88	.000
Taking out garbage	2.50	2.62	.119	3.90	.000
Planning household budget	3.65	3.76	.118	3.24	.000
Paying bills, banking	3.73	3.71	.817	3.25	.000
Caring for children	3.76	3.89	.049	2.67	.000
Supervising school work	3.35	3.35	.934	2.33	.000
Caring for dependent adults	2.58	2.86	.050	2.22	.046

There were no significant differences in the amount of time devoted to homemaking activities between female RNs and RNAs, but female RNs reported significantly more hours than their male counterparts — a mean of 24.13 hours compared with 16.40 hours a week for men (p=.000).[5] When the respondents were asked how much free time they had after sleeping, working, doing chores around the house etc., there were less pronounced differences in their responses, perhaps because women were more likely to be employed in part-time work (among the RNs, 20 percent of women and 4 percent of men worked for 20 hours a week or less; p=.000). Female RNs estimated 16.09 free hours, female RNAs 15.57 hours and male RNs reported 18.18 hours a week (p=.003).

When we look at the concerns respondents experienced with respect to their home responsibilities, similar but less pronounced patterns emerge. They were asked to rate their concerns about home responsibilities, with a score of one representing "not at all a concern" and a score of four representing "an extreme concern." Table 2 presents the mean ratings. Among female RNs and RNAs, the latter reported a significantly greater degree of concern about the lack of challenge in their home responsibilities, not contributing enough to the family income, not being appreciated for all their work and having little control over the family budget. Their main shared concerns are workload issues: having to "divide themselves up in pieces and juggle things"; not having enough time for themselves; not having enough time for their families; and having to plan or restructure their time. Similar concerns were expressed by male RNs. However, female RNs expressed significantly greater concern than the men about having to divide themselves up, feeling a lack of appreciation for all the work they do, that they were too available to other people, that they didn't have enough time for themselves and that they disliked housework.

Table 2 Concerns About Home Responsibiities by Occupation and Sex

Home Responsibilities: Concerns	Women			Men	
	RN	RNA	t sig	RN	t sig
A lack of challenge	1.60	1.83	.000	1.54	.200
Not being able to set your own goals	1.61	1.69	.055	1.62	.820
Not enough free time for family	2.26	2.37	.016	2.30	.386
Not enough free time for yourself	2.37	2.43	.219	2.23	.008
Having to restructure or plan your time	2.24	2.26	.682	2.12	.019
Lack of appreciation of all the work you do	2.12	2.28	.002	1.73	.000
Having to divide yourself up in pieces and juggle things	2.56	2.54	.722	2.14	.000
Being too available to other people	1.92	1.98	.202	1.75	.001
Having little control over the family budget	1.39	1.51	.003	1.14	.490
Not contributing enough to the family income	1.38	1.57	.000	1.39	.883
Disliking housework	2.12	1.97	.002	1.84	.000

The women in the sample felt that they had a comparatively high degree of control over their home life — maybe because this is typically seen as women's primary sphere of responsibility. Table 3 shows mean rankings for four aspects of home life, where one represents "none/hardly any" and four "almost complete control." There were no significant differences between female RNs and RNAs, but compared with male RNs, the women experienced a greater degree of control over the use of household income, setting their own goals, the use of their own time and managing competing demands.

Table 3 Control Over Home Life by Occupation and Sex

Control Over Home Life	Women			Men	
	RN	RNA	t sig	RN	t sig
Use of household income	3.25	3.19	.108	3.04	.000
Use of your time	2.96	2.97	.782	2.78	.000
Setting your own goals	3.21	3.19	.759	3.03	.000
Managing competing demands	2.97	2.98	.819	2.86	.017

Table 4 presents data on the extent to which the respondents perceived their home responsibilities as rewarding, with a score of one indicating that home responsibilities are "not at all rewarding" and a score of four indicating that they are "extremely rewarding." The relative consistency of responses among RNs and RNAs, and men and women, is remarkable. Among the main shared rewards were: a sense of competence, of being good at what they do; having enough time and enough energy to enjoy their children/partner; and being able to pursue their own interests.

The section of the questionnaire that focussed on home responsibilities also posed a number of questions about social support. In particular, we asked about the respondents' relationships with their partners/spouses: "To what extent do you talk to him/her about things that worry you?" "To what extent do you feel you can talk to him/her quite easily?" "To what extent does he/she understand the demands of your work?" "How well do you and your partner get along in general?" (In each case, one represented the most negative response and five the most positive.)

The data are presented in Table 5. There were differences among the women respondents. RNAs appeared to have somewhat less supportive relationships, saying their partners were less likely to understand the demands of their work and giving a lower rating to how well they and

Table 4 Rewards of Home Responsibilities by Occupation and Sex

Home Responsibilities: Rewards	Women			Men	
	RN	RNA	t sig	RN	t sig
Being free to make your own schedule	2.95	2.93	.687	2.83	.014
Having enough time and enough energy to enjoy your children/partner	3.10	3.05	.271	3.07	.656
Doing creative things around the house	2.87	2.90	.583	2.81	.217
Having the amount of responsibility you can handle	2.99	2.92	.086	2.91	.107
Keeping the house looking nice and cared for	2.99	3.15	.000	2.98	.799
The appreciation you get from your family	2.97	2.99	.655	3.08	.030
A sense of competence, of being good at what you do	3.27	3.37	.010	3.35	.064
Being able to pursue your interests	3.04	3.00	.299	3.10	.234
Having other people enjoy your home	2.91	2.99	.060	2.88	.614
Being available to do things for others	2.89	3.06	.000	2.81	.102

Table 5 Aspects of Relationship with Partner/Spouse by Occupation and Sex

Partner/Spouse	Women			Men	
	RN	RNA	t sig	RN	t sig
To what extent do you talk to him/her about things that worry you?	3.89	3.80	.145	3.70	.004
To what extent do you feel you can talk to him/her quite easily?	3.96	3.84	.071	4.03	.302
To what extent does he/she understand the demands of your work?	3.46	3.32	.036	3.88	.000
How well do you and your partner/spouse get along in general?	4.23	4.12	.036	4.25	.759
To what extent do you wish you could confide in him/her?	4.29	4.36	.155	4.33	.449

their partner got along together. Comparing female and male RNs, we see that the women were significantly more likely to say that they could talk to their partner about things that worried them, while the men reported a significantly greater degree of understanding of the demands of their work on the part of their partner. Generally, respondents saw their relationships as supportive — most of the means were close to or above 3.80.

Paid Work

Table 6 shows the mean ratings for nurses' concerns with respect to their current job. The respondents were asked: "In thinking about your current job, to what extent, if any, is each of the following a concern?" (a score of one represented "not at all a concern" and a score of four indicated "an extreme concern"). The scores of the RNAs were generally higher than those of the female RNs and they expressed significantly higher levels of concern about being in a dead-end job and being exposed to hazards in their work. Female RNs were more concerned about sexual discrimination or harassment.

Several of these dimensions of work experience were a concern for male RNs too, though the men were significantly more likely to express concerns about being in a dead-end job and to say that the job did not meet their expectations. They were more bothered by sex discrimination and harassment, as well as discrimination because of race or ethnicity. They also expressed greater concern about poor supervision and about workload.

To focus only on sex and job differences would ignore important common themes in nurses' responses. Indeed, if we look at the aspects of work which were of greatest concern there was a remarkable degree of

Table 6 Job-related Concerns by Occupation and Sex

Concerns	Women			Men	
	RN	RNA	t sig	RN	t sig
Overload					
Having too much to do	2.39	2.32	.152	2.35	.469
The job's taking too much out of you	2.17	2.22	.305	2.28	.041
Having to deal with emotionally difficult situations	2.27	2.18	.027	2.42	.002

Concerns	Women			Men	
	RN	RNA	t sig	RN	t sig
Conflict with Physicians					
Having to do things on your job that are against your better nursing judgement	1.75	1.75	.988	1.88	.014
The pace of work being too fast	1.94	2.04	.045	1.82	.025
Not meeting the standards for professional practice	1.48	1.54	.177	1.59	.014
Dead-end Job					
Having little chance for advancement	2.07	2.55	.000	2.30	.000
The job's not using your skills	1.54	2.23	.000	1.77	.000
The job's monotony, lack of variety	1.32	1.78	.000	1.52	.000
Limited opportunity for professional or career development	1.99	2.40	.000	2.20	.000
The job not meeting your expectations	1.53	1.72	.000	1.72	.000
Hazard Exposure					
Being exposed to illness or injury	2.12	2.36	.000	2.26	.015
The physical conditions of your job — noise, crowding, temperature, etc.	2.00	2.19	.000	2.02	.719
The job being physically strenuous	1.96	2.58	.000	1.87	.078
Adjusting to changing shifts	2.33	2.17	.013	2.40	.296
Poor Supervision					
Lack of support from your supervisor for what you need to do your job	2.07	2.11	.411	2.30	.000
Your supervisors' lack of competence	1.68	1.62	.298	1.93	.000
Your supervisors' lack of appreciation of your work	1.83	1.86	.492	2.04	.000
Your supervisor having unrealistic expectations of your work	1.81	1.89	.126	1.94	.020
Discrimination					
Facing discrimination or harassment because of your sex	1.27	1.16	.001	1.63	.000
Facing discrimination or harassment because of your race or ethnic background	1.12	1.11	.814	1.32	.000

similarity. Issues regarding overload were important. Both RNs and RNAs and men and women voiced strong concerns about having too much to do, the job taking too much out of them, and having to deal with emotionally difficult situations. They were bothered by their exposure to hazards, in particular, by the physical conditions of the job, by being exposed to illness and injury, and by the problems associated with changing shifts. They also expressed concern about the lack of support they felt they received from their supervisor(s) for what they needed to do their jobs.

Another way of looking at nurses' concerns is to explore job-related stress. With respect to each of 59 possible sources of stress they were asked: "For each situation you have encountered in your present work setting, would you indicate how stressful it has been for you?" (A score of one indicated "never stressful" and a score of four indicated that the situation was "extremely stressful.") Table 7 shows the mean ratings nurses assigned to these potentially stressful aspects of their work. While the magnitude of the stress differed at times, all nurses emphasized the stress associated with two broad aspects of their jobs: workload problems and dealing with death and dying. They also experienced stress as a result of having to deal with violent patients.

There were also many significant differences between female RNs and RNAs. The aspects of work which the RNs experienced as more stressful centred around conflicts with physicians, uncertainty concerning appropriate treatments, being blamed for things that go wrong and some of the

Table 7   Sources of Job-related Stress by Occupation and Sex

Sources of Job-related Stress	Women			Men	
	RN	RNA	t sig	RN	t sig
Death and Dying					
Performing procedures that patients experience as painful	2.38	2.43	.184	2.29	.024
Feeling helpless in the case of a patient who fails to improve	2.41	2.32	.026	2.22	.000
Listening or talking to a patient about his/her approaching death	2.24	2.20	.343	2.08	.001
The death of a patient	2.46	2.37	.035	2.25	.000
The death of a patient with whom you developed a close relationship	2.62	2.69	.166	2.36	.000
Physician(s) not being present when a patient dies	1.93	1.72	.000	1.76	.002
Watching a patient suffer	2.78	2.92	.001	2.64	.006

Sources of Job-related Stress	Women			Men	
	RN	RNA	t sig	RN	t sig
Conflict with Physicians					
Criticism by a physician	2.54	2.34	.000	2.39	.003
Conflict with a physician	2.35	2.08	.000	2.28	.158
Disagreement concerning the treatment of a patient	2.26	2.10	.000	2.18	.052
Making a decision concerning a patient when the physician is unavailable	2.30	2.09	.000	2.17	.006
Having to organize doctors' work	2.23	2.03	.005	2.15	.139
Inadequate Preparation: Emotional					
Feeling inadequately prepared to help with the emotional needs of a patient's family	2.08	2.08	.998	2.25	.077
Being asked a question by a patient for which you do not have a satisfactory answer	2.01	2.06	.136	.189	.002
Feeling inadequately prepared to help with the emotional needs of a patient	2.33	2.32	.765	2.00	.030
Inadequate Preparation: Practical					
Feeling inadequately trained for what you have to do	1.83	1.70	.002	1.80	.607
Being in charge with inadequate experience	2.10	1.97	.124	1.98	.080
Lack Of Support: Peers					
Lack of opportunity to talk openly with other personnel about problems in the work setting	2.23	2.30	.134	2.22	.806
Lack of opportunity to share experiences and feelings with other personnel in the work setting	1.95	1.88	.111	1.88	.123
Lack of an opportunity to express negative feelings towards patients to other personnel on the unit	1.64	1.68	.287	1.64	.996
Difficulty in working with a particular nurse (or nurses) outside immediate work setting	1.85	1.82	.525	1.86	.825
Difficulty in working with a particular nurse (or nurses)	2.30	2.41	.016	2.32	.713
Difficulty in working with nurses of the opposite sex	1.15	1.16	.844	1.37	.000

Sources of Job-related Stress	Women			Men	
	RN	RNA	t sig	RN	t sig
Lack of Support: Supervisors					
Lack of support by immediate supervisor	2.16	2.01	.007	2.24	.160
Lack of support by nursing administrators	2.41	2.48	.288	2.60	.002
Lack of support by other health care administrators	2.25	2.21	.469	2.43	.001
Conflict with a supervisor	2.30	2.22	.119	2.36	.307
Criticism by a supervisor	2.09	1.96	.005	2.09	.994
Criticism by nursing administration	2.24	2.26	.822	2.35	.069
Being held responsible for things over which you have no control	2.53	2.45	.156	2.62	.099
Work Load					
Unpredictable staffing and scheduling	2.65	2.67	.777	2.67	.759
Too many non-nursing tasks required, such as clerical work	2.63	2.53	.038	2.64	.904
Not enough time to provide emotional support to the patient	2.49	2.68	.000	2.29	.000
Not enough time to complete all of your nursing tasks	2.53	2.60	.190	2.31	.000
Not enough time to adequately cover the unit	2.72	2.81	.057	2.73	.830
Not enough time to respond to the needs of patients' families	2.37	2.41	.275	2.27	.027
Demands of Patient Classification System	2.16	2.05	.054	2.06	.093
Having to work through breaks	2.34	2.18	.001	2.23	.039
Having to make decisions under pressure	2.28	2.11	.000	2.20	.064
Uncertainty Concerning Treatment					
Inadequate information from a physician regarding the medical condition of a patient	2.50	2.31	.000	2.40	.036
A physician ordering what appears to be inappropriate treatment for a patient	2.44	2.36	.094	2.36	.125
A physician not being present in a medical emergency	2.60	2.35	.000	2.46	.018

Sources of Job-related Stress	Women			Men	
	RN	RNA	t sig	RN	t sig
Not knowing what a patient or a patient's family ought to be told about the patient's condition and its treatment	2.14	2.19	.212	2.05	.060
Fear of making a mistake in treating a patient	2.22	2.07	.000	2.20	.659
Being exposed to health and safety hazards	2.43	2.52	.098	2.50	.260
Uncertainty regarding the operation and functioning of specialized equipment	2.15	1.90	.000	2.05	.052
Patients and their Families					
Patients making unreasonable demands	2.57	2.78	.000	2.61	.494
Patients' families making unreasonable demands	2.54	2.75	.000	2.54	.912
Being blamed for anything that goes wrong	2.43	2.18	.000	2.40	.599
Being the one that has to deal with patients' families	2.21	2.24	.475	2.14	.095
Having to deal with violent patients	2.74	2.98	.000	2.75	.969
Having to deal with abusive patients	2.56	2.91	.000	2.64	.156
Having to deal with abuse from patients 'families	2.39	2.54	.002	2.37	.681
Not knowing whether patients' families will report you for inadequate care	1.73	1.80	.140	1.81	.147
Sex Discrimination					
Being sexually harassed	1.74	1.85	.172	1.60	.067
Experiencing discrimination on the basis of sex	1.62	1.44	.009	1.87	.000
Other Problems					
Experiencing discrimination because of race or ethnicity	1.51	1.43	.301	1.70	.011
Floating to other units/services that are short-staffed	2.79	2.48	.000	2.64	.048
Breakdown of computer	1.93	1.81	.128	1.85	.172

workload issues. On the other hand, RNAs focussed on issues concerning patients — having to watch a patient suffer, not having enough time to provide emotional support to patients, or having to deal with several different types of problems with patients and their families. When asked how often the different types of stressful situations occurred, as Table 8 indicates, RNAs were significantly more likely to say they had to deal with death and dying, and it was the problem they were most likely to encounter. Though they were not among the most frequently experienced problems, female RNs were more likely to report stress associated with conflicts with physicians, being accountable but not having control, uncertainty concerning treatment and sexual discrimination.

There were also sex differences in sources of work-related stress. As can be seen in Table 7, male RNs were more likely to focus on problems associated with social support: the lack of support of nursing and other health care administrators; experiencing discrimination on the basis of sex; and finding it difficult to work with women nurses. In contrast, female RNs were more likely to emphasize the stress arising from dealing with death and dying and issues linked with heavy workloads — for example, not having enough time to provide emotional support to patients and not having enough time to complete all their nursing tasks. When asked how often the various sources of stress occurred in their work setting, Table 8 shows that male RNs reported significantly more experience of the various aspects of lack of support (conflict with physicians and with nurses, and lack of support), being accountable without having control, sexual discrimination and sexual harassment.

In Table 9 we show mean scores for the rewards that nurses derived from their work. They were asked: "In thinking about your current job, to what extent, if any, do you find each of the following rewarding?" (One represented "not at all rewarding" and four represented "extremely rewarding.") For RNs and RNAs, men and women, the most rewarding feature of work was being able to help others. The various aspects of helping others, as well as aspects of decision authority, received the highest mean scores in all three groups. There were also some pronounced job and sex differences. Female RNs were more likely to emphasize the rewards of challenging work and of relatively good incomes, while the RNAs were more likely to stress the importance of being needed by others and of liking their immediate supervisor(s). Comparing women and male RNs, we see that the women were significantly more likely to find rewards in collegial support, the priority being given to patient care and the challenges they experienced in their work.

We also asked the respondents about the degree of control they felt they exercised over various aspects of their work. The mean scores are shown in Table 10. (One represented "hardly any," while four indicated

Table 8   Frequency of Types of Work Stressors by Occupation and Sex

Present Work Environment	Women			Men	
	RN	RNA	t sig	RN	t sig
Death and dying	2.38	2.65	.000	2.29	.103
Conflict with physicians	1.89	1.49	.000	2.02	.003
Lack of support	1.95	1.88	.097	2.20	.000
Conflict with other nurses	1.66	1.70	.235	1.83	.000
Problems with patients and their families	2.07	2.10	.501	2.15	.111
Problems with workload	2.43	2.44	.854	2.37	.244
Feeling inadequately prepared	1.62	1.54	.024	1.62	.898
Uncertainty concerning treatment	1.71	1.54	.000	1.83	.003
Accountability without control	1.88	1.59	.000	2.08	.000
Health and safety hazards	1.89	1.83	.147	1.95	.288
Sexual harassment	1.20	1.28	.044	1.29	.030
Ethnic or racial discrimination	1.23	1.26	.579	1.31	.088
Sexual discrimination	1.27	1.15	.003	1.58	.000

Table 9   Job-related Rewards by Occupation and Sex

Rewards	Women			Men	
	RN	RNA	t sig	RN	t sig
Helping others at work					
Helping others	3.40	3.50	.002	3.32	.048
Being needed by others	2.96	3.20	.000	2.84	.009
Having an impact on other people's lives	3.13	3.19	.129	3.05	.061
Decision authority					
Being able to make decisions on your own	3.25	3.12	.002	3.12	.329
Being able to work on your own	3.28	3.23	.301	3.22	.224
Having the authority you need to get your job done without having to go to someone else for permission	3.09	3.07	.791	3.11	.691

Rewards	Women			Men	
	RN	RNA	t sig	RN	t sig
The freedom to decide how you do your work	3.12	3.15	.573	3.10	.646
Challenge					
Challenging or stimulating work	3.15	2.88	.000	3.06	.046
Having a variety of tasks	3.07	2.88	.000	2.97	.021
The sense of accomplishment and competence you get from your job	3.18	3.18	.950	3.03	.001
The job's fitting your interest and skills	3.07	2.82	.000	2.92	.002
The opportunity for learning new things	2.95	2.80	.001	2.85	.039
Supervisor support					
Your immediate supervisor's respect for your abilities	2.70	2.78	.096	2.65	.387
Your supervisors' concern about the welfare of those under them	2.47	2.56	.061	2.41	.338
Your supervisors' encouragement of your professional development	2.44	2.53	.125	2.39	.412
Liking your immediate supervisor(s)	2.59	2.78	.000	2.45	.010
Recognition					
The recognition you get	2.49	2.51	.723	2.50	.869
The appreciation you get	2.57	2.67	.048	2.51	.253
Satisfaction with Salary					
The income	2.60	2.33	.000	2.55	.250
Making good money compared to other people in your field	2.24	2.08	.001	2.32	.162
Collegial Support					
Becoming assertive as nurses	2.66	2.62	.279	2.54	.013
Nurses standing by each other	2.72	2.78	.172	2.46	.000
People you work with are significant in your life	2.48	2.50	.636	2.30	.000
The competence of other nurses	2.84	2.89	.164	2.71	.009
Other					
The image your profession has	2.35	2.45	.020	2.24	.038
The priority given to patient care	2.97	3.08	.013	2.80	.001

"almost complete" control.) There was barely any variation between the female and male RNs. The most obvious differences were between female RNs and RNAs, with the former being significantly more likely to experience control in almost all dimensions of their work.

Table 10 Control Over Aspects of Work by Occupation and Sex

Amount of Control	Women			Men	
	RN	RNA	t sig	RN	t sig
Influence over the planning of work	2.60	2.31	.000	2.66	.255
Influence over the setting of the pace of work	2.22	2.21	.811	2.31	.133
Influence over how time is used in work	2.49	2.35	.004	2.55	.329
Influence over the planning of work breaks	2.40	1.93	.000	2.51	.068
Influence over the planning of vacations	2.66	2.33	.000	2.65	.929
Flexible working hours	2.14	1.87	.000	1.90	.000
Freedom to receive a phone call during working hours	2.94	2.52	.000	3.00	.258
Freedom to receive a private visitor at work	2.45	2.18	.000	2.41	.495
Varied task content	2.38	1.92	.000	2.42	.416
Varied work procedures	2.30	1.88	.000	2.32	.730
Possibilities for on-going education as part of the job	2.03	1.92	.019	2.02	.931
Influence over the selection of supervisor(s)	1.16	1.06	.003	1.18	.552
Influence over the selection of co-worker(s)	1.37	1.24	.004	1.48	.003

There were no sex or job differences in the level of job satisfaction reported by respondents, or in how stressful they considered their lives to be. In general, they reported high levels of job satisfaction: on a four point scale, 3.71 for female RNs, 3.63 for RNAs and 3.61 for the men. However, a small minority expected they would make job-related changes in the near future or else were undecided about whether they would do so. Both RNAs (23 percent "yes" and 25 percent "undecided"; p=.000) and male RNs (25 percent "yes" and 21 percent "undecided"; p=.000) were significantly more likely than female RNs to be thinking of going back to school. The men were thinking of changing their job in nursing (18 percent "yes" and 21 percent "undecided"; p=.002) and leaving nursing (9 percent "yes" and 18 percent "undecided"; p=.004). Female RNs were more likely than the men to be considering changing the number of hours they worked (15 percent "yes" and 15 percent "undecided"; p=.000) and stopping work (5 percent "yes" and 10 percent "undecided"; p=.003). Perhaps this was because of the greater total number of hours worked by the women.

DISCUSSION

Our primary aim in this first stage of the research was to explore ways in which occupational roles and sex are associated with concerns, rewards, control and sources of stress in both paid and unpaid work. The results suggest that sex is particularly important in the domestic sphere. Both sex and occupational roles were associated with respondents' experiences in their paid work. These sex differences may be interpreted in various ways. They may be a result of biology, though feminists have shied away from such explanations because of the ways in which they have been used against women (Fausto-Sterling, 1985). They may also stem from patterns of socialization, societal definitions of appropriate roles for women and men, structured constraints on the choices women and men can make and the associated discrimination against women. All these are likely to interact with each other. Though research into such relationships is still in its infancy, we emphasize the importance of gender in the sense of structurally and culturally determined ideas of appropriate roles for women and men and the related constraints on their paid and unpaid work roles.

Roles within the home continue to be shaped by gender. It is remarkable that even in this relatively highly educated sample, domestic roles are so clearly gendered. Women continue to perform the tasks traditionally assigned to them — those associated with daily reproduction which have a distinct pattern of regular demands on their time. In contrast, men assume responsibility for maintenance work, which, with the exception of emergencies, will have more flexible timing. The greater and more structured workload of women is externally generated, responding to the needs of others, and so it is understandable that the women were more likely to feel that they had to "divide themselves up in pieces and juggle things." They felt that they were too available to other people and not appreciated enough — a theme echoed in the literature on women's invisible work and the lack of recognition that is accorded to women's multifaceted caring roles (Armstrong and Armstrong, 1984; Charles and Kerr, 1988; Daniels, 1987; DeVault, 1991; Luxton and Rosenberg, 1986).

With respect to their paid work roles, some issues stand out as common to all nurses. Foremost among these is the problem of workload, a problem that has undoubtedly become more intense as nursing has been rationalized and public sector cutbacks have affected the health care sector and hospitals in particular (Armstrong et al., 1994; Campbell, 1987; Walters and Haines, 1989). The concerns nurses voiced about the lack of support from their supervisors may also be linked to the implementation of cost saving measures — and the tensions being experienced in this, the most immediate authority relation. At the same time, the work of nurses is physically and emotionally demanding and shiftwork compounds these demands. In more positive terms, nurses shared the rewards of an occupation that has traditionally been defined in terms of its caring role; helping others stood out as a major reward. The importance of the decision-making authority they enjoyed was another shared rewarding element.

The most marked differences between female RNs and RNAs were occupational. RNAs are more likely than RNs to be involved in providing direct patient care and they are closest to what still appear to be definitions of "real" nursing. The increased rationalization of nursing care has led to a decrease in the emphasis on the basic care aspects of the work of RNs and created a space for the development of the RNA position (Campbell 1994; 1987; Coburn, 1988). RNAs are most likely to be exposed to the hazards of direct patient care — lifting, illness and injury, violence from patients and sexual harassment. It is understandable that they were more likely to emphasize patient care as a source of stress as well as a source of important rewards. They were also more likely to be worried about not being able to provide enough emotional support to patients. In their subordinate position, they are less likely to experience control over their work, and with lower educational qualifications and lower incomes, they are more likely to see the job as a "dead end."

In contrast, RNs have achieved greater independence from medicine and attained a greater degree of professional autonomy (Coburn, 1988). Yet medical dominance remains strong and nurses are still subject to medical authority as well as being subordinate within the administrative hierarchy of the hospital. Nursing has experienced the apparently contradictory processes of professionalization and proletarianization (Coburn, 1988; Carroll and Warburton, 1989) and such contradictions find expression in the responses of the RNs in this study. They reported a relatively high degree of control in their work setting yet they experienced stress as a result of conflicts with doctors and expressed concerns about accountability and uncertainty. This juxtaposition of a subordinate status and control/responsibility is a potentially stressful mixture. In more positive terms, their work presents them with challenges and tangible financial rewards. In these respects the rewards, concerns and sources of stress experienced by nurses are shaped by their occupational roles.

There were also some striking differences between female and male RNs, illustrating some of the influences of gender in the workplace. Some of the more characteristic elements of women's work in caring appear to be central features of women's experiences in the workplace. Female RNs were more likely to experience stress in connection with the death of patients, and were concerned about not being able to provide sufficient emotional support to patients. They also emphasized the priority given to patient care. A general concern with the nature of relationships in their workplace was also evident in the rewards that women derived from other nurses — whether through helping others or the rewards of support from their peers. It may be that these various aspects of nursing are more important to women or else that women are more likely to be doing such caring work.

In one of the few studies which compares women and men in nontraditional occupations, Williams (1989) has noted that male nurses are often characterized as being stronger, more aggressive, more demanding and career minded. Some of these features emerged in men's responses in our study. The issues which were of greatest concern to the men centred around career paths and discrimination. They saw nursing as a dead-end job; it had not met their expectations. While the female RNs were more likely to be thinking of stopping work or changing their hours, the men were more often thinking of leaving the profession or changing their job in nursing. In part, this may reflect the dissatisfaction of men working in a female profession; men may attribute the problems of nursing to its domination by women (Williams, 1989:129). They were also more likely to feel that they were subject to discrimination. They experienced difficulties in working with female nurses, were concerned about poor supervision and experienced stress as a result of lack of support from nursing and health care administrators. Williams (1989:118) reports that male nurses tend to separate themselves from informal networks, distancing themselves from women, and they are especially alert to the potential for discrimination, even though there was little evidence in her study that it occurred. In our sample, it is interesting that such concerns were voiced despite the fact that the men were more likely to be in management positions (29 percent of male vs. 19 percent of female RNs; $p=.000$). Gender may shape their expectations and their perceptions of discrimination. Their responses may also have been influenced by race, because they were significantly more likely to identify themselves as a member of an ethnic or racial minority (28 percent of male vs. 18 percent of female RNs; p=.000). At this point it is impossible to disentangle the effects of gender and race and ethnicity.

Finally, it is important to highlight other patterns in the data. With respect to both their job and home responsibilities, respondents expressed relatively low levels of concern, while the rewards they experienced were comparatively high. As Barnett et al. (1991) have suggested, the reward of helping others is important and this, together with elements of decision-making authority and control, may help to counteract some of the more demanding aspects of nurses' paid and unpaid work roles. Social support may also be important — the more extensive support networks of women may mediate the demands of work and home. For men, the experience of discrimination may have important effects. For female and male RNs, conflicts with physicians may compound the impact of other demands in the workplace. Our next step is to trace the associations between these many facets of respondents' lives, in order to explore in more detail what influences their levels of health and well being. In so doing, we hope to achieve a fuller understanding of the complex links between gender and paid and unpaid work which are implied in this present analysis.

ACKNOWLEDGEMENTS

The research reported here was funded by grants from the Social Sciences and Humanities Research Council and the Quality of Nursing Worklife Programme of McMaster University and University of Toronto. We thank Janet Mayr and Paul Roberts for their help with the computer analysis, and Rhonda Lenton for her comments on the analysis.

NOTES

1. A Registered Nurse (RN) is a graduate of a three-year programme in nursing at a College of Applied Arts and Technology or a four year undergraduate programme in nursing at a university, and has completed successfully the registration examinations administered by the regulating body. The RN is a member of a self-regulating group whose members are recognized by legislation as being independent practitioners who are accountable for their actions. RNs work in a variety of settings. A Registered Nursing Assistant (RNA), now referred to as a Registered Practical Nurse, is a graduate of an eight- to twelve-month practical training programme provided through a vocational training stream in a High School or at a Community College,

and who has completed successfully the registration examinations administered by the regulating body. RNAs work primarily in institutional settings. In Ontario, The College of Nurses of Ontario has responsibility for regulating RNs and RNAs.

2. This paper is largely descriptive. This is a first step in the analysis of our data and, while it is important to present findings in this form, it is also problematic. Bivariate analysis raises more questions than it can answer and it is important to resist "overinterpretation" of the data. In our subsequent work, we are using multivariate analyses to explore the labour market experiences of men and women RNs, as well as the links between paid and unpaid work and nurses' health and well-being.

3. As Egeland and Brown (1988) have noted, there are "islands of masculinity" in nursing. Male RNs in our study were more likely than female RNs to be working in a psychiatric hospital (24 percent vs. 3 percent; p=.000) while women RNs were more likely to be employed in a general hospital (60 percent vs. 49 percent; p=.000). This means that the differences between women and men reported in this analysis may be more job related than might appear.

4. Initially, we requested a sample of 5,200 female nurses distributed proportionally across the regions, plus all male nurses registered in Ontario. We received a total of 6,650 names and addresses. Unfortunately, our funding would not stretch to a survey of this size and so we excluded every fourth female RN and RNA and every tenth male. This yielded a sample of 5,205 nurses: 2,400 female RNs, 1,500 female RNAs and 1,305 men.

5. These differences may be in part a result of differences in family structure and responsibilities. Female RNs were significantly more likely to have children 13 years and over and to be caring for a dependent adult. There were no significant differences in whether or not they had a partner and in whether they had children under 13 years of age.

REFERENCES

Armstrong, P., J. Choiniere, G. Feldberg and J. White. *Voices From The Ward*. Occasional Paper. North York, Ontario: York University Centre for Health Studies, 1994.

Armstrong, P., and H. Armstrong. *The Double Ghetto: Canadian Women and Their Segregated Work*, Revised Edition. Toronto: McClelland & Stewart, 1984.

Barnett, R.C., H. Davidson and N.L. Marshall. "Physical Symptoms and the Interplay of Work and Family Roles." *Health Psychology* 10, 2 (1991). pp. 94-101.

Campbell, M. "The Structure of Stress in Nurses' Work," in *Health, Illness and Health Care in Canada*, Second Edition. B. Singh Bolaria and H. Dickinson (eds.). Toronto: Harcourt Brace, 1994.

Campbell, M.L. "Productivity in Canadian Nursing: Administering Cuts," in *Health and Canadian Society: Sociological Perspectives*. D. Coburn, C. D'Arcy, G. Torrance and P. New (eds.). Toronto: Fitzhenry & Whiteside, 1987.

Carroll, W.K., and R. Warburton. "Feminism, Class Consciousness and Household-work Linkages Among Registered Nurses in Victoria." *Labour/Le Travail* 24 (1989). pp. 131-45.

Charles, N., and M. Kerr. *Women, Food and Families*. Manchester: Manchester University Press, 1988.

Coburn, D. "State Authority, Medical Dominance, and Trends in the Regulation of the Health Professions: The Ontario Case." *Social Science and Medicine* 37, 2 (1993). pp. 129-38.

— "The Development of Canadian Nursing: Professionalization and Proletarianization." *International Journal of Health Services* 18 (1988). pp. 437-56.

Daniels, A.K. "Invisible Work." *Social Problems* 34 (1987). pp. 403-15.

DeVault, M.L. *Feeding the Family: The Social Organization of Caring as Gendered Work*. Chicago: University of Chicago Press, 1991.

Egeland, J.W., and J.S. Brown. "Sex Role Stereotyping and Role Strain of Male Registered Nurses." *Research in Nursing and Health* 11 (1988). pp. 257-67.

Fausto-Sterling, A. *Myths of Gender: Biological Theories About Women and Men*. New York: Basic Books, 1985.

Frankenhauser, M., U. Lundberg and M. Chesney. *Women, Work and Health: Stress and Opportunities*. New York: Plenum Press, 1991.

Gans, J.E. "Men's Career Advantages in Nursing: The Principle of the Peter." *Current Research on Occupations and Professions* 4 (1987). pp. 181-98.

Gray-Toft, P., and J.G. Anderson. "The Nursing Stress Scale: Development of an Instrument." *Journal of Behavioural Assessment* 3, 1 (1981). pp. 11-23.

Hall, E.M. "Double Exposure: The Combined Impact of the Home and Work Environments on Psychosomatic Strain in Swedish Women and Men." *International Journal of Health Services* 22, 2 (1992). pp. 239-60.

Karasek, R., and T. Theorell. *Healthy Work: Stress, Productivity, and the Reconstruction of Working Life*. New York: Basic Books, 1990.

Lowe, G.S. *Women, Paid/Unpaid Work, and Stress*. Ottawa: Canadian Advisory Council on the Status of Women, 1989.

Luxton, M., and H.G. Rosenberg. *Through the Kitchen Window: The Politics of Home and Family*. Toronto: Garamond, 1986.

Messing, K. *Occupational Safety and Health Concerns of Canadian Women*. Ottawa: Labour Canada, 1991.

Michaelson, W. *From Sun to Sun: Daily Obligations and Community Structure in the Lives of Employed Women and their Families*. Totowa, New Jersey: Rowman and Allanheld, 1985.

Tierney, D., P. Romito and K. Messing. "She Ate Not the Bread of Idleness: Exhaustion is Related to Domestic and Salaried Working Conditions Among 539 Hospital Workers." *Women and Health* 16, 1 (1990). pp. 21-42.

Villeneuve, M.J. "Recruiting and Retaining Men in Nursing: A Review of the Literature." *Journal of Professional Nursing* 10, 4 (1994). pp. 217-28.

Walters, V., and T. Haines. "Workload and Occupational Stress in Nursing." *The Canadian Journal of Nursing Research* 21, 3 (1989). pp. 49-58.

Williams, C.L. *Gender Differences at Work: Women and Men in Nontraditional Occupations*. Berkeley: University of California Press, 1989.

D. Lynn Skillen

Nurses' Work Hazards
in Public Health Units

En 1992, une recherche a été effectuée à partir d'une problématique des dangers du travail comme relevant de l'organisation plutôt que des individus. Les sujets de cette recherche étaient des travailleuses professionnelles de la santé issues d'organisations à prédominance féminine. Cinquante-sept infirmières professionnelles (cadre et non-cadre) de cinq organismes de santé publique de l'Alberta ont participé à cette étude. Des questionnaires auto-administrés, des entrevues semi-dirigées et des groupes de discussion avec modérateur ont servi à documenter les perceptions des employées relativement aux dangers (à la santé et la sécurité) présents dans leur travail, ainsi qu'aux facteurs organisationnels qui leur sont associés. La collecte et l'analyse des données furent menées de façon simultanée, selon la démarche de la théorie ancrée de Glaser & Strauss (1967). Les infirmières en santé publique nous ont décrit des dangers à la santé et la sécurité de type biologique, ergonomique, physiques et psychosociaux. L'analyse indique que les facteurs organisationnels sont inséparables des dangers du travail que les sujets ont relevés dans leur environnement physique et psychosocial. Quatre éléments pour une théorie de la surveillance environnementale du milieu ont émergé des données: les conditions propices à la collégialité, l'inspection des lieux, les structures organisationnelles de surveillance des dangers, et le transfert d'informations concernant les dangers. L'auteure met l'accent sur les conditions de collégialité, conditions particulièrement importantes pour les travailleuses d'organisations à prédominance féminine. L'étude a permis aux professionnelles d'un secteur socio-économique, jusque-là négligé, de faire une évaluation des risques environnementaux pour leur santé et leur sécurité, tout en mettant en relief les relations complexes entre organisation et facteurs sociaux affectant la sécurité au travail des femmes dans le secteur des services.

Reconceptualization of work hazards as a problem of the organization rather than of the individual guided an exploratory study, completed in 1992, on female health care workers employed in a predominantly female organization. Fifty-seven staff and managerial public health nurses in five autonomous public health units across the province of Alberta participated in the study. Self-administered questionnaires, semi-structured interviews and moderated focus groups were used to document employee perceptions of their work hazards and the organizational factors associated with them. Data collection and analysis proceeded simultaneously using the constant comparative method of grounded theory (Glaser and Strauss, 1967). Public health nurses described safety, psychosocial, biological, ergonomic and physical hazards. Results indicate that organizational factors are inseparable from the hazards respondents perceived in their physical and psychosocial work environments. Four elements that influence organizational hazard surveillance emerged from the data: conditions for collegiality; control over the physical plant; the structures for surveillance; and hazard information transfer. The conditions for collegiality have particular relevance for women workers in a predominantly female organization and are presented here. The research assisted women in a neglected sector of the workforce — public health professionals — to assess their work environments for hazards to their health and safety. It illuminated the complex relationship between organizational and systemic social factors and the work hazards of women in a human service organization.

I have the right to be as healthy leaving as I am coming. I have a right to a healthy environment.

— (Public Health Nurse, 1991).

Nurses as workers have the right to expect their work environment to be safe and the people to whom nurses provide care have the right to expect that nurses take into consideration the possible causal relationship of their jobs to their health problem.

— (Brown, 1981:172).

INTRODUCTION

Organizations have a moral and ethical responsibility to minimize work hazards (Krause, 1977; Sass, 1986; 1989), a social responsibility to promote health and safety (Shaw, 1990), and a legislated responsibility to control identified work hazards (Province of Alberta Occupational Health and Safety Act, 1980). Healthy environments are a mechanism for promoting individual and collective health (Epp, 1986; Health and Welfare Canada, 1990; Perkins, 1991; Premier's Commission on Future Health Care for Albertans, 1989; World Health Organization, Health and Welfare Canada and Canadian Public Health Association, 1986). At provincial, federal and international levels, normative documents recognize the salience of physical, social, economic, political and spiritual environments for the promotion of health at work and leisure. These documents state explicitly that institutions responsible for health care must assume a significant role in health promotion for their *employees* as well as for the public, an emphasis not apparent in the past. Furthermore, all levels are expected to be involved in the promotion of health within a health care facility, from governing boards and senior management to staff. It is incumbent upon senior management to conduct assessments of organizational strengths and weaknesses and seek input from staff in order to achieve environments supportive to health and well-being (Health and Welfare Canada, 1990). Federal guidelines for health promotion state clearly that *staff* of health care facilities are to be enabled to influence their physical environment both inside and outside the facility (Health and Welfare Canada, 1990).

Research on a predominantly female health care organization, the public health unit, encouraged staff and managers to consider their work hazards (Skillen, 1992). This research incorporated a liberal feminist approach which focusses on women's equal access to opportunities available to men in society (McLaren, 1988; Saunders, 1982). It addressed three neglected areas in occupational health: occupational hazards of health care workers (HCWs), organizational factors associated with exposure to work hazards, and occupational hazard surveillance for women. This paper presents a summary of the perceived work hazards of public health nurses (PHNs) and a discussion of the organizational conditions necessary for collegiality, one of the organizationally generated conditions associated with work hazards for these women.

RESEARCH DESIGN

One subunit of public health units was selected for study. Ten managerial and 47 staff public health nurses, from five autonomous public health units in northern, central, and southern regions of Alberta, participated. All respondents were female. The sample included both full- and part-time workers, living in urban and rural communities, employed in both unionized and non-unionized health units.

The study proceeded inductively and deductively, guided by four major research questions: (1) What are the actual or potential biological, chemical, ergonomic, physical, psychosocial, reproductive, and safety hazards that public health nurses[1] perceive in their work environments?; (2) What organizational factors underlie the hazards perceived by public health nurses in their work environments?; (3) What factors in the external environment of each health unit underlie the hazards that public health nurses perceive in their work environments?; (4)What are the organizationally related strategies that informed public health nurses generate for reducing the hazards they perceive in their work environments? A descriptive component to the research provided an account of the perceived hazards; an exploratory component maximized identification of the organizational factors. Data were collected in two stages. Self-administered questionnaires addressed the *types* or *nature* of work hazards; semistructured interviews explored the *organizational* structures and contexts underlying the hazards; and moderated focus groups capitalized on the interactive group process to generate ideas for reducing hazards in the work environment.

PERSPECTIVES UNDERLYING THE RESEARCH
Organizational Factors and Occupational Hazards

The dominant paradigms in the occupational health field (lifestyle, environmental and epidemiological) have failed to scrutinize the organizational dimensions of work hazards (Skillen, 1992). By focussing on individual responsibility for protecting health through individual behaviours, the lifestyle perspective neglects the organizational context of those behaviours (Castillo-Salgado, 1987; Feagin, 1986; McKee, 1988; McLeroy, Gottlieb and Burdine, 1987; Sass, 1986; Wikler, 1987; Winett, King and Altman, 1989). By emphasizing acceptable exposure limits for biological, chemical, ergonomic and physical hazards at the worksite, the environmental approach ignores psychosocial hazards and the organizational context. The epidemiological perspective provides surveillance of hazard outcomes (disease and injury by industry after the fact), but neglects the organizational factors underlying exposures (Skillen, in press; Walters, 1985). Conventional applications of these perspectives have avoided assessment of organizationally generated hazards and stressors. Consequently, an exploratory research design was indicated to identify organizational factors associated with the work hazards of PHNs.

Occupational Health and Safety for Women

Women's occupational health and safety issues have been neglected (Messing, 1991; 1994; Skillen, 1992). Historically, researchers in occupational health and safety have studied male workers, a practice established before the influx of women into the paid labour force. In addition, researchers have concentrated on hazards in the physical work environment (House and Jackman, 1979; Karasek and Theorell, 1990; Weinstein, 1985), a pattern introduced because of the highly visible and dangerous occupations of mining, forestry and construction. To be certain, accidents and insidious hazards to health in high risk goods-producing industries should not be ignored (Robinson, 1987). At the same time, however, psychosocial stressors and the service sector should not be avoided. The service sector now comprises over 70 percent of the labour force (Krahn, 1992) and merits attention for "less tangible, but equally debilitating" hazards (Weinstein, 1985:53). Psychosocial work stressors are particularly severe in human service organizations and may be organizationally, as well as occupationally, generated (Fletcher, Jones and McGregor-Cheers, 1991; Parasuraman and Hansen, 1987; Sprout and Yassi, this volume; Walcott-McQuigg and Ervin, 1992). Research links psychosocial stressors at work to occupational morbidity and mortality (Glowinkowski and Cooper, 1986; Karasek and Theorell, 1990; Klitzman, House, Israel and Mero, 1990; Levi, 1990; Lowe, 1989; Stewart and Arklie, 1994). Lippel (this volume) has observed that compensation for the effects on health of psychosocial stressors favours male workers.

The fact that women are occupationally segregated would appear to have a bearing on the surveillance of hazards to their health and safety. It is in the service sector, in traditional and predominantly female occupations, that the majority of Canadian women aged 15 years and over are employed (Ghalam, 1993; Sprout and Yassi, this volume). In 1991, almost three-quarters of employed women were located in five occupations: clerical, sales, service, teaching and nursing or related health professions (Ghalam, 1993). Because of occupational segregation, it must be recognized that women may be exposed to different work hazards than men, yet researchers often draw inferences about women's work-related risks from research on male workers (Haw, 1982; Messing, 1991; 1994). Limited support for change in workplace hazard surveillance for women has been found in two important and related movements: the women's health movement and the occupational health movement (Chavkin, 1984). While addressing the stressors of household and public work, feminist literature has provided little guidance for examining factors underlying a healthful environment for women's work in the public sphere. To illustrate, Reskin and Hartmann (1991) consider occupational segregation to be but one manifestation of unequal opportunities for women in paid work, along with wages, benefits and sexual harassment. They do not address unequal opportunities with respect to surveillance of occupational hazards to women's health.

Although occupational stressors for women have been scrutinized (Lowe, 1989), organizational level responses to those stressors do not appear to have been subjected to a feminist critique. Feminists have focussed on gender inequality in the workplace as a result of limited access to wages, benefits, occupational mobility and occupational choice, but not as a result of limited access to hazard surveillance for the protection of health (Aitkenhead and Liff, 1991; Armstrong and Armstrong, 1988; Beechey, 1987; Butter, Carpenter, Kay and Simmons, 1987; Epstein, 1988; Kanter, 1977; Kaufman, 1989; Lowe, 1989; Renzetti and Curran, 1989; Reskin and Hartmann, 1991; Walby, 1990). Kanter (1977), for example, demonstrated that the numerical distribution of women and men in the organization affected their interaction and favored the men, who enjoyed numerical dominance. Women's "rarity and scarcity" (p. 207) therefore negatively influenced their working environment. Skillen (1992), however, noted that men in a numerical minority were still able to retain powerful interaction patterns when women predominated in health units. The feminist literature appears less likely to address hazard surveillance for working women and more likely to deal with corporate exclusionary practices relating to reproductive health, occupational mobility or sexual harassment (Bramwell and Davidson, 1991; Crull, 1984; Scott, 1984; Stockdale, 1991).

Hazards for Health Care Workers

Work hazards of HCWs were neglected for decades (Coleman and Dickinson, 1984; Emmett and Baetz, 1987; Rogers, 1989; Yassi and Guidotti, 1990). An in-depth review of four bodies of literature (occupational health, public health, organizational analysis, industrial sociology) illuminated a paradox: the very professionals expected to promote and protect health might constitute vulnerable populations and be employed in unhealthy, unsafe work environments. Concentrating on the provision of quality health care for the Canadian public, the health care delivery system has overlooked the health and safety of its employees. This is due in part to the marginalization of occupational health professionals within mainstream health care. The neglect also stems from professional ideologies of caring which concentrate on the care recipient; occupational health specialists who focus on male workers in the goods-producing sector; and legislation in the occupational health field which fails to provide adequate direction for identifying vulnerable workers.

In recent years, the environmental perspective, one of the dominant paradigms in the occupational health field, has been applied to hospital-based, but not community-based, nurses. It is now recognized that employees in hospitals may be exposed to unhealthy physical work environments (Astbury and Baxter, 1990; Estryn-Behar et al., 1990; Hadley, 1990; Hipwell, Tyler and Wilson, 1989; Lipscomb and Love, 1992; Messing, 1991; Orr, 1988; Triolo, 1989a; 1989b).

Another dominant paradigm, the lifestyle or individualistic perspective, has been applied to community-based health professionals in the limited published studies. Alberta Health (1991) revealed occupational health and safety issues to be the second most important source of dissatisfaction for PHN informants, but the broad scope of the study limited the number of questionnaire items to only psychosocial and safety hazards. The other published Alberta studies involving PHNs (Birk, 1988; Ebert and MacAlister, 1970; Field, 1980; Hoskin, 1987; Moore, 1977; Morrison, 1983; Tenove, 1981) did not address occupational hazards per se, but did illustrate methodological issues for consideration in this research. Other Canadian studies placed work conditions among the top ten critical issues for PHNs, identified noise as a hazard for PHNs, provided insights into organizational factors and identified psychosocial hazards for urban and rural PHNs (Clarke, Beddome and Whyte, 1990; Hache-Faulkner and MacKay, 1985; North York Department of Health, 1984; Stewart and Arklie, 1994; Woodcox, Isaacs, Underwood and Chambers, 1994). International studies further emphasized psychosocial hazards for PHNs (Davison, 1987; Fletcher, Jones and McGregor-Cheers, 1991; Goodwin, 1983; 1987; Walcott-McQuigg and Ervin, 1992; West, Jones and Savage, 1988; West and Savage, 1988a; 1989b), but neglected the physical work environment and focussed on the individual. In short, prior to this research, no comprehensive examination of the work hazards of PHNs had been conducted and no study had explicitly addressed the organizational context for such hazards.

An Interactionist Approach

I adopted an exploratory research design based on an interactionist approach to obtain a better understanding of the organizational context of PHNs' work hazards. When the basic social processes or structures of phenomena are poorly understood, interpretations by researchers require grounding in the actors' reported experiences. Although PHNs have personal experience with hazards, these have not been studied from their perspective. In organizations, employees use their interpretations of everyday life experiences as a basis for subsequent action (Gephart, 1987; Kinlaw, 1988; Krackhardt, 1990; Prus, 1990). Employees' knowledge of their own occupation and its context is specific and rich, but they respond to perceptions of their world, not objective facts (Berger and Luckman, 1967; Hinkin and Schriesheim, 1988). Although participants' definitions of the situation may not be accurate in an objective sense, they are essential to a grounded, context-sensitive understanding of reality (Prus, 1990). "If men [sic] define situations as real, they are real in their consequences" (Thomas and Thomas, 1928:572). Consequently, PHNs' perceptions of both their physical and psychosocial work environments were examined.

RESULTS: WORK HAZARDS
Psychosocial Work Environments

Public health nurses considered psychosocial hazards to be their most significant work hazards. Using the term "stressor" to refer to hazards in the psychosocial domain, they located the origins of these stressors in both the external and internal environments of health unit organizations. Externally located stressors were associated with the provincial government, client populations, community agencies and institutions. Internally located stressors were related to administration, clerical work, collegial relations, workload and Boards of Health.

According to 83 percent of the sample, the major external stressor was the provincial government. Cutbacks and hiring freezes had caused staff shortages, programme changes, the addition of prenatal classes to workloads and threats of lay-offs. Inconsistent applications of budget cuts across health units had given PHNs the task of placating a displeased public. Public health nurses were concerned about the implications of government-supported regionalization of health services and dissolution of health units (which became a reality in April 1995 in Alberta). They identified the potential loss of good administrators, power struggles, and job losses for PHNs who were not degree-prepared as potential results of these initiatives. A more frequently mentioned government stressor was the decision makers' apparently uninformed attitude towards preventive services. Inconsistencies in government directives, a lack of policies and standards of practice for the whole province, and differences between federal and provincial jurisdictions were also identified as stressors.

Almost three-quarters (74 percent) of the sample reported client-related stressors. These stressors included: client response to the health unit or service, the nature of the client problem or situation (e.g., poverty and neglect, culture, family violence, communicable disease) and PHNs' unmet expectations for impartial, professional and confidential service for their clients from other service providers. Approximately one-half of the sample described stressors related to community agencies and institutions. Most were concerned with communication and coordination between agencies, but PHNs also referred to the reduced accessibility of services and personnel within social agencies and the demands made upon health units by agencies and institutions. Just under one-third of the sample reported physician-related stressors, including physicians in government departments who provided inconsistent directives for case management and community-based physicians who appeared to resent PHNs' autonomy. Twenty-eight percent described union-related stressors linked to union philosophy and confrontations or negotiations. Others identified the absence of a union as a stressor.

According to 74 percent of the sample, the major internal stressor was administration. Most referred to the behaviours and decisions of management, but respondents also called attention to paperwork, including the province-wide nursing activity reporting system. Almost two-thirds reported stressors related to the clerical aspects of their work. A large majority described just getting clerical work done as the stressor, either because of the time required or because of obstacles to obtaining clerical assistance.

Over half of the respondents referred to collegial stressors, including personality clashes, colleagues' professional performance and colleagues' affect. The principal collegial stressors, however, were such negative behaviours as a failure to cooperate, accept professional differences or share the workload equitably. Stressors also included budgetary, conceptual and staffing differences between two nursing subunits: Home Care and Public Health. Workload (including staffing issues) was a significant stressor. Forty-five PHNs reported a workload increase during the past year. Thirty described work overload and 23 identified work pace as a stressor. Twenty-two PHNs reported feeling under pressure often. For nine, the pressure was a serious problem.

Finally, the majority of respondents reported stressors originating with Boards of Health composed of elected officials without health profession backgrounds. To a minor extent, stressors derived from their allocation of resources for salaries, inservice, continuing education or programs. A major stressor was the Boards' lack of vision in relation to preventive health services. In sum, the internally and externally located stressors in the psychosocial work environments of PHNs were inextricable from organizational factors. The data implicated organizational complexity, authority structure and formalization, in addition to organizational technology, environment and goals (Skillen, 1992).

Physical Work Environments

In their physical work environments, PHNs considered safety and physical hazards to be the most important, while acknowledging ergonomic and biological hazards and discounting chemical and reproductive hazards. Whether part-time or full-time, urban or rural, unionized or non-unionized, respondents were in agreement about the hazards. The vast majority (97 percent) perceived risks to their safety, identifying dogs and road travel most often. Working alone and unprotected were important concerns. Public health nurses reported verbal and physical abuse by clients. As well, they reported work injuries, including motor vehicle accidents, needle sticks and dog bites. They commonly used personal protective equipment such as car seat belts and surgical gloves; however, the cost of the gloves influenced their availability and use. Although health units had some written safety policies and procedures, fewer than half of the respondents reported a committee dedicated to the health and/or safety of employees.

Physical hazards were the second significant concern of the PHNs. Temperature extremes, inadequate ventilation and air quality were identified by the majority. More than one-third of the sample described exposures to noise and dust. Exposures to building and vehicle vibration, inadequate illumination and cramped workspaces were reported less frequently. Video display terminals (VDTs) — used by one-third of the sample, but less than weekly by the majority of respondents — were not a concern.

Public health nurses recognized biological and ergonomic hazards in their work environments, but were less concerned about these. Most handled vaccines, were exposed to human body fluids or waste and encountered bacteria, viruses and parasites in their work environments. A very large majority of PHNs (88 percent or more) reported immunity for polio, diphtheria, tetanus, rubella, red measles and mumps. Only about one-half of the sample was protected against hepatitis B and tuberculosis. Just three health units provided the costly vaccine against hepatitis B for their PHN employees. Over half the respondents had experienced a needle stick injury, 10 in the previous year. When handling used syringes, most but not all PHNs followed recommended procedures. A large majority reported carrying heavy equipment or materials at work. Close to one-half indicated that providing direct services to clients or performing service-related activities required uncomfortable positions or repetitive movements. More than one-quarter described having to use uncomfortable furniture.

Chemical and reproductive hazards were not a serious concern, although respondents did report exposure to tobacco smoke, disinfectants and cleaning agents or solvents. In three health units, they had not been informed by their employers about the Workplace Hazardous Materials Information System (WHMIS), legislation dealing with designated chemical and biological substances. To conclude, safety, physical, ergonomic and biological hazards in the physical work environments of respondents were interrelated with organizational factors.

Findings from both physical and psychosocial domains of PHNs' work provided evidence that PHNs' work hazards demand an organizational analysis and response if work hazards are to be recognized, evaluated and controlled or eliminated. Perceived hazards are linked to various organizational interdependencies (i.e., dependencies within and between organizations and institutions). To illustrate, the availability of safe, well-maintained vehicles for PHNs was a responsibility of general administration. Maintenance of the heating, ventilation and air conditioning (HVAC) system was contracted out by general administration. Clarification of clerical responsibilities was the jurisdiction of general administration. Purchase of adjustable furniture and equipment was subject to recognition of the physical variations among employees by personnel responsible for purchasing. Nursing administrators were dependent upon colleagues in lateral positions on the organizational chart to reduce hazards for their staff. Without budgetary control, they were dependent upon colleagues for decisions to pay for hepatitis B vaccine for their staff. Interdependence of the organization with another institution, the government, was exemplified by government control over funding to hire prenatal instructors at the health unit level. In short, organizational factors cannot be separated from PHNs' work hazards. Collective efforts are required when biological, ergonomic, physical, psychosocial and safety hazards are identified in the workplace (Skillen, 1992). Individuals alone cannot bring about the necessary changes.

RESULTS: ORGANIZATIONAL CONDITIONS FOR COLLEGIALITY

Reconceptualization of the problem of work hazards permitted organizational patterns in these five health units to be viewed from a new perspective. Analysis of the data generated four major categories of organizational conditions that facilitated or restricted hazard surveillance: conditions for collegiality, control over physical plant, structures for surveillance and hazard information transfer.[2] I will discuss the data concerning the organizational conditions for collegiality here because of its relevance for women's occupational health and safety. The notion of an environment for collegiality derives from a liberal feminist perspective and draws attention to variations in physical proximity and gender equality that are relevant to the surveillance of work hazards.

Analysis of the interview data indicated that physical proximity and gender equality influence interdependencies within the organization, creating an environment for collegial interchange the nature of which either facilitates or hinders hazard identification and control. Collegiality, or collegial relationships, require respect and equality. Without conditions for collegiality, observations and feelings about hazards might not be articulated and acknowledged beyond an intrapersonal level. An environment conducive to discussion is important for the exchange of concerns and information about work hazards.

Physical Proximity

During the research, it became clear that health unit personnel were dispersed within and between not only buildings, but also geographical areas and political jurisdictions. Spatial complexity creates stressors and hinders hazard resolution. The health units' mandate to service geographically dispersed populations necessitated suboffices (regional, district, or outlying offices). A manager admitted, "it would be easier if we were all under one roof but that's not practical in terms of [the] distance that they [PHNs] would have to travel." When health unit personnel were located in one building, administrative and professional subunits, and subunits of subunits, were dispersed over different floors. The seat of authority for a health unit might be in one geopolitical site, but personnel could be located in two buildings with professional and administrative subunits distributed across the two locations.

The implications of spatial complexity for work hazard reduction were highlighted by respondents' observations. Personnel dispersal made it difficult to network. One PHN stated: "It's harder to pick up the phone and talk to somebody about a work stressor. It would have to definitely be in writing." In one unit, a PHN commented that being in a suboffice limits communication with administration. "With head office, we're not as visible ... Oftentimes our concerns and issues are minimized because we're not visible ... Senior management isn't seeing them [hazards] themselves every day." A suboffice PHN commented, "I don't think that they have ... realized some of the physical hazards that we deal with. You know, with the driving conditions, the road conditions." One PHN described what suboffices have had to do:

We wrote letters to our administration department, our ... administrator for the health unit ... He's the man who pays the bills, who signs the contracts with the various agencies, pays the rent on the building, gets all the maintenance stuff, gets the windows fixed when they are broken ... but which again takes months and months and months and months of phoning [location of] head office, writing letters, begging, borrowing and stealing and nagging to get basic building care done.

In contrast, monthly meetings arranged on-site at suboffices by and with a managerial PHN in two of the health units provided PHNs with opportunities for discussing concerns.

Respondents linked having more than one main office to the creation of "division and stress." One PHN suggested that having a single main building would allow a mid-manager to "talk to someone that's a mid-manager as well." By contrast, a PHN in the health unit with a consolidated main office stated, "it gives us a better perspective of the health unit functioning as a whole ... even though we're individual programs ... it's nice to be here to be more aware of what's going on in the other programs ... Suboffices don't have that as much."

Where one existed, a coffee room could provide opportunities for collegial interaction among employees within and between subunits. Both social and professional interchanges could occur in the coffee room. Respondents in some suboffices observed, "In our office, because we're a smaller office, we share a lot." For the fifth health unit, the dispersion of personnel highlighted the importance of the coffee room. "This health unit was at one time all in one building by itself and they all coffeed together," explained one PHN. Another related, "and then something as simple as taking our coffee room away from us, you know, because ... the administration felt we were too clicky, the nurses, so away went our coffee room." A PHN in one unit commented: "At coffee ... if there's a work stressor ... people are usually fairly vocal." At another site, PHNs reported, "we have coffee with the people [in Environmental Health] every day"; "we get along really well ... everything is divulged in there [our coffee room]."

The spatial conditions for collegiality could change in main offices. "We don't even hardly know those people over there ... We're in and out all the time but you don't know them [Home Care, Speech, Nutrition] like you do when you have coffee with them" and "because basically 75 percent to 90 percent of the staff in this place is female, they [Environmental Health] ... never coffee with us." For two units, the on-site coffee room was used to discuss or reduce stressors. In the unit without a coffee room, PHNs and secretaries found an alternative location for coffeeing together — a nearby cafeteria.[3]

Communication about the nature of hazards and communication to those responsible for addressing hazards appears to be contingent upon the geographical location (physical proximity) of organizational personnel. By increasing physical proximity, the individuals or subunits with the influence to make changes are brought closer to the perceived hazard. For example, reducing the distance between individuals exposed to a hazard in the physical work environment and individuals in positions of authority over maintenance and cleaning services might promote effective management of physical resources (e.g., equipment, facilities, property).

Gender Equality

Gender equality is another organizational condition for collegiality. Walby (1991) defines patriarchy as "a system of social structures and practices in which men dominate, oppress and exploit women" (p. 20). Walby's notion of social structures and practices is particularly useful for analyzing variations in PHNs' experience with collegiality and hazard surveillance. It opens up for scrutiny the privilege of males in non-hierarchical organizational positions with respect to PHNs.

Just as the spatial complexity of organizations has implications for employees' physical proximity, the structural dimension of gender configuration has relevance for gender equality. The term "configuration" refers to both the numbers and positions of men and women in these organizations. "Without structures that potentially benefit all organization members more broadly," problems of gender equality cannot be resolved (Kanter, 1977:266). The health units in the sample ranged from almost totally female organizations to organizations with male management and male subunit employees (e.g., Environmental Health, Finance) that were still predominantly female. Although chairpersons of the Boards of Health were female as well as male, few females were members of the governing Boards. Because the assignment of men and women to operational positions in the organizations was not consistent across the sample, male domination and female subordination could not be taken for granted. For example, there were extremely few men in the employ of one unit and no managerial positions among them. In another, the large numbers of PHNs appeared to take precedence over any gender effect; the responsibilities of the male medical officer of health were shared with a female administrative assistant. Others had all-female management or predominantly male management. In short, the sexual division of labour varied across the five units.

Gender relations also varied across units. These variations became apparent as PHNs described avenues for identifying and evaluating perceived work hazards and reported differences among subunits in terms of their control over hazards. Individual interviews shed light on PHNs' limited access to resources for investigating perceived work hazards and various milieux for voicing concerns.

To place PHNs' perceptions of gender relations in context, the majority lacked a specific educational background for assessing their occupational hazards. Only three out of 57 PHNs (five percent) had certification in occupational health nursing and just 16 reported participation in some form of continuing education in occupational health; therefore, most had to seek information and resources. When responses were coded for the focus group question "What is the most useful thing you have learned from this?" 60 percent of the responses referred to an increased awareness. Public health inspectors were an obvious resource to PHNs by virtue of their mandate to conduct environmental inspections and investigations under the Public Health Act (1984). For example, they were familiar with relevant legislation, including WHMIS. This was the *first* conjuncture with patriarchal attitudes, as male co-workers in non-hierarchical positions discounted PHN concerns, effectively creating obstacles for hazard surveillance.

The *second* conjuncture was located within the hierarchy of authority when PHNs attempted to deal with actual or potential hazards such as the condition of health unit vehicles, availability of surgical gloves or HBV vaccine, purchase of cellular phones for isolated home visiting in rural areas, assessment of the HVAC (heating, ventilation, air conditioning) system and security in isolated buildings. By de-emphasizing their concerns, controlling economic resources and determining communication networks, males in one or more levels of management (e.g., professional management, administration, as chairs of the Board of Health, as members on the Board) contributed to the denial of access to strategies for prevention or intervention in PHNs' perceived hazards at work.

Public health nurses had limited access to specialized occupational health resources. They occasionally reported consulting with occupational health specialists in the government regarding employee exposures, but only with respect to some inadequacy in the HVAC system. For example, respondents commented, "When we were concerned about the air quality, we ... went the route through the organization and that didn't work so then people personally phoned [the government]." They also acknowledged opportunities to bring forward health and safety concerns to their collective bargaining unit and to their negotiating or liaison committee. However, occupational health and safety concerns and the importance of documentation had only been discussed in union meetings and at the negotiating table; they were not covered by collective agreements. "We fill in incident reports," explained one PHN, who stated that the reports go to the personnel officer. Without a background for analysis of the reports, it might be expected that a person in this position would do little follow-up. In non-unionized units, only non-binding routes for collective action were available for dealing with concerns regarding work hazards. In one unit, for example, "the negotiating committee is made up of people from the different departments and if you had concerns, they would collectively go to the Board." In another, a PHN stated, "Because it's a female profession I really don't think they [the Board] listen." To illustrate, a letter written collectively by PHNs regarding psychosocial hazards was destroyed by the chairperson and not transmitted to the Board. "He tore it up in front of the director and said 'this is not my problem.'"

With little access to occupational health resources, PHNs turned to related professionals. When hazards are suspected, one PHN explained, "I would probably talk with the Environmental Health people in the organization ... to verify whether this is really a concern. I wouldn't necessarily stop there if I really felt it was a concern." Not all respondents reported cooperation from the Environmental Health Program. Some stated: "We do use Environmental Health [the inspector], but she's female too and she listens"; but others reported: "public health inspectors are traditionally very closed mouth ... they don't give us too much information." Members of one unit commented, "That's viewed as a different department that's above the nurses and when we take a concern to them [Environmental Health], it's treated ... like we're being silly." In contrast, for a PHN in another unit, the Environmental Health division was the most appropriate resource. She explained:

> If you check with the health inspector she can get all the facts straight and then she can approach it from that point of view rather than a community health nurse trying to be on to an environmental health issue. Really it's ... the health inspector's ball park. It's not really a community health nurse ball park issue I think.

In addition to describing the health inspectors' responses to their concerns, some PHNs also portrayed an organizational subunit that has more control over its work hazards than that experienced by PHNs, because of gender make-up. Their comments included: "They are all male except for one. And, well I think they have more ear to the top [access to management]" and "I think the men have a little more ... leeway maybe or say in some things." A colleague stated, "They also have the ear of the MOH [medical officer of health] more than we do [whispers] because they're men [laughs] ... They're persistent ... We're second-rate." Regarding a safety hazard perceived by PHNs, one commented, "Really, really serious problem but the men don't think of it that way. They don't see it as a problem."

In the fifth unit, PHNs commented: "the old boy network has been very detrimental to this health unit" and "there's lack of communication and there is a very strong ... sense that 'those women are bitching again.'" A colleague described feeling at times that "we just don't get any respect as a nurse," and another stated, "sometimes we do feel like ... they just think we're a bunch of ... cackling old hens."

Counterposing the above are comments made in another unit: "it's a bonus [laughs] that our entire organization is female"; "the lady we have as CEO, she could run circles around anybody"; and "if our Board ever changes, especially our Board chairman, we don't know what we'll get. She's excellent." In a different unit, respondents said, "Generally I would say the group is listened to and respected"; "as you go up from management ... [they] are open to and receptive to what the Community Health nurse, for instance, has to say about our issues that we've [PHN and interviewer] discussed"; and "we have had a pretty understanding Board."

The words of the PHNs in the sample attest to men's perpetration of stereotypical female images in their workplaces: "When we take a concern to them, it's treated ... like we're *being silly*"; "we're *second-rate*"; "those women are *bitching* again"; "they felt that ... we were *being emotional* and ... *worried too much*"; and "this is *stupid*" [italics added]. The use of affective terminology not only resonates with stereotyping, but also serves as a reinforcement or counterfoil for the masculine norm of rationality (Kanter, 1977). Whether explicit or implicit, this language reinforced male superiority and trivialized PHNs' concerns.

The men responsible for the reported reactions were essentially applying a "gender" not "job" analytical model to the situation (Feldberg and Glenn, 1979; Northcott and Lowe, 1987) and failing to acknowledge the working conditions that framed PHNs' perceptions. Feldberg and Glenn demonstrate that sex-segregated models of analysis for the workplace effectively devalue job-related perceptions of female workers, attributing them instead to personal characteristics. By focussing on individual factors, the "gender" model precludes collective efforts to address structural conditions in either the physical or psychosocial work environments. The male actors in this situation experienced power as a result of the social relations they generated.

In summary, physical proximity and gender equality for employees and management reflect two structural dimensions of organizations (spatial complexity and gender configuration and gender relations) that affect organizational hazard surveillance through their influence on collegiality. By promoting collegiality, some health units provided a mechanism for employees to raise, share and resolve concerns regarding hazards in the workplace. By neglecting collegiality, others were more likely to maintain the status quo.

LIMITATIONS OF THE STUDY

Although the study is limited in its generalizability because it used a small sample in one Canadian province, the precautions taken during sample selection regarding organizational and nurse characteristics open up the possibility of cautious generalization. First, inclusion of the obvious organizational differences in the sample of five units ensured representation of the known characteristics shared by health units across the province. Next, pretesting with health units from within and outside the sample population permitted any additional differences to surface. Third, inclusion of non-study participants in the focus groups provided opportunities to dispute the results. In addition, a limitation of the study normally would be that it studied a sample of women only. Because 96 percent of all nurses are women, this sample was representative of the population of interest. Since all health units in the Province of Alberta shared the same mandate under the existing legislation, it was reasonable to expect commonalities among Alberta organizations. Finally, the study's generalizability was enhanced by multiple triangulation, as more than one autonomous organization was studied, obvious organizational differences were included in the sample, multiple informants in each organization contributed their perspectives and more than one data gathering technique was used.

CONCLUSION

When these data were collected in 1991, employees in the community-based health care system had not engaged in a comprehensive assessment of their work hazards, and organizations in the community-based health care system had not undergone a critical assessment of their role in the production and reproduction of work hazards. As employees, managers and service providers, PHNs are in a position to reduce work-related exposures for themselves and the populations they serve. Consideration of their own hazards contributed to their knowledge about women's occupational hazards and provided data on an understudied sector in the service industry. Both feminist and organizational subunit perspectives add credence to the importance of social structural factors in setting the stage for work hazards to develop. A gender-informed analysis of the conditions for collegiality has shown that organizational factors are inseparable from work hazards.

ACKNOWLEDGEMENTS

This research was supported by Project Grants from the Alberta Foundation for Nursing Research (AFNR) and the Alberta Association of Registered Nurses (AARN) 75th Anniversary Competition. Neither AFNR nor AARN are necessarily supportive of the research findings.

NOTES

1. The original research questions used the term "Community Health Nurse" to identify the individual nurse who focusses on health promotion and disease prevention in the population served by the public health unit. To distinguish that nurse from the Home Care Nurse who provides treatment for an identified patient in the community, the term now being used more often is "Public Health Nurse." The words are changed here to reflect the change in practice.

2. The process used to discover the four categories is discussed elsewhere (Skillen, in press). When grounded theory methodology is used, category generation derives from observed regularities (Marshall and Rossman, 1989).

3. What was management indicating to employees who had to find an off-site location for interaction? Did that distance management from employees? Was management also contributing to reduced communication about work hazards among its professional employees by its structuring of employee locations?

REFERENCES

Aitkenhead, M., and S. Liff. "The Effectiveness of Equal Opportunity Policies," in *Women at Work: Psychological and Organizational Perspectives*. J. Firth-Cozens and M.A. West (eds.). Buckingham: Open University Press, 1991.

Alberta Health. *Perceptions of Nursing Worklife: A Community-based Study — Analysis and Results*. Edmonton: Alberta Health, 1991.

Armstrong, P., and H. Armstrong. "Women's Work in the Labour Force," in *Gender and Society: Creating a Canadian Women's Sociology* A.T. McLaren (ed.). Toronto:

Copp Clark Pitman Ltd., 1988.

Astbury, C., and P.J. Baxter. "Infection Risks in Hospital Staff from Blood: Hazardous Injury Rates and Acceptance of Hepatitis B Immunization." *Journal of the Society of Occupational Medicine* 40 (1990). pp. 92-3.

Beechey, V. *Unequal Work.* London: Verso, 1987.

Berger, P.L., and T. Luckmann. *The Social Construction of Reality.* Toronto: Anchor Books, 1967.

Birk, H.A. *Initiating Outreach Home Visits: PHN Approaches.* Unpublished Master's thesis. Clagary: University of Alberta, 1988.

Bramwell, R.S., and M.J. Davidson. "Reproductive Hazards at Work," in *Women at Work: Psychological and Organizational Perspectives.* J. Firth-Cozens and M.A. West (eds.). Buckingham: Open University Press, 1991.

Butter, I.H., E.S. Carpenter, B.J. Kay and R.S. Simmons. "Gender Hierarchies in the Health Labor Force." *International Journal of Health Services* 17, 1 (1987). pp. 133-49.

Castillo-Salgado, C. "Promotion of Health in the Workplace: The Relative Worth of Lifestyle and Environmental Approaches," in *Dominant Issues in Medical Sociology.* H.D. Schwartz (ed.). New York: Random House, 1987.

Chavkin, W. "Introduction," in *Double Exposure: Women's Health Hazards on the Job and at Home.* W. Chavkin (ed.). New York: Monthly Review Press, 1984.

Clarke, H.F., G. Beddome and N.B. Whyte. *Vision for Tomorrow: A Public Health Nurse Driven Future for Public Health Nursing.* Vancouver: Registered Nurses' Association of British Columbia, 1990.

Coleman, L., and C. Dickinson. "The Risks of Healing: The Hazards of the Nursing Profession," in *Double Exposure,* op. cit.

Crull, P. "Sexual Harassment and Women's Health," in *Double Exposure,* op. cit.

Davison, D. "Burnt Out Cases? ... Occupational Stress in Health Visitors in an Inner City." *Health Visitor* 60, 2 (1987). p. 51.

Ebert, B., and M. MacAlister. "A Study of the Activities of Nursing Personnel in Ten Health Units and One City Health Department in the Province of Alberta." *Canadian Journal of Public Health* 61 (1970). p. 126-31.

Emmett, E.A., and J.H. Baetz. "Health in the Health Care Industries." *Occupational Medicine: State of the Art Reviews* 2, 3 (1987). pp. ix-xv.

Epp, J. *Achieving Health for All: A Framework for Health Promotion.* Ottawa: National Health and Welfare Canada, 1986.

Epstein, C.F. *Deceptive Distinctions: Sex, Gender, and the Social Order.* New York: Yale University Press and Russell Sage Foundation, 1988.

Estryn-Behar, M., M. Kaminski, E. Peigne, N. Bonnet, E. Valchere, C. Gozian, S. Azoulay and M. Giorgi. "Stress at Work and Mental Health Status Among Female Hospital Workers." *British Journal of Industrial Medicine* 47, 1 (1990). pp. 20-8.

Feagin, J.R. *Social Problems: A Critical Power-conflict Perspective,* Second Edition. Englewood Cliffs, NJ: Prentice-Hall Inc., 1986.

Feldberg, R.L., and E.N. Glenn. "Male and Female: Job Versus Gender Models in the Sociology of Work." *Social Problems* 26, 5 (1979). pp. 524-38.

Field, P.A. *An Ethnography: Four Nurses' Perspectives of Nursing in a Community Health Setting*. Unpublished Ph.D. dissertation. Edmonton: University of Alberta, 1980.

Fletcher, B.C., F. Jones and J. McGregor-Cheers. "The Stressors and Strains of Health Visiting: Demands, Supports, Constraints and Psychological Health." *Journal of Advanced Nursing* 16 (1991). pp. 1078-89.

Gephart, R.P. Jr. "Organization Design for Hazardous Chemical Accidents." *Columbia Journal of World Business* 22, 1 (1987). pp. 51-8.

Ghalam, N.Z. *Women in the Workplace*. Ottawa: Statistics Canada, Housing, Family and Social Statistics Division, 1993.

Glaser, B.G., and A. Strauss, *The Discovery of Grounded Theory*. Chicago: Aldine Publishing Company, 1967.

Glowinkowski, S.P., and C.L. Cooper. "Organizational Issues in Stress Research." *Journal of Managerial Psychology* 1, 1 (1986). pp. 3-11.

Goodwin, S. "Caring for the Carers: Coping with Stress Part 2." *Health Visitor* 56, 2 (1983). pp. 46-8.

— "Stress in Health Visiting." *Recent Advances in Nursing* 15 (1987). pp. 99-111.

Hache-Faulkner, N., and R.C. Mackay. "Stress in the Workplace: Public Health and Hospital Nurses." *Canadian Nurse* 81, 4 (1985). pp. 40-2.

Hadley, M. "Background Paper Regarding Abuse of Nurses in the Workplace." *AARN Newsletter* 46, 9 (1990). pp. 6-9.

Haw, M.A. "Women, Work and Stress: A Review and Agenda for the Future." *Journal of Health and Social Behaviour* 23, 2, (1982). pp. 132-44.

Health and Welfare Canada. *A Guide for Health Promotion by Health Care Facilities*. Ottawa: Minister of Supply and Services, 1990.

Hinkin, T.R., and C.A. Schriesheim. "Power and Influence: The View from Below." *Personnel* 65, 5 (1988). pp. 47-50.

Hipwell, A.E., P.A. Tyler and C.M. Wilson. "Sources of Stress and Dissatisfaction Among Nurses in Four Hospital Environments." *British Journal of Medical Psychology* 621 (1989). pp. 71-9.

Hoskin, P.L.A. *The Health of Nurses: Their Subjective Well-being, Lifestyle/Preventive Practices and Goals for Health*. Unpublished Master's thesis. Lethbridge, Alberta: University of Lethbridge, 1987.

House, J.S., and M.F. Jackman. "Occupation Stress and Health," in *Toward a New Definition of Health: Psychosocial Dimensions*. P.I. Ahmed and G.V. Coelho (eds.). New York: Plenum Press, 1979.

Kanter, R.M. *Men and Women of the Corporation*. New York: Basic Books, 1977.

Karasek, R., and T. Theorell. *Health Work: Stress, Productivity, and the Reconstruction of Working Life*. New York: Basic Books, 1990.

Kaufman, D.R. "Professional Women: How Real are the Recent Gains?" in *Women: A Feminist Perspective*. J. Freeman (ed.). Mountainview, CA: Mayfield Publishing Co., 1989.

Kinlaw, D.C. "What Employees 'See' is What Organizations 'Get.'" *Management Solutions* 33, 3 (1988). pp. 38-42.

Klitzman, S., J.S. House, B.A. Israel and R.P. Mero. "Work Stress, Nonwork Stress, and Health." *Journal of Behavioral Medicine* 13, 3 (1990). pp. 221-43.

Krackhardt, D. "Assessing the Political Landscape: Structure, Cognition, and Power in Organizations." *Administrative Science Quarterly* 35 (1990). pp. 342-69.

Krahn, H. *Quality of Work in the Service Sector.* Ottawa: Statistics Canada, 1992.

Krause, E.A. *Power and Illness: The Political Sociology of Health and Medical Care.* New York: Elsevier, 1977.

Levi, L. "Occupational Stress: Spice of Life or Kiss of Death?" *American Psychologist* 45, 10 (1990). pp. 1142-5.

Lipscomb, J.A. and C.C. Love. "Violence Toward Health Care Workers: An Emerging Occupational Hazard." *AAOHN Journal* 40, 5 (1992). pp. 219-28.

Lowe, G.S. *Women, Paid/Unpaid Work, and Stress: New Directions for Research.* Background paper. Ottawa: Canadian Advisory Council on the Status of Women, 1989.

Marshall, C., and G.B. Rossman. *Designing Qualitative Research.* London: Sage Publications, 1989.

McKee, J. "Holistic Health and the Critique of Western Medicine." *Social Science and Medicine* 26, 8 (1988). pp. 775-84.

McLaren, A.T. *Gender and Society: Creating a Canadian Women's Sociology.* Toronto: Copp Clark Pitman Ltd., 1988.

McLeroy, K.R., N.H. Gottlieb and J.N. Burdine. "The Business of Health Promotion: Ethical Issues and Professional Responsibilities." *Health Education Quarterly* 14, 1 (1987). pp. 91-109.

Messing, K. "Women's Occupational Health and Androcentric Science." *Canadian Woman Studies* 14, 3 (1994). pp. 11-6.

— "Occupational Safety and Health Concerns of Canadian Women." Background paper. Ottawa: Women's Bureau, Labour Canada, 1991.

Moore, J.E. *Community Health Nursing in Alberta: Current Manpower and Programs.* Edmonton: Alberta Social Services and Community Health, 1977.

Morrison, P.M. *A Descriptive Study of the Administrative Behavior of Alberta Community Health Nursing Managers.* Unpublished Master's thesis. Edmonton: University of Alberta, 1983.

Neuberger, J.S., A.M. Kammerdiener and C. Wood. "Traumatic Injuries Among Medical Centre Employees." *AAOHN Journal* 36, 8 (1988). pp. 318-25.

North York Department of Public Health. *A Management Study of the Department of Public Health.* North York, Ontario: North York Department of Public Health, 1984.

Northcott, H.C., and G.S. Lowe. "Job and Gender Influences in the Subjective Experience of Work." *Canadian Review of Sociology and Anthropology.* 24, 1 (1987). pp. 117-31.

Orr, J. "We Don't Need Dead Heroines … Aggression and Violence are Everyday Hazards for Health Professionals." *Nursing Times* 84, 36 (1988). p. 22.

Parasuraman, S., and D. Hansen. "Coping with Work Stressors in Nursing." *Work and Occupation* 14, 1 (1987). pp. 88-105.

Patterson, N.B., D.E. Craven, D.A. Schwartz, E.A. Nardell, J. Kasmer and J. Nobe. "Occupational Hazards to Hospital Personnel." *Annals of Internal Medicine* 102 (1985). pp. 658-80.

Perkins, F. "Supportive Environments for Health: The Sundsvall Statement." *Alberta Public Health Association Newsletter* 6 (October 1991). p.6.

Premier's Commission on Future Health Care for Albertans. *The Rainbow Report: Our Vision for Health.* Edmonton: Queen's Printer, 1989.

Province of Alberta. *Occupational Health and Safety Act.* Edmonton: Queen's Printer, RSA, 1980.

— *Public Health Act.* Edmonton: Queen's Printer, RSA, 1984.

Prus, R. "The Interpretive Challenge: The Impending Crisis in Sociology." *Canadian Journal of Sociology* 15, 3 (1990). pp. 355-63.

Renzetti, C.M., and D.J. Curran. *Women, Men, and Society: Sex Segregation on the Job.* Toronto: Allyn and Bacon, 1991.

Reskin, B.F., and H. Hartmann. "Women's Work, Men's Work: Sex Segregation on the Job," in *The Sociology of Gender.* L. Kramer (ed.). New York: St. Martin's Press, 1991.

Robinson, J.C. "Worker Responses to Workplace Hazards." *Journal of Health Politics, Policy and Law* 12, 4 (1987). pp. 665-79.

Rogers, B. "Establishing Research Priorities in Occupational Health Nursing." *AAOHN Journal* 37, 12 (1989). pp. 493-500.

Sass, R. "Workplace Health and Safety: Report from Canada." *International Journal of Health Services* 8, 2 (1986). pp. 213-34.

— "The Implications of Work Organization for Occupational Health Policy: The Case of Canada." *International Journal of Health Services.* 19, 1 (1989). pp. 157-73.

Saunders, E. "Theoretical Approaches to the Study of Women," in *Social Issues: Sociological Views of Canada.* D. Forcese and S. Richer (eds.). Scarborough, Ontario: Prentice-Hall Canada, 1982.

Scott, J.A. "Keeping Women in their Place: Exclusionary Policies and Reproduction," in *Double Exposure,* op. cit.

Selevan, S.G., M.L. Lindbohm, R.W. Hornung and K. Hemminki. "A Study of Occupational Exposure to Antineoplastic Drugs and Fetal Loss in Nurses." *New England Journal of Medicine* 313, 19 (1985). pp. 1173-8.

Shaw, M. "Building Consensus in the '90s." *At The Centre* 9 (1990). p. 3.

Skillen, D.L. *An Organizational Analysis of Work Hazards in Community Health.* Unpublished Ph.D. dissertation. Edmonton: University of Alberta, 1992.

— "Toward a Social Structural Understanding of Occupational Hazards in Public Health." *International Journal of Health Services* (forthcoming).

Stewart, M.J., and M. Arklie. "Work Satisfaction, Stressors and Support Experienced by Community Health Nurses." *Canadian Journal of Public Health* 85, 3 (1994). pp. 180-4.

Stockdale, J.E. "Sexual Harassment at Work," in *Women at Work: Psychological and Organizational Perspectives.* J. Firth-Cozens and M.A. West (eds.). Buckingham: Open University Press, 1991.

Tenove, S.C. *Procedures and Criteria Used by Alberta Health Units in Selecting Community Health Nurses.* Unpublished Master's thesis. Edmonton: University of Alberta, 1981.

Thomas, W.I., and D.S. Thomas. *The Child in America: Behavior Problems and Programs.* New York: Alfred A. Knopf, 1928.

Triolo, P.K. "Occupational Health Hazards of Hospital Staff Nurses. Part I: Overview and Psychosocial Stressors." *AAOHN Journal* 37, 6 (1989a). pp. 232-7.

— "Occupational Health Hazards of Hospital Staff Nurses. Part II: Physical, Chemical, and Biological Stressors." *AAOHN Journal* 37, 7 (1989b). pp. 274-9.

Walby, S. *Theorizing Patriarchy.* Oxford: Basil Blackwell, 1990.

Walcott-McQuigg, J.A., and N.E. Ervin. "Stressors in the Workplace: Community Health Nurses." *Public Health Nursing* 9, 1 (1992). pp. 65-71.

Walters, V. "The Politics of Occupational Health and Safety: Interviews with Workers, Health and Safety Representatives and Company Doctors." *Canadian Review of Sociology and Anthropology* 22, 1 (1985). pp. 57-9.

Weinstein, M.S. "Health Promoting Work." *Canadian Journal of Public Health* 76, Supplement 1 (1985). pp. 52-5.

West, M.A., A. Jones and Y. Savage. "Stress in Health Visiting: A Quantitative Assessment." *Health Visitor* 61, 9 (1988). pp. 269-71.

West, M.A., and Y. Savage. "Stress in Health Visiting: Qualitative Accounts." *Health Visitor* 61, 10 (1988a). pp. 305-8.

— "Coping with Stress in Health Visiting." *Health Visitor* 61, 12 (1988b). pp. 366-8.

Wikler, D. "Who Should be Blamed for Being Sick?" *Health Education Quarterly* 14, 1 (1987). pp. 11-25.

Wineman, S. *The Politics of Human Services: Radical Alternatives to the Welfare State.* Montreal: Black Rose Books, 1984.

Winett, R.A., A.C. King and D.G. Altman. *Health, Psychology and Public Health.* Toronto: Pergman Press, 1989.

Woodcox, V., S. Isaacs, J. Underwood and L.W. Chambers. "Public Health Nurses' Quality of Worklife: Responses to Organizational Changes." *Canadian Journal of Public Health* 85, 3 (1994). pp. 185-7.

World Health Organization, Health and Welfare Canada, and Canadian Public Health Association. "Ottawa Charter for Health Promotion." *Canadian Journal of Public Health* 77, 6 (1986). pp. 425-30.

Yassi, A., and T.L. Guidotti. "Occupational Health Services for Hospital Workers." *Healthcare Management Forum* 3, 3 (1990). pp. 20-2.

Making
Issues
Visible to
Researchers

Rendre les
enjeux visibles
aux milieux de
recherche

Karen Messing

Chicken or Egg

Biological Differences and the Sexual Division of Labour

Cet article examine l'influence des différences biologiques entre les femmes et les hommes sur l'interaction travail-santé. Ces différences sont examinées à même des recherches effectuées à la demande de regroupements de travailleuses. D'abord, le design industriel du milieu de travail se fait souvent en fonction d'un gabarit masculin. Les femmes qui tentent d'utiliser des outils ou de l'équipement trop grands risquent de se blesser. Deuxièmement, les femmes et les hommes sont souvent assignés à des tâches différentes. Quand un emploi expose son titulaire à des risques, on tend à exclure les femmes de cet emploi ou alors on nie l'existence de risques particuliers. Troisièmement, les rôles (biologique et social) des femmes dans la reproduction se distinguent habituellement de ceux des hommes. Les mesures et pratiques en milieu de travail ne tenant pas compte des responsabilités familiales, les femmes y sont désavantagées. Quatrièmement, des conditions physiques ou organisationnelles extrêmement difficiles posent des risques pour les travailleuses comme pour les travailleurs. Mais la division sexuelle du travail tend à occulter certains besoins d'intervention. De plus, elle pose des difficultés d'analyse pour les chercheurs et chercheures, puisqu'elle engendre une sorte de paradoxe. Les conditions de travail et les capacités physiques n'étant pas complètement différenciées selon le sexe, il n'est donc pas approprié d'utiliser le sexe comme unique catégorie d'analyse dans des études en santé au travail. En revanche, comme les milieux de travail et de vie nous poussent à traiter (à tort ou à raison) les deux sexes de façon séparée, il est nécessaire de tenir compte de la variable «sexe» dans de telles études. Afin de découvrir les modes exacts d'interaction entre l'emploi, le sexe et la santé, on a besoin d'une connaissance intime des facteurs en jeu dans les milieux de travail, laquelle peut être acquise par l'observation du travail réel.

This paper asks how biological differences between women and men influence the effects of the workplace on their health. These differences are considered in various ways that are the result of research projects carried out in collaboration with women workers. First, physical design of the workplace is often conceived in relation to the dimensions of male bodies. Women attempting to work with tools and equipment too large for them may be at extra risk. Second, women and men are usually assigned to jobs with different requirements. When a job involves risks, women may be excluded or the risks may be rendered invisible by denial or misrepresentation. Third, women and men have different reproductive roles. Since workplace policies and practices are designed in relation to a lifestyle usually found among males, women may be disadvantaged. Finally, extreme physical or organizational conditions in many jobs create risks for workers of both sexes. The sexual division of labour may distract the attention of practitioners from these risks. In addition, this division creates problems for researchers. Since working conditions and physical capacities do not vary strictly according to gender, it is impossible to treat gender as a simple independent variable in occupational health studies. However, because many employers, workers and families treat the two genders in stereotyped ways, gender cannot be ignored in occupational health research. Discovering the exact ways that gender, job assignments and health interact in the workplace requires intimate knowledge of practices in each workplace, which can only be attained by observing the real work environment.

INTRODUCTION

Once I attended a seminar in occupational health lasting several months. I found myself getting angry quite frequently — whenever I felt that gender was not being taken into consideration in the proper way. Two different situations provoked my wrath: when women were treated separately in analyses; and when women were not treated separately. Afraid I was going insane, I discussed my problem with a friend. Luckily, I chose Margrit Eichler, an expert on feminist research.[1] She explained to me that I was probably right in both cases: I got angry when women were lumped in with men, but it annoyed me when women were treated as though we were intrinsically different from men and functioned in strange, exotic ways. As a geneticist, I am particularly sensitive to false allocation of male/female differences to a genetic component. I have always told my students that it is impossible to unravel genetic and environmental determinants of socially defined characteristics like sex differences.

This confusion is not abstract: it has implications for prevention strategies. If we believe that women and men react very differently to the workplace, we may justify sex-typed task allocation. There are also implications for research. If we think that "sex" is in itself a determinant of health in the same way as tobacco consumption, we will control for sex in relating working condition to health effects.[2] If we think that sex is a surrogate for living or working conditions, we will be forced into more complex analyses.

For example, we at CINBIOSE are in the process of analyzing some data in collaboration with French researchers. In 1987, Marie-Josèphe Saurel-Cu-bizolles and Monique Kaminski and collaborators collected data from inter-views and medical examinations of 878 women and 592 men employed in 17 poultry slaughterhouses and canneries.[3] Among them, women have signifi-cantly more leaves for health problems and work accidents than men (43 percent cf. 33 percent, p <0.001). Table 1 shows some associations between working conditions and medical leave for respiratory problems for women and men.[4] These associations differ by sex: women workers have more problems when the temperature is variable and when they have young children; men have fewer problems when the temperature is variable and do not seem to be affected by the presence of children. As we continue the analysis, we find that the factors associated with respiratory problems in a logistic regression equation differ by sex.

We are interested in knowing why. Is this due to biological differences? There are many differences between men and women's bodies which may cause them to react differently to the same workplace.[5] Women may regulate temperature differently from men. Or is the disparity attributable to the different social roles ascribed to men and women in the home? A large number of studies show that women do most housecleaning, childcare and domestic chores. For example, women in the French study do four times as much housework as men.

These are just two types of male/female differences which can affect health in the workplace. There are many other differences between women and men, in their biology and in their social situation. These can be relative differences such as those relating to height, weight, childcare practices and smoking behavior, or genetically determined absolute dif-ferences such as those concerning the reproductive system. However, what happens in the workplace is an interaction between individuals and their work situation, and women's working conditions also differ from those of men. For example, women in the French study were more likely to do repetitive work, work quickly, work in the cold and have a work station poorly adapted to their size, while men were more likely to lift weights, to work with wet hands, wet feet and wet clothes and to have irregular schedules.[6]

Table 1   Sick Leave for Respiratory Problems Among Poultry Slaughterhouse and Cannery Workers

	Women			Men		
	No sick leave during the year	Took sick leave during the year	Total	No sick leave during the year	Took sick leave during the year	Total
Has children under 6	253	56 (18%)	309	173	20 (12%)	193
Has no children under 6	514	54 (10%)	568	359	40 (10%)	399
Total	767	110	877	532	60	592

For women: $p < 0.001$, chi^2
For men: n.s., chi^2

	Women			Men		
	No sick leave during the year	Took sick leave during the year	Total	No sick leave during the year	Took sick leave during the year	Total
Work temperature constant	490	60 (11%)	550	217	32 (13%)	249
Work temperature variable	276	52 (16%)	328	312	27 (8%)	339
Total	766	112	878	532	60	588

For women: $p < 0.05$, chi^2
For men: $p < 0.05$, chi^2

The relationship between individuals and their work has been represented by ergonomists as a series of complex interactions (Figure 1, drawn from Guérin et al.).[7] According to this representation, occupational illness occurs when there is incompatibility between job demands and the capacities of the person assigned to it. In the following discussion, I will suggest that the sexual division of labour is both a determinant and an effect of this incompatibility. I will use data from our own and other studies to explore the different ways the workplace interacts with men's and women's bodies, jobs and lifestyles.

The argument can be summarized as follows:

Task assignment often represents a prediction about the compatibility of demands and capacities, and task assignments by sex thus result from representations of the capacity of each. In this context, statistical differences between the average woman and the average man are represented in the workplace as norms, sometimes of questionable accuracy, and are used to justify excluding women from jobs entailing a high risk of injury in the short term, while exposing men to a high perceived risk.

Figure 1

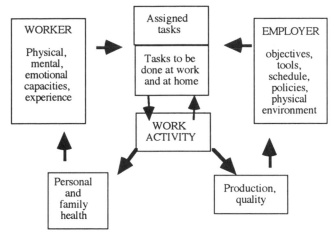

Adapted from: Guérin, F., et al., p. 85, by addition of family responsibilities.

These assignments may not promote health, but they do expose women and men to different health risks. The health risks in women's jobs are usually hidden, both because visible risks are a reason for exclusion and because women's health problems are often ascribed to weakness or hysteria. However, women are often assigned to jobs entailing invisible, long-term risk, including repetitive, boring and tiring work, entailing economic deprivation and material insecurity. The physical demands of women's jobs have not been well characterized, and can be quite heavy.

In addition, the sexual division of labour in paid labour is in itself a risk factor, since it contributes to fragmentation of the labour process and thus to repetitive strain injury and depersonalization of work. By incarnating a sexist view of human capacities, it justifies exposing men to injury and women to low pay and boring, repetitive and taxing working conditions. The sexual division of unpaid labour constitutes another risk factor, since it contributes to an artificial dichotomization of human experience. Both men and women are forced to perform exploits of juggling in order to maintain the fiction that they are constantly available for paid work and that their family responsibilities can be fulfilled no matter what their professional obligations.

These sexual divisions of labour are a response to the fact that many jobs are so exacting that they can only be done by a small proportion of the population with extreme physical or social characteristics: all but the tallest, the most agile or those with no family responsibilities may be excluded de facto. Until jobs are redesigned and the workplace is humanized for all workers, the sexual division of labour appears to many in the workplace as the only reasonable way of avoiding occupational illness, even if its success in health protection cannot be demonstrated.

The current situation creates problems for researchers. Since working conditions and physical capacities do not vary strictly according to sex, it is impossible to treat sex as a simple independent or dependent variable in occupational health studies. However, because many employers, workers and families treat the two genders in stereotyped ways, sex cannot be ignored in occupational health research. Discovering the exact ways that gender, job assignments and health interact in the workplace requires intimate knowledge of practices in each workplace, which can only be attained by contact with the real work environment.

THE SEXUAL DIVISION OF LABOUR AS A REACTION TO PERCEIVED RISK

FIRST OBSERVATION **relating to the sexual division of labour and occupational health:** When a task is perceived to be at risk for injury, there are concerns about men's occupational health, whereas women may be excluded.

Men, Women and Accidents

In Quebec, men have three times as many compensated workplace injuries and illnesses as women.[8] Information from other jurisdictions gives even higher ratios.[9] If we take these data at face value, discounting for the moment the fact that women's occupational health problems have been underreported and undercompensated, they suggest that men are much more apt to be in jobs that are ill-fitted to their capacities.

Anecdotal evidence suggests an explanation. Vilma Hunt,[10] former head of the United States Environmental Protection Agency, tells the story of how men at Three Mile Island indignantly refused her suggestion that they wear lead jock straps when they entered the reactors during the cleanup. Paradoxically, they felt that their masculinity would be threatened if they protected their genitals from radiation.

Similarly, a Canadian train employee was interviewed on the radio after containers holding poisonous materials turned over near a town in the prairies. The town was temporarily evacuated, but the employee explained to the interviewer that he wasn't afraid to participate in the cleanup: "I'm young and strong."

Women also support this view that men should be willing to take risks without fear. Sex-typed jobs in a Quebec textile factory with a 90 percent male workforce were eliminated following the enactment of human rights legislation. Changes in the collective agreement abolished seniority by sex and made all jobs accessible to all workers. A single seniority list replaced the separate male and female lists, and all workers were asked to follow the same career path. These changes coincided with heavy cuts in employment due to automation. Since many of the women's jobs on an assembly line were cut, they found themselves "bumped" to entry-level jobs. One of these jobs involved driving a motorized cart with 10 300-pound (135 kilogram) rolls of fabric. The rolls had to be manipulated onto the cart and the back end of the cart had to be directed manually, with a lever placed in an awkward position. Many women objected to doing this job and were laid off, one by one, until 90 percent of the layoff list was female. The women said that the job was impossible for a woman and demanded restoration of the segregated seniority lists. The union women's committee and the company pointed out in vain that the man who had done this job successfully for the previous two years was five feet three inches (139 cm) tall and weighed 130 pounds (60 kilograms). The women retorted that they would not accept the risk of back problems.

Similar stories are told to us by hospital workers. A woman fought to gain access to a kitchen worker's job, then laid a grievance against lifting the heavy kitchen pots. In many hospital departments, the hospital sets informal guidelines so that a given number of men are on duty at one time to control violent patients or to lift heavy weights.

It seems that a high risk of immediate injury is considered to be acceptable for men but not women. In other words, risk of injury is an occupational health problem for men, but a reason for exclusion of women.[11] Thus, if we accept historical definitions of occupational illness, it appears that men are forced by stereotyping to accept increased risk of acute physical injury. The sexual division of labour then appears to be protective of women's health.

However, feminists question this view, asking whether it is really helpful to exclude women from non-traditional jobs and whether the work assigned to women is truly protective of their health.[12] We must ask whether the sexual division of labour in manual jobs corresponds to the physical capacity of each sex, and thus constitutes an adaptive response to the requirements of the workplace. At CINBIOSE, we have been examining the health effects of women's jobs in segregated workplaces where manual tasks are performed.

THE SEXUAL DIVISION OF LABOUR AS A DETERMINANT OF SPECIFIC RISKS

SECOND OBSERVATION relating to the sexual division of labour and occupational health: Tasks assigned to women are probably responsible for a large number of chronic health problems.

CINBIOSE has been involved in several studies of the sexual division of labour in factory work. Nicole Vézina has described the differing constraints of work in poultry slaughterhouses (see her paper in this book). Lucie Dumais, Ana Maria Seifert, Julie Courville, Nicole Vézina and I have identified elements of women's and men's work in a cookie factory, where men's and women's jobs are very different, as regards the amount of weight lifted and the frequency of movements.[13] We are now characterizing women's and men's jobs in the service sector.

Cleaners

We have studied a cleaning service assigned to suburban trains in France, employing 19 men and 17 women. We recall this study briefly because it has been published.[14] Toilet cleaning by three workers was observed systematically for a total of 10 hours using paper and pencil or Psion Organiser II programmed with the Kronos programme (patented by Alain Kerguelen). We recorded postures, time per lavatory, the state of the lavatory and the state of the water supply. One of the researchers, a physician, conducted health examinations, which were complemented by observations of the work activity and examination of absence and accident data furnished by the company.

RESULTS: The sexual division of labour in itself gave rise to health effects.
There was a rigid sexual division of labour, in which the task of lavatory cleaning was exclusively assigned to women. Interviews and observations revealed a number of physical constraints associated with the work, and particularly with lavatory cleaning, which involved trajectories of over nine miles (20 kilometres) per day and maintaining uncomfortable

postures. Twenty-five percent of time during the actual cleaning was spent in a crouched position. Women employees suffered from many musculoskeletal problems. Men's jobs involved occasional to very occasional lifting of heavy weights and some work accidents had occurred. Older men, however, were assigned to a job (chrome polishing) which required little energy expenditure or force. We concluded that the inability to rotate jobs due to sex-typed job assignment was associated with specific health and safety risks for both sexes, and that the physical cost of women's jobs was undervalued. We also observed that older men were assigned to very easy tasks while older women were forced to clean lavatories, even when they had medical advice saying that the job was too hard for them.

Studies in Progress: Characterizing Risk Factors in Jobs Assigned to Women

We are currently studying cleaners in Quebec hospitals[15] and cleaning done by municipal workers.[16] Céline Chatigny, Julie Courville and I observed cleaning in one hospital.[17] Light work, done primarily by women, involves dusting, cleaning toilets and disinfecting beds. Lifting the end of the bed during disinfection is very difficult; the end weighs 55 pounds (25 kilograms) and tends to block workers' movements. The number of disinfections varies according to the ward and the hospital but can be up to three or four a day. No other especially heavy manipulation is involved, but other constraints involve cramped, bent postures, prolonged scrubbing and high reaching. In several hospitals women have to dust in very awkward positions due to a hospital rule that states: "Women are not allowed to climb stepladders. If a woman climbs a stepladder the hospital's liability insurance no longer applies." The insurance policy may be fictional but the rule is in effect in several hospitals.

Men's cleaning jobs involve mopping floors, operating floor polishers and vacuum cleaners, and sometimes window washing and emptying garbage cans. In one hospital under study, workers of both sexes and supervisors agreed that "light" work was more difficult than "heavy" work. Still, women workers by and large refused to do "heavy work," on the grounds that they did not like to climb ladders, that the mops were too heavy or that the men were hostile to the idea. Both sexes suffered from a relatively high rate of work illnesses and injuries (one worker in four per year is compensated).

The emotional cost of doing cleaning work is also high for both men and women. Workers described the lack of respect they receive as the hardest part of their job. Contempt for cleaners translates into low priority for cleaning equipment, ignorance of cleaning constraints when planning hospital schedules and offensive remarks. One woman described her humiliation when the hospital used its public address system to forbid patients to talk to her, while another explained how she always worked in a dress, stockings and high heels in order to maintain her self-respect. In these circumstances, it is possible that hostility between the sexes is exacerbated by the emotional cost of doing cleaning work.

We are now selecting dimensions on which to analyze "light" and "heavy" cleaning systematically. Our major problem is that none of the grids currently available in ergonomics can be applied, since the task components which make women's jobs difficult remain unrecognized.

For example, we are looking for "objective" correlatives of meticulousness, mentioned by hospital cleaners and municipal cleaners alike as an important characteristic of women's work in cleaning. We will observe the amplitude of movements and the number of times the same surface is gone over. Rubbing and scrubbing incidents will be recorded as indicators of precision.

We are also participating in an attempt to use women's knowledge of their own jobs in order to characterize the work load. In collaboration with the women's committees of the three major Quebec labour unions (the Centrale des Enseignants du Québec, the Confédération des Syndicats Nationaux and Fédération des Travailleurs du Québec), we will be working with bank tellers, secretaries and primary school teachers in order to look at mental, emotional and physical aspects of their work. It will be easier to relate these characteristics to health effects once they have been carefully described and assessed.

THE SEXUAL DIVISION OF LABOUR ENTAILS HEALTH COSTS FOR WOMEN AND MEN

THIRD OBSERVATION: The sexual division of labour may itself constitute a health risk. We have observed that the sexual division of labour assigns different types of risks to women and to men. It supports sexist representations of men's and women's capacities and contributes to perpetuation of risks for both sexes.

In the above examples, the sexual division of labour is part of a system of work organization ("taylorization") which fragments the work process and has its own mental and physical health costs.[18] Ursula Franklin has described other disadvantages of this type of work organization for the workers: loss of control and ownership of the finished product.[19] We would add that the sexual division of labour, by restricting women to few operations, intensifies the repetitive nature of work for women and condemns them to reusing the same muscles and articulations over periods of years.

Most of the costs of repetitive work have been borne by women workers and the struggle for recognition of cumulative trauma disorders has been largely waged by feminist researchers.[20] However, the costs of the sexual division of labour for male workers should not be ignored; as we saw in the first section, they may be forced by stereotyping to incur risks of injury.

FAMILY RESPONSIBILITIES AND OCCUPATIONAL HEALTH

FOURTH OBSERVATION relating to the sexual division of labour and occupational health: The sexual division of unpaid labour is based on differences in reproductive roles but goes beyond biological differences. This division of labour may also contribute to health problems.

The sexual division of labour operates both in the paid workplace and in allocating family responsibilities. Just as the physical requirements of tasks may act to select out workers of a particular size or shape, organizational components of tasks may keep out workers with family responsibilities. Barrère-Maurisson reports that, within a large company, certain functions were always carried out by young, single men, others by married women, still others by older men with non-working wives.[21] In a CINBIOSE study, women in non-traditional municipal jobs were significantly less likely than men to be living with children, possibly due to the difficulty of reconciling family life with extremely irregular work hours.

In the data from the French slaughterhouses and canneries, men average many fewer hours of domestic work than women. On the other hand, men's mean paid work week was two hours longer and they were more apt to have irregular schedules. The health effects of the differing schedules have rarely been examined, although, not surprisingly, Quebec hospital workers who combine a full work week with 20 or more hours of domestic work report more fatigue and insomnia than those doing less domestic work.[22]

Study in Progress

CINBIOSE is currently involved in a study of how men and women with young children balance family responsibilities. Louise Vandelac and

Andrée-Lise Méthot interviewed 23 women and four men about techniques used to balance professional and family responsibilities. This exploratory study is being continued in four workplaces with a combination of methods: survey questionnaire, in-depth interviews and ergonomic analysis.[23] Preliminary results from 23 interviews suggest that, at the birth of a child, company policies and pay differentials make it desirable for women to reduce their hours or take unpaid leave while men work extra hours to make up the difference in pay.[24] Still, the combined paid and unpaid work week of women greatly exceeded that of men.

The researchers are examining the costs of this situation for workers of both sexes. They suggest that current work organization segments human existence into two non-interpenetrating spheres. Workers are expected to leave their desires and needs at the door of the workplace. Their home life is not supposed to affect their capacity to work. In occupational health jurisprudence, a domestic determinant of a health problem is an accepted reason for denial of compensation.[25] The workplace, however, is allowed to impinge on all areas of the workers' lives by requiring shift work, overtime, and schedule irregularities and by inducing fatigue and health symptoms which follow the worker home.[26]

The unequal separation of domestic responsibilities within families has been a response to these extreme demands of the workplace. Currently, the sexual division of labour within the workplace and between workplace and home has been challenged by feminists. This point has been extensively discussed by other writers, has been recently reviewed[27] and will not be further discussed here.

However, this idea that extreme job demands may be a reason to maintain sexual segregation emerges also from a CINBIOSE examination of the sexual division of labour in a workplace during attempts at integration.

THE ESTABLISHMENT OF A SEXUAL DIVISION OF LABOUR IN AN INTEGRATED JOB

FIFTH OBSERVATION **relating to the sexual division of labour and occupational health:** Some jobs are so difficult for women that sex-based task assignments are seen as the only viable solution.

Lucie Dumais, Julie Courville, Ana Maria Seifert, Micheline Boucher and I have collected data on work accidents and job content among blue collar employees of a large Quebec municipality, in which women were being integrated as a result of an equal-opportunity programme. We selected jobs which respected the following criteria: (1) the job involved physical exertion; (2) the job was non-traditional for women, that is, fewer than one-third of workers were women (the Statistics Canada definition); (3) there was at least one work accident in this job during the two-year period beginning on January 1, 1989.

There are a total of 201 job titles, of which women are employed in 22. Two were eliminated from consideration on the basis of the first criterion, one on the basis of the second and five others, involving very few workers, on the basis of the third criterion. The final sample consisted of 14 job titles.

The municipality organizes work in order to profit from maximum flexibility. The permanent employee has a job title, but may be asked to do work corresponding to another job title. The temporary employee may be asked to do work corresponding to any job title for which he or she has qualified. Most women have been hired since 1987 (at the beginning of the affirmative action programme) and have not yet become permanent.

In addition to their job titles, employees are assigned to given activities. Thus, a "cleaner" may be assigned to "maintenance of arenas" or to "cleaning of municipal buildings." The final sample included all 1,589 new accidents in the 14 job titles and 43 activities in 1989-1990.

Table 2 The Number of Accident Claims Filed for 14 Jobs Held by Municipal Workers by Sex and Employment Status, 1989-1990 (from Seifert, Chatigny, Boucher, Dumais, Messing)

	Permanent		Temporary	
	Number (%) of accidents	Number (%) of employees	Number (%) of accidents	Number (%) of employees[1]
Women	40 (6.1)	97 (4.9)	74 (32.2)	239 (39.3)
Men	619 (93.9)	1808 (95.1)	156 (67.8)	369 (60.7)
Total	659 (100.0)	1905 (100.0)	230 (100.0)	608 (100.0)

[1]Number of employees nominally assigned to the 14 job titles.

RESULTS: **Women's accidents were not randomly distributed.** Women temporary workers were underrepresented among accident victims (Table 2). However, calculating denominators for accident claims posed problems, since no figures were available for the number of hours people actually worked. Women generally were less senior than men, and temporary women workers probably worked fewer hours than men.[28] Thus, we could not tell by simple examination of statistics whether the accident rates differed by sex, although some differences appeared in types of accidents; women gardeners may have had more accidents where excessive effort was involved.

Interviews

The likelihood that women and men differed in regard to occupational accidents and health symptoms was explored in interviews. Sixty women holders of the 14 job titles were randomly selected; half of them were temporary workers. They were paired with the 30 permanent and 30 temporary male workers, hired at the date closest to the date at which the women had been hired, with the same job title. Workers were interviewed by one of three interviewers, all women, using a questionnaire covering various aspects of the work and of the domestic situation. Workers were also asked to describe all tasks done during the previous work week and to indicate on an outline of the human body the sites of pain and fatigue felt at the end of the workday during the previous week. In order to determine whether members of a pair did the same tasks, the task descriptions were compared. Workers were asked to describe physical difficulties with their jobs. In order to decide which member of a pair had more physical difficulty with the job, a person who had not participated in the interviews compared blindly the number of difficulties reported by each member of a pair.

Seven workers were: no longer employed by the city (three); on long-term leave (two); could not be contacted (one); or refused (one). Fifty-eight women and 55 men comprised the final sample. Of these, there were seven unpaired workers and 53 pairs. The average age for women was 34.5 years, and for men, 34.6.

Results: **The sexual division of labour was re-established in these jobs.** The most surprising finding was that we had not succeeded in finding women and men who did the same jobs by our technique of pairing people hired with the same job title at the same time. At the time of the interview (about six years after hiring), 19 of the 53 pairs of men and women were no longer assigned to the same jobs. Males in the final sample were assigned to 20 jobs and females to 14. Even among the 34 "true" pairs who held the same job title, only half gave similar job descriptions.

Workers were also specifically asked whether, in their teams, men and women were assigned to the same tasks. Because the workforce was overwhelmingly male, many men did not have any women in their work teams and could not answer the question. When the women's responses were considered, over half (27/52) of the women who answered reported that they did not do the same tasks as their male colleagues. The reasons given were varied: choice of the supervisor, the team or the individual, or lack of appropriate-sized equipment. The principle used to constitute this sexual division of labour was characterized in two ways: 10 women (mostly cleaners) said women did work which required more care or which had to be done to a higher standard and 17 (mostly gardeners) said that men did the jobs requiring more physical strength. According to interviews with both women and men gardeners reporting a sexual division of labour, women were more likely to do weeding and planting and pruning bushes. Men were more likely to do "heavier" tasks such as pushing loaded wheelbarrows uphill, pruning trees and using forks and picks. Men were also more likely to use machines such as the cultivator.

Thus, many of the 50 percent of workers who reported a sexual division of labour suggested that a reason for this was an attempt to assign workers to tasks appropriate for their body type. Among gardeners (the group who reported their work to be the most physically strenuous), 68 percent of women reported a sexual division of labour. This argument is borne out to some extent by the data on height and physical difficulty (Tables 3a and 3b).

Does the sexual division of labour prevent pain or difficulties with the task? Women in the municipal jobs reported more pain and fatigue than the men. Overall the 58 women reported 216 pain and fatigue sites after work compared to 160 for the 55 men (3.7 sites/person cf. 2.9). Six women (10 percent) and 13 men (24 percent) reported no symptoms of pain or fatigue. Gardeners reported the most pain: 76 percent of women and 67 percent of men reported some pain after work, with women averaging twice as many pain sites as men.

Among the 18 pairs where both members had the same job title and were assigned to roughly similar tasks, the woman often reported more physical difficulties and pain and fatigue symptoms than the man (Table 4). However, some of these symptoms were attributed to inappropriate equipment; for example, several women complained of sore feet from badly fitting work boots and sore hands from too-large secateurs, while no men complained of sore hands or feet. Thus, redesign of equipment might make it easier for women to do these jobs.

Table 3a   Height of Municipal Blue Collar Workers Interviewed

Sex (N)	Mean Height	% <73" (161 cm)	% >80" (176 cm)
Women (58)	73" (161 cm)	53%	0%
Men (55)	80" (176 cm)	0%	50%

Table 3b   Physical Difficulty According to Height Among Municipal Workers

	% of Women <73" (161 cm) N=30	% of Women ≥73" (161 cm) N=27	% of Men <80" (176 cm) N=27	% of Men ≥80" (176 cm) N=27
Reports difficulty handling weights	33	37	33	15

Table 4   Physical Difficulties and Number of Sites of Pain and Fatigue Reported by Paired Men and Women Doing the Same Tasks

	Number of "true" pairs where …		
	… the woman reports more problems	… the woman and the man report equal numbers of problems	… the man reports more problems
What do you find physically difficult?	7	10	1
Number of symptoms of pain and fatigue?	11	4	2

Pain and fatigue sites were distributed differently over the body, with women reporting proportionately more pain in the upper limbs (Table 5, $chi^2 = 8.78$, $p < 0.001$ comparing men and women with and without upper limb pain). It is possible that the excess upper limb pain among women is due to the fact that sexual dimorphism in lifting capacity is greatest for the upper limbs. But it is also possible that the tasks assigned to women imposed a greater strain on their arms. One thing is clear: Sex-typed job assignments based on physical capacity did not appear to be protective, since women reported about the same overall amount of pain whether or not they had sex-typed job assignments.

Table 5 Pain Sites Reported by Male and Female Workers in a Municipality

	N	Number (%1) reporting pain, any site	Number (%) with pain in upper limbs	Number (%) with pain in lower limbs	Number (%) with pain in back	Number (%) with pain in other sites
Gardeners						
Women	25	19 (76%)	8 (32%)	6 (24%)	13 (52%)	4 (16%)
Men	18	12 (67%)	1 (6%)	6 (33%)	8 (44%)	2 (11%)
Total Sample						
Women	58	39 (67%)	125 26%)	12 (21%)	28 (48%)	4 (7%)
Men	55	27 (49%)	3 (5%)	10 (18%)	17 (31%)	9 (16%)

[1]Percentages do not add to 100% because individuals reported multiple symptoms.

We cannot decide in this instance whether sexual dimorphism disqualifies women from the full range of tasks involved in gardening. We can, however, observe that both women and men find gardening extremely difficult. Micheline Boucher is currently observing gardening tasks to see how they can be made easier. She found, for example, that a short worker used her spade in an awkward position because it was too tall for her to grasp it easily.[29]

It is difficult to study selective effects by workplace-based research techniques, since the excluded workers disappear from the study sample. However, we suspect that there may be selective effects operating against women workers in the municipality.

These may not be confined to the physical aspects of the job, but may also include organizational constraints. In interviews, temporary workers complained of the difficulty of adapting to constantly varying work schedules and work areas, since they could be assigned to any part of the city. Women were much more likely to mention schedules as a difficult aspect of their task (16 percent of women cf. 6 percent of men), and 42 percent of women mentioned having had trouble in obtaining daycare. Among the workers who were interviewed, only 29 percent of the women lived in couples compared to 43 percent of the men, which could be a result of selection. In this sense, the preferential allocation of women to part-time work in Canada (75 percent of part-time workers are women) is a response to the difficulties of balancing work with family responsibilities in the absence of adequate provisions for childcare and housework.

These results suggest that perpetuation of the sexual division of labour may be a response to heavy physical and organizational requirements, compounded by tools and equipment ill adapted to the bodies of average women. At the same time, this division does not appear to solve the problem, since the tasks assigned to women do not seem to protect them from health problems.

EXTREME CONDITIONS IN THE WORKPLACE MAY FAVOUR PERPETUATION OF A SEXUAL DIVISION OF LABOUR

We observed in several studies that the sexual division of labour is current in jobs with a manual component and in allocation of domestic tasks. We note that there is heavy resistance to change in this situation. We attribute some of this resistance to selective forces operating in the workplace: physical and organizational constraints which exclude the average woman's body or lifestyle. We suggest that the sexual division of labour may be a not-so-inappropriate response to excessive requirements of some workplaces.

We do not know whether there would be excess health costs if the "average" woman persisted in doing the tasks done by men in factories; women in non-traditional jobs with no change in task requirements are a small, highly selected group. But neither do we know whether men would be "fit" to do the high-speed repetitive tasks done by women, followed by evenings and weekends occupied by domestic tasks. The concept of fitness has been limited to women's attempts to enter non-traditional fields. Perhaps because job applications have been lacking, no attention has been paid to the fitness of men to do women's traditional work.[30] The concept of physical strength, for example, usually includes weightlifting rather than work speed. Endurance may be a requirement for women who combine a long, paid work day with long hours of childcare and domestic work, but this has not been studied.

One anecdote may illustrate these issues. In a poultry processing plant, both women workers and the employer objected when we suggested that the women could do some of the heavier jobs assigned to men. They agreed that the women could do the jobs, but pointed out that the jobs assigned to women would also have to be desegregated. All present agreed that men would not be able to do the inspecting and sorting jobs and that women would just have to do them over again. Talk of integrating women into men's jobs was abandoned.

Thus, people in the workplace agreed that some jobs are beyond the capacity of most men or most women. In biological terms, some jobs are situated in the non-overlapping portions of the curves of male and female abilities. However, when constraints are sufficient to exclude one sex, they are often at the limit of the capacity of the other. In the municipal jobs, only the largest workers found the job to be within their capacity. In hospitals, men have complained that the jobs women escape by virtue of their sex pose just as many problems for men.

In fact, many jobs done by both sexes appear to require extreme physical exploitation: the 26,000 pounds (12,000 kilograms) per day handled by the postal workers; the 7,800 cookie packages per day of the assembly line workers. Organizational constraints can be similarly exaggerated: Only 15 percent of French slaughterhouse workers know at the beginning of work the time at which they will finish;[31] the municipal workers do not know where they will be working from one week to the next. Quebec women with young children average 72 hours per week of combined domestic and professional work.[32]

We must ask whether, in some industries, employers have an economic interest in maintaining jobs close to the human limit. Nicole Vézina[33] tells of the package sorting plant that installed soundproofing only until the legal limit of 90 decibels was attained and then stopped, although only half the conveyors were soundproofed. We were consulted by a group of cleaners who were forced to carry their vacuum cleaners in harnesses on their backs while cleaning stairs and hallways on the night shift: The weight of 12 pounds (5 kilograms), the 105° F (40° C) temperature of the exhaust (expelled onto the back) and the noise of 89.6 decibels were all within the limits of legality even though the cumulative effect was exhaustion.[34]

Such extremely difficult working conditions may reinforce the sexual division of labour by making it appear to be the only way for women to protect themselves. But this does not mean that sex-typed job assignments protect women's health. They appear on the contrary to confine women in tasks with specific risks to their mental and physical health.

SOLUTIONS
Integrating Jobs Traditionally Held by Men

Two types of solutions have been proposed for the integration of women into non-traditional jobs with a strong physical component. One is pre-employment testing, to make sure that only the strongest women and those most able to do the job are hired (see paper by Stevenson, in this book). But the philosophy of pre-employment screening must also be questioned. Fitness is a static concept which does not take into account the workers' capacity to change or adapt their jobs. Neither does it take into account that, where sexism is not a problem, many workplaces succeed in finding places for a variety of physical types. Places for older or shorter men have always been found in factories where there is a tradition of retaining workers. In an era of high unemployment, severely selective screening may be feasible. But this approach does nothing to counter the effects of extreme job conditions on even the strongest workers. It reinforces the sexual division of labour over the long run, by supporting rigid job definitions.

The second solution is to change the workplace so that more jobs can be done without risk to health. This "ideal" solution would include attention to organizational parameters such as fragmentation of the work process and humanistic scheduling as well as task height, equipment and tools. For this type of solution to receive support in the workplace, research would have to demonstrate its feasibility and demand for change would have to be strong. Also, costs of perpetuating the present situation would have to be calculated.

One type of change can often be introduced at little or no cost, however. Women entering a new job can be encouraged to develop new ways to do the job which respect their physical parameters. For example, Quebec ambulance drivers found that it was better to work in single-sex teams because women tended to lift stretchers in two movements (floor to knees, knees to waist) while men did it all at once; mixed teams had a tendency to roll the patient off the stretcher while lifting. In another study, a mechanic found that a longer wrench permitted her to tighten bolts more quickly than the wrench used by her taller colleague.[35] Thus, treating the body and the work environment as dynamic rather than static components of work activity may lead to new approaches to the question of "fitness" of each sex to do jobs usually held by the other.

Gender-inclusive Analysis

If we return to the original question — how to do gender-inclusive research in occupational health — we see that analyses of occupational risk are not easy, in the face of complex relationships among sex, biology, job assignment and working conditions. In order to analyze workplace forces in a gender-sensitive way, we must rid our minds of several well-entrenched assumptions: that risk is a reason for exclusion of women but not men from workplaces; that biology is an important determinant of fitness for work; that there is only one good way to do a task; that women's traditional tasks in the home and the workplace are easy; that occupational health problems be recognized as such only under the impossible condition that there be no interaction between the workers' problems and their extraprofessional lives. We must take into account the effects of tasks assigned to each sex, possible poor adaptation of working conditions to the specificities of one sex or the other, selective effects, and family responsibilities as well as biological differences.

Simply comparing the sexes or controlling for sex is not adequate to take into account the very different realities of each. Since working conditions are different for the two sexes in the same job, comparisons may be inappropriate. Since working conditions and physical capacities do not vary strictly according to sex, it is impossible to treat sex as a simple independent variable in occupational health studies. Controlling for sex is one inappropriate way to treat sex as a determinant of health in itself rather than a surrogate for exposure (see paper by Mergler, in this book).

Figure 2

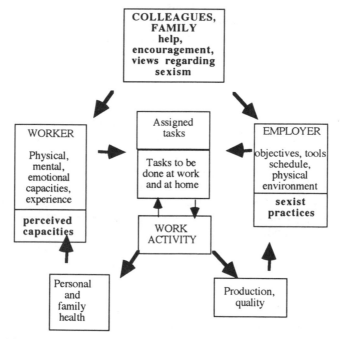

Adapted from: Guérin, F., et al., p.85, by addition of family responsibilities.

One way of being sure that sex is treated appropriately is to pay a great deal of attention to characterizing exposure. If all the components of workplace exposure are taken into account, sex will not be treated as a surrogate for exposure. However, it is also necessary to know more about the effects of other components of women's lives, such as the double work day.

Once all this groundwork has been done, the only sex-specific problems which should be left are reproductive effects such as cycle irregularity and dysmenorrhea. However, because many employers, workers and families treat the two genders in stereotyped ways, sex cannot be ignored in occupational health research. Sexism is an unidentified factor which confuses the interaction between worker's bodies and work activity (Figure 2). Discovering the exact ways in which gender, job assignments and health interact in the workplace requires intimate knowledge of practices in each workplace, which can only be attained by contact with the real work environment.

ACKNOWLEDGEMENTS

I am grateful for support from the Social Sciences and Humanities Research Council of Canada, from the Equality Fund of Labour Canada, from the Conseil Québécois de la recherche sociale and from the Institut de recherche en santé et en sécurité du travail du Québec. I thank Lucie Dumais for her helpful comments.

NOTES

1. Eichler, M., *Non-sexist Research Methods: A Practical Guide*, (Winchester, Mass.: Allen and Unwin, 1987).

2. Donna Mergler will discuss controlling for sex in a subsequent paper.

3. The methods and many results are presented in Saurel-Cubizolles, M-J, M. Bourgine, A. Touranchet and M. Kaminski, *Enquête dans les abattoirs et les conserveries des régions Bretagne et Pays-de-Loire, Conditions de travail et santé des salariés, Rapport à la Direction Régionale des Affaires Sanitaires et Sociales des Pays-de-Loire*, (Villejuif, France: INSERM Unité 149, 1991).

4. These are from unpublished data collected by Marie-Josèphe Saurel-Cubizolles and Monique Kaminski of INSERM Unité 149, Paris, which we are analyzing in collaboration with them. We are grateful for technical help from France Tissot and Marie-Aude Le Berre.

5. Messing, K., *Occupational Health and Safety Concerns of Canadian Women: A review/Santé et sécurité des travailleuses: un document de base*, (Ottawa: Labour Canada, 1991); Courville, J., "Les obstacles ergonomiques à l'intégration des femmes dans les postes traditionnellement masculins," Masters Thesis, (Montreal: UQAM, 1990).

6. Saurel-Cubizolles et al., op. cit.; Le Berre, M-A, "Etude des conditions et des arrêts de travail dans les abattoirs de volaille et des conserveries," Status Report, (Montreal: CINBIOSE and Département de Statistique, IUT Vannes, 1993). This analysis is based on data from Saurel-Cubizolles et al.

7. Guérin, F., A. Laville, F. Daniellou, F. Duraffourg and A. Kerguelen, *Comprendre le travail pour le transformer,* (Montrouge, France: Éditions de l'ANACT, 1991).

8. Laurin, G., *Féminisation de la main d'oeuvre: Impact sur la santé et la sécurité du travail,* (Montreal: Commission de la santé et de la sécurité du Québec, 1992).

9. Bell, C.A, N.A. Stout, T.R. Bender, C.S. Conroy, W.E. Crouse and J.R. Myers, "Fatal Occupational Injuries in the United States, 1980 through 1985," *Journal of the American Medical Association* 263 (1990), pp. 3047-50; Cone, J.E, D. Makofsky and R. Harrison, "Fatal Injuries at Work in California," *Journal of Occupational Medicine* 33 (1991), pp. 813-7; Hough, A., "Comparison of Losses due to Accidents Reported by Males and Females," *Journal of Occupational Health and Safety* (Aust., N.Z.) 5 (1989), pp. 237-42; Laurin, G., op. cit.; Robinson, J.C., "Trends in Racial Equality and Inequality and Exposure to Work-related Hazards, 1968-1986," *AAOHN Journal* 37 (1989), pp. 56-63.

10. Personal communication.

11. In the past, the higher pay men received for sex-segregated jobs compensated them for the risk of injury. When the pay differential is abolished, we hear men ask "Why should I be treated like a beast of burden?"

12. Armstrong, P., and H. Armstrong, *Theorizing Women's Work,* (Toronto: Garamond Press, 1991), Chapter 1.

13. Dumais, L., K. Messing, A-M Seifert, J. Courville and N. Vézina, "Make Me a Cake as Fast as You Can: Determinants of Inertia and Change in the Sexual Division of Labour of an Industrial Bakery," *Work, Employment and Society* 3 (1993), pp. 363-82.

14. Messing, K., C. Haëntjens and G. Doniol-Shaw, "L'invisible nécessaire: l'activité de nettoyage des toilettes sur les trains de voyageurs en gare," *Le travail humain* 55 (1992), pp. 353-70; Messing, K., G. Doniol-Shaw and C. Haëntjens, "Sugar and Spice: Health Effects of the Sexual Division of Labour Among Train Cleaners," *International Journal of Health Services* 23 (1993), pp. 133-46.

15. Messing, K., C. Chatigny and A-M Seifert, "L'entretien 'sanitaire' l'est-il pour les gens qui l'assurent? Une démarche collective en ergonomie," *ACFAS* 61 (1993), p. 360.

16. Seifert A-M, C. Chatigny, M. Boucher, L. Dumais and K. Messing, "L'entretien ménager, métier non-traditionnel pour les femmes," *ACFAS* 61 (1993), p. 125.

17. Chatigny, C., J. Courville and K. Messing, "Projet de l'institut de cardiologie de Montréal/UQAM sur l'entretien sanitaire, rapport et recommandations," 1994.

18. Lowe, G.S., and H.C. Northcott, *Under Pressure: A Study of Job Stress,* (Toronto: Garamond Press, 1986); Vinet, A., M. Vézina, C. Brisson and P-M Bernard, "Piecework, Repetitive Work, and Medicine Use in the Clothing Industry," *Sociology of Science and Medicine* 28 (1989), pp. 1283-8; Brisson, C., A. Vinet, M. Vézina and S. Gingras, "Effect of Duration of Employment in Piecework on Severe Disability Among Female Garment Workers," *Scandinavian Journal of Work, Environment and Health* 15 (1989), pp. 329-44.

19. Franklin, U., *The Real World of Technology,* (Toronto: CBC Enterprises, 1990).

20. Punnett, L., J.M. Robins, D.H. Wegman and W.M. Keyserling, "Soft Tissue Disorders in the Upper Limbs of Female Garment Workers," *Scandinavian Journal of Work, Environment and Health* 11 (1985), pp. 417-25; Silverstein, B.A, L.J. Fine and T.J. Armstrong, "Occupational Factors and Carpal Tunnel Syndrome," *American*

Journal of Industrial Medicine 11 (1987), pp. 343-58; Stock, S., "Workplace Ergonomic Factors and the Development of Musculoskeletal Disorders of the Neck and Upper Limbs: A Meta-analysis," *American Journal of Industrial Medicine* 19 (1991), pp. 87-107.

21. Barrère-Maurisson, M-A, *La division familiale du travail: La vie en double*, (Paris: PUF, 1992).

22. Tierney, D., P. Romito and K. Messing, "She Ate not the Bread of Idleness: Exhaustion is Related to Domestic and Salaried Work of Hospital Workers in Quebec," *Women and Health* 6 (1990), pp. 21-42.

23. Messing, K., "L'application d'une méthodologie ergonomique à la conciliation des responsabilités professionnelles et familiales," communication at the 61st annual meeting of the Association canadienne française pour l'avancement des sciences. To be published in Corbeil, Christine, and Francine Descarries (eds.), *Cahiers de recherches féministes*.

24. Vandelac, L., and A-L Methot, *Concilier l'inconciliable*, (Montréal: Fédération des travailleuses du Québec, 1993).

25. Nicole Vézina tells for example of the woman with shoulder problems which were attributed not to her repetitive task, but to the fact that her cupboard shelves at home were too high. Industrial deafness cases invoke the worker's ski-doo or presence at a disco as reasons to deny compensation.

26. Workers are not compensated for loss of quality of life due to symptoms, only for illnesses and injuries.

27. Armstrong, P., and H. Armstrong, *Theorizing Women's Work*, (Toronto: Garamond Press, 1991).

28. Note that this points up a general problem in accident statistics for women: accidents are rarely calculated per number of hours worked, but rather by the number of workers. Male/female comparisons may underestimate women's accident rates because of this. This point is discussed in detail in Messing, K., J. Courville, M. Boucher, L. Dumais and A-M Seifert, "Can Accident Rates be Compared by Gender?" *Safety Science* 18 (1994), pp. 95-112.

29. We have previously observed other situations where task dimensions posed special difficulties for women's bodies. In a post office, women appeared to suffer many more work accidents in a job where workers handled packages weighing a total of 26,000 pounds (12,000 kilograms) per day, at a speed of one two-pound (900-gram) package every three seconds. The work station imposed an extra burden on shorter workers, who had to handle the packages with the shoulder joint quite extended. The proportion of women in this job decreased with seniority, possibly due to a selective effect operating against shorter workers. (Courville, J., N. Vézina and K. Messing, "Analyse des facteurs ergonomiques pouvant entraîner l'exclusion des femmes du tri des colis postaux," *Le travail humain* 55 (1992), pp. 119-34.)

30. This situation appears to be changing with the rise in unemployment among young men. Women's committees complain that men are moving into assembly line jobs usually held by women.

31. Le Berre, M-A, *Étude des conditions et des arrêts de travail dans des abattoirs de volaille et des conserveries*, (Montreal: CINBIOSE, 1993). Report of a project in collaboration with INSERM Unité 149.

32. Vandelac et Méthot, op. cit.

33. Personal communication.

34. Report submitted by a consulting firm to the Quebec Health and Safety Commission, 1992.

35. Courville, J., N. Vézina and K. Messing, "Analysis of Work Activity of a Job in a Machine Shop Held by Ten Men and One Woman," *International Journal of Industrial Ergonomics 7* (1991), pp. 163-74.

Catherine Teiger

Les barrières cachées à l'intégration sécuritaire des femmes au travail

"Mental barriers" are important "hidden obstacles" to the safe integration of women into the workplace. Because they are hidden, these barriers may be harder to eradicate than physical, technical or even social barriers. This paper argues that the ergonomic analysis of work may serve to deconstruct some of these hidden obstacles. As a starting point, two major assumptions about health and work should be borne in mind. First, safety and health need to be seen as dynamic, a basis for the full development of the individual. Second, work is composed of official duties as well as unofficial, unaccounted-for tasks and skills. The latter refer to the mental or cognitive activity deployed daily by the worker. These are seldom recognized as important by supervisors or, often, by the workers themselves. Such non-recognition seems to be more common in women's jobs (for instance, in clerical work or in quality control jobs). As a result, risks to women's health are overlooked. These risks are likely to unduly augment "muscular fatigue" and lead to "nervous fatigue," as well as professional or personal devaluation. Ergonomics can help to reveal hidden demands on workers but, as shown through a brief history of ergonomics in France, this does not guarantee social recognition of mental work. Ergonomists and trade unionists may gain support for this recognition by working together. However, ergonomic analysis sometimes raises questions about traditional union practices, especially as these concern gender relations.

Quand on parle de «barrières cachées» à l'intégration sécuritaire des femmes au travail, on fait généralement référence aux «barrières mentales». Parce qu'elles sont cachées, elles peuvent être plus difficiles à éliminer que les obstacles physiques, techniques ou sociaux. Nous suggérons que l'analyse ergonomique du travail permet de déconstruire certaines de ces barrières cachées. Deux postulats fondent notre argumentation. D'abord, tel que suggéré par l'OMS et C. Dejours, le travail et la santé sont conçus comme dynamiques, à la base du développement intégral de l'individu. Ensuite, le travail n'est pas seulement ce qu'on en dit officiellement dans une description de tâches; il se compose aussi de nombreuses procédures, activités et qualifications qui restent implicites. Ces dernières font justement référence aux activités «mentales» ou «cognitives» déployées par les travailleurs et travailleuses, bien qu'elles soient rarement prises en compte comme telles par les contremaîtres ou par les travailleurs eux-mêmes. Cette «invisibilité», cette «non-reconnaissance», semble plus aiguë dans les emplois féminins (par exemple, le travail clérical ou le contrôle de qualité). Il se pourrait donc que les risques à la santé des femmes au travail ne soient pas pris en compte adéquatement. Cela entraînerait une augmentation de la «fatigue musculaire» et déclencherait également un processus de «fatigue nerveuse», et contribuerait, aussi, à la dévalorisation personnelle et professionnelle des femmes. L'ergonomie peut mettre au jour les exigences cachées du travail des femmes. Bien que l'ergonomie ne garantisse pas à elle seule la reconnaissance sociale du travail mental, tel que nous le décrivons brièvement pour le cas de la France, ergonomes comme syndicalistes pourraient bénéficier d'une mise en commun de leurs travaux et objectifs. En revanche, gardons à l'esprit que l'analyse ergonomique peut aller jusqu'à remettre en question certaines pratiques traditionnelles des syndicats, notamment dans leurs rapports avec les hommes et les femmes.

INTRODUCTION

Puisque le titre général de ce colloque est *Les barrières sociales, techniques et physiques à l'intégration sécuritaire des femmes au travail* et que j'avais proposé, dans un premier temps, de parler des exigences cachées du travail et de la façon dont les femmes y faisaient face, mon intervention portera plutôt, en associant les deux idées, sur *les barrières cachées à l'intégration sécuritaire des femmes au travail*. J'entends par là, *les barrières mentales* qui sont encore plus difficiles à éliminer, parfois, que les barrières sociales, techniques et physiques, par ce fait même qu'elles sont cachées, et ce dans tous les sens du terme. J'essayerai de montrer en quoi l'analyse ergonomique du travail peut servir — du moins on l'espère! — à déconstruire certaines de ces barrières.

On considérera ici que «l'intégration sécuritaire» se réfère aux relations travail-santé, la santé étant prise au sens large (santé physique, mentale et sociale, selon la fameuse définition de l'Organisation Mondiale de la Santé, en 1947), et envisagée plutôt comme un idéal à atteindre dans une optique de développement des individus (Dejours, 1993), c'est-à-dire comme un processus dynamique plutôt que comme un état à conserver.

Mais avant d'entrer dans le vif du sujet, je voudrais dire combien je suis heureuse d'être ici aujourd'hui et de poursuivre ainsi des relations déjà anciennes avec le Québec qui m'ont amenée, en particulier, à travailler il y a une dizaine d'années, à l'Institut de recherches appliquées au travail de Montréal (IRAT), avec la sociologue Colette Bernier, que plusieurs parmi vous connaissent. Nous avons travaillé, en tentant d'associer la démarche sociologique et la démarche ergonomique, sur un projet général consistant à analyser quels étaient — à l'époque, en 1984-85 — les effets de l'informatisation sur la qualification des employés dans le secteur tertiaire (Bernier, 1990; Bernier et Teiger, 1985a, b et c; 1987; 1988; 1990a et b; Teiger et Bernier, 1990; 1991; 1992). Comme toutes les recherches menées à l'IRAT, celle-ci avait été réalisée avec la participation des organisations syndicales des secteurs concernés. Une des études avait porté, par exemple, avec la Centrale de l'Enseignement du Québec (CEQ), sur des employés de soutien de l'Université du Québec à Montréal (UQAM) (registraire, bibliothèque, etc.). Cette recherche a grandement contribué à l'élaboration des réflexions présentées ici. Je prendrai donc des exemples tirés de ces études dont certains résultats, je crois, restent d'actualité bien qu'ils datent d'une dizaine d'années.

J'aimerais aussi préciser qu'il était important que Danièle Kergoat parle en premier, car le point de vue sociologique donne un cadre général qui permet de mettre en perspective les phénomènes. Ce qui est spécialement précieux pour nous, ergonomes, qui nous attachons à l'analyse de situations particulières et avons, de ce fait, des difficultés à savoir ce qui est généralisable ou pas dans nos résultats. Il est donc très important pour les ergonomes, afin de bien situer leur travail dans son contexte, de travailler directement avec des sociologues ou, du moins, de se tenir au courant de leurs recherches.

Enfin, je tiens à mentionner que mes recherches n'ont pas porté uniquement sur le travail des femmes, et cela volontairement. Non par volonté d'avoir un point de vue universel sur le travail, ce que je ne crois pas possible, mais par volonté de chercher à la fois ce qui est commun aux situations des travailleurs, qu'ils soient hommes ou femmes, et ce qui est différent, dû au fait que des problèmes communs prennent parfois des formes effectivement différentes ou sont présents à des degrés divers dans les situations de travail selon que ce sont des hommes ou des femmes qui sont concernés, ou dû au fait qu'il s'agisse de problèmes spécifiques aux uns ou aux autres.

METTRE EN ÉVIDENCE LES BARRIÈRES CACHÉES
Le travail: de quoi parle-t-on? Mythes et/ou réalités?

En premier lieu, je voudrais rappeler qu'il y a travail et travail — ce qui est maintenant une banalité parmi les ergonomes — et que le travail conçu par les ingénieurs, prévu par les organisateurs, imaginé par les entrepreneurs, en général, n'est jamais celui que les salariés réalisent à leur poste de travail. Le travail à faire (souvent dénommé «la tâche») comporte des exigences dont une bonne partie est inapparente pour qui les considère de l'extérieur, mais auxquelles les travailleurs sont confrontés, auxquelles ils doivent faire face en permanence, et dont ils doivent tenir compte dans l'activité qu'ils déploient s'ils veulent l'accomplir. Le premier titre proposé pour cet exposé contenait cette question de savoir comment faire face aux exigences cachées du travail et quelles sont les conséquences, elles aussi souvent cachées — ce qui ne veut pas dire anodines! — de cet état de fait. Cet écart entre le travail théorique, prévu, attendu (la tâche) et le travail tel qu'il est réellement effectué (l'activité concrète) est inéluctable, il existe partout, pour tout le monde, dans toutes les situations de travail. Qu'il s'agisse des situations prétendument les plus élémentaires telles que le travail à la chaîne, répétitif et parcellisé des secteurs de la production de masse, que l'on exécute, croit-on, toujours de la même façon ou des situations très sophistiquées telles que le contrôle de processus informatisés, on s'aperçoit, à l'analyse fine, que les exigences du travail réel, concret, sont tout à fait différentes de ce qui a été prévu. Et donc que les travailleurs, qu'ils soient hommes ou femmes, mettent en jeu, de ce fait, un grand nombre de compétences qui, elles non plus, ne sont pas prévues dans les profils d'emploi, par exemple, mais sans lesquelles le travail n'existerait pas, c'est-à-dire ne serait pas fait, sans lesquelles la production ne sortirait pas (Boël et al., 1985; Daniellou et al., 1982; Teiger, 1982; 1993b).

Ce constat fut l'un des premiers résultats issus des études faites dans les entreprises, sur les postes de travail, lorsque — au début des années 1960, en France du moins — les chercheurs ont commencé à sortir des laboratoires. On a pu montrer alors que les idées courantes sur le travail industriel ouvrier, fondées sur ce que le taylorisme avait essayé de faire croire — à savoir que les travailleurs n'avaient pas besoin de leur intelligence pour travailler puisqu'on avait prévu et organisé le travail pour eux, qu'ils avaient juste à faire ce qu'on leur disait de faire et comment on leur disait de le faire et à le répéter de façon identique — n'étaient bien évidemment pas exactes. Elles étaient si peu exactes que, lors des grandes grèves des O.S. (ouvriers spécialisés de la production de masse) — qui ont eu lieu fin des années 1960 — début des années 1970, et dont a parlé

Danièle Kergoat — les premières grandes actions de protestation ont consisté, entre autres, tout simplement à faire «la grève du zèle», c'est-à-dire à appliquer absolument à la lettre les consignes données par l'organisation du travail. Et l'on s'apercevait que très, très vite, les chaînes de production s'arrêtaient ... Ce n'était pas compliqué et c'était très efficace!

Bien qu'il s'agisse là d'une preuve par l'absurde en quelque sorte, cela prouvait bien à quel point, d'habitude, quand le système de production fonctionnait, c'était grâce à tout ce que les travailleurs faisaient sans qu'ils aient théoriquement à le faire, sans que personne ne sache qu'ils le faisaient, hormis les travailleurs eux-mêmes, qui n'en parlaient jamais. Car cela va de soi, pour la plupart des travailleurs, de faire tout ce qui est possible pour que le travail soit fait, et même bien fait! Il s'agit bien, dans ce cas, d'un travail inapparent pour lequel les travailleurs ne sont pas «payés». Ce travail est réalisé grâce au déploiement de cette activité incessante qu'on appelait *activité mentale* à l'époque, qu'on appellerait *cognitive* aujourd' hui; la mise en oeuvre de l'intelligence étant indispensable pour apprécier la situation, au fur et à mesure, déceler les anomalies, les aléas, pallier les incidents, répondre à tout ce qui est imprévu, tout ce qu'il est d'ailleurs et de toute façon impossible de prévoir de façon régulière, contrairement à ce que d'aucuns peuvent rêver ou laisser croire (Teiger et Laville, 1972).

Ces résultats obtenus, d'abord, dans des situations industrielles classiques (travail à la chaîne) puis, moins classiques à l'époque (contrôle de processus), se sont révélés également exacts à propos du travail des employés de bureau. Par exemple, au cours de l'entrevue que nous avions réalisée, C. Bernier et moi, au début de l'étude concernant le travail des employées (femmes) du registraire avec le responsable du service (homme), ce dernier nous avait expliqué que le travail consistait juste à recopier, en les entrant dans l'ordinateur, des données portées sur les dossiers d'inscription des étudiants. Et il nous avait dit : «Pff ! Pourquoi est-ce que vous voulez étudier ce travail-là? Franchement, y a rien là; elles lisent les dossiers, puis "y a qu'à pitonner!" Il n'y a pas de problème !» «Y a qu'à! ...» : cette expression fait une belle carrière dans les discours tout faits sur le travail qui paraît si simple à ceux qui ne le font pas qu'il peut se faire apparemment «sans même y penser». En l'occurrence, le responsable du service estimait que les employées se contentaient d'appuyer sur les touches du clavier quasiment automatiquement! Et nous avons ajouté: «Bon, Y a qu'à pitonner! ... peut-être, mais nous on aimerait voir comment elles pitonnent et aussi pouvoir en parler avec elles». Et pour voir «comment elles pitonnaient», on a commencé par effectuer ce travail nous-mêmes pendant une semaine et nous avons eu bien du mal à y comprendre quelque chose et nous avons fait beaucoup d'erreurs! Et, bien sûr, nous nous sommes aperçues que non seulement il n'y avait pas «qu'à pitonner» mais que les employées connaissaient, en fait, toute l'organisation de l'université, les diplômes, les filières d'enseignement, etc, alors que leur responsable prétendait qu'elles ne savaient rien sur l'organisation de l'enseignement et surtout qu'elles n'avaient besoin de rien savoir pour accomplir leur tâche.

Tout ce que les employées avaient appris, elles l'avaient appris par l'expérience et grâce à l'entraide collective, très importante, questions et réponses fusant et s'entrecroisant continuellement tout au long de la journée, alors qu'en théorie elles n'avaient pas l'autorisation de parler entre elles. Plusieurs mois étaient nécessaires aux nouvelles embauchées pour «se sentir un peu à l'aise» et plusieurs années pour maîtriser à peu près les multiples difficultés du travail. Elles étaient à même, ainsi, de corriger les erreurs que faisaient éventuellement les étudiants sur leurs dossiers d'inscription, ou celles des employées du service en amont, ce qui évitait de retourner les dossiers à ce service et permettait, entre autres, de gagner du temps. Elles avaient acquis, d'elles-mêmes également, et en observant le technicien, des connaissances sur le système informatique et sur les procédures leur permettant de résoudre certains incidents, sans dépendre de la disponibilité du technicien, ce qui non seulement n'était pas prévu, mais n'était pas autorisé! Elles exécutaient ainsi, de fait, tout un travail très qualifié de correction, de contrôle, de réparation qui ne faisait absolument pas partie de leur définition d'emploi et qui était totalement *méconnu*, et par conséquent, *non reconnu* et non rémunéré. Il s'agit bien, dans ce cas, de travail *masqué* dont les réelles exigences et caractéristiques demeurent cachées derrière les barrières mentales (cachées elles aussi) constituées par la représentation faussée de ce travail qu'en ont ceux qui ne le considèrent que de l'extérieur, à partir d'idées *a priori*; à commencer par les responsables hiérarchiques eux-mêmes (Bernier et Teiger, 1990; Teiger et Bernier, 1992).

C'est d'abord ce type de barrières, les barrières mentales, qui s'oppose à l'intégration des femmes, de façon sécuritaire, dans le milieu de travail. Parce que la méconnaissance de ces aspects non visibles du travail, de toute cette part d'activité mentale considérable, car indispensable, quelle que soit la tâche à faire — même si ce n'est pas toujours sous la même forme — souvent fatigante et coûteuse pour les travailleurs et travailleuses ... constitue vraiment une barrière à l'amélioration de la situation. Parce que l'on ne peut pas améliorer quelque chose qui n'existe pas, que cette méconnaissance, d'ailleurs, soit due à l'ignorance ou au refus de reconnaître ces aspects, on ne peut rien transformer tant qu'on ne reconnaît pas l'existence du problème.

Et il faut bien reconnaître que le travail réalisé par la main-d'oeuvre féminine se trouve en bonne place dans ce domaine des représentations faussées, comme le montrent les travaux de sociologues comme D. Kergoat. Le plus grave étant que, parfois, les travailleurs et travailleuses eux-mêmes intériorisent ces représentations erronées de leur travail qui sont dévalorisantes pour eux et fonctionnent aussi chez eux comme des *barrières cachées*, aussi longtemps qu'on n'en parle pas. J'y reviendrai plus loin.

Le premier travail que l'on peut faire, quand on est ergonome, est de mettre au jour cette réalité-là. De la faire exister, tout simplement, en la décrivant et en la faisant reconnaître comme telle par tous les acteurs de la situation étudiée, et, au-delà d'elle, par les acteurs sociaux. Mais cette démarche, qui semble évidente et simple, ne se fait pas toute seule parce qu'on est face au même phénomène que celui dont D. Kergoat a parlé à propos des bagarres qu'il lui a fallu mener pour imposer un point de vue nouveau sur le travail féminin. Rien que pour faire reconnaître la réalité du travail, pour faire admettre cette réalité cachée — j'insiste encore une fois parce qu'évidemment elle n'est pas apparente, on ne voit pas ce qu'il y a dans la tête des gens, on ne voit donc pas tout ce que ça leur demande de réaliser leur travail — il faut mener des batailles, symboliques certes, mais néanmoins de vraies batailles.

Ignorance ou refus de savoir?

Pourquoi est-ce si difficile? Comme je viens de l'indiquer rapidement, il faut bien savoir que, parmi les interlocuteurs concernés par ces questions, certains, non seulement ignorent — ce qui est un moindre mal, car lorsqu'on est ignorant on peut toujours apprendre! — mais refusent de reconnaître l'évidence. Dans ce dernier cas, par contre, il est très difficile d'apprendre et de changer de point de vue! Donc, cette méconnaissance du travail, dans le monde social, est due à la fois à l'ignorance, mais aussi, souvent, au refus de connaître et au refus de savoir ainsi qu'à la dénégation de cette réalité qui dérange. Et, à l'heure actuelle, en raison précisément du contexte socio-économique de l'intensification du travail, de la dégradation des conditions de travail, des problèmes du chômage — les blocages sont encore plus importants.

Depuis les débuts de l'ergonomie en France (dans les années 1960) on a rencontré grosso modo trois phases, dans les réactions des entreprises. Il y a 25 ans, quand les travaux de recherche sur le terrain ont commencé, il s'est effectivement produit, dans les directions d'entreprises, un blocage, un refus de reconnaître beaucoup des résultats mis en évidence par les études. Cette attitude s'explique par la photographie du travail industriel proposée, jugée trop choquante par rapport à la vision taylorienne ambiante, que contestaient vigoureusement, par ailleurs, les organisations syndicales, comme nous l'avons déjà dit. Puis, il en suivit une phase de prise en considération de cette réalité, et même de demande d'aide de la part des entreprises pour transformer des situations critiques et surtout pour mettre en place de façon plus satisfaisante, du point de vue des travailleurs, les situations nouvelles entraînées par l'extension de l'automatisation et surtout par le début de l'informatisation massive; cela afin d'éviter les problèmes sociaux, notamment. Actuellement on a l'impression d'assister à un retour en arrière; c'est-à-dire, de nouveau, à un refus de connaître et de reconnaître la réalité. Peut-être parce qu'elle est trop difficile à prendre en compte, qu'elle remet trop de choses en question. À la limite, on assiste à des situations où règne ce qu'on peut appeler du déni et l'on touche alors, non plus seulement au domaine de l'ergonomie ou de la sociologie, mais à celui de la psychopathologie du travail.

En effet, nos collègues psychopathologues (ou psychodynamiciens) du travail se situent exactement sur ce terrain-là en ce moment; ils cherchent à mettre en évidence comment, dans les lieux de travail, on refuse les réalités et quelles sont les conséquences de ce refus sur les personnes et sur les collectifs de travail (Dejours, 1992). Ces conséquences peuvent aller très loin et être très graves étant donné qu'à chaque niveau de la hiérarchie chacun fait comme s'il n'y avait pas de problèmes ou refuse de les voir et d'en faire état; du coup on ne peut plus les traiter, on ne peut même plus en parler. Ainsi, par exemple, dans des situations à haut risque, là où il y a des dangers vraiment très importants, des dangers physiques qui peuvent être mortels pour les travailleurs et aussi pour l'environnement — comme dans les centrales nucléaires, les usines chimiques — et où il se produit fatalement des incidents, d'inévitables dysfonctionnements techniques, une usure des équipements et du matériel, chacun à son niveau masque les choses. Les ouvriers masquent les problèmes qu'ils rencontrent, et se «débrouillent» pour éviter les problèmes avec leurs supérieurs. Les ingénieurs, de leur côté, savent très bien que les ouvriers cachent des choses, mais font, eux aussi, comme s'il ne se passait rien et ne transmettent rien à la direction. Quant à la direction, au bout de la ligne, on ne sait trop si elle sait ou non ce qui se passe mal à la base, mais en tous les cas, elle fait comme si tout se passait très bien. Ainsi, du haut en bas de la hiérarchie de l'entreprise, chacun est piégé par la consigne implicite et intériorisée: «Il faut que tout baigne dans l'huile!»

Cette expression familière pour dire que tout va bien provient, entre autres, probablement du désir de ne pas affoler les populations environnantes ...

Le mythe de la perfection de la technique et ses conséquences

D'où viennent ces phénomènes? En partie du fait que l'on vit toujours, en France du moins, avec le mythe positiviste (au sens de «croyance dans le progrès») de la perfection de la technique; alors que toutes les études de terrain remettent complètement en question cette vision mythique — et par conséquent mystificatrice — de la réalité: la technique n'est pas parfaite. Mais au lieu de prendre cette constatation comme un principe de réalité à prendre en compte: «la technique n'est pas parfaite? Qu'est-ce qu'on peut faire, justement, pour pallier cela, tant sur le plan technique qu'organisationnel et individuel», on persiste à penser: «la technique est parfaite, elle peut et doit être parfaite» donc on ne fait rien ou peu de choses pour essayer d'imaginer, de prévenir à l'avance les dysfonctionnements techniques sinon par une autre solution technique ou par des avalanches de consignes et procédures. Quand ils surgissent et ne peuvent être attribués à la fameuse «erreur humaine», les dysfonctionnements inévitables sont donc considérés comme des mises en échec des responsables techniques, ce qui est insupportable; à chaque niveau, on fait alors comme si les dysfonctionnements n'existaient pas. Les salariés savent pertinemment qu'ils font «comme si» et cette situation provoque, comme l'ont montré des études récentes de psychopathologie du travail, une souffrance dissimulée et une angoisse très grande portant sur la question de savoir « combien de temps cela va tenir ainsi, et quand cela va-t-il éclater»? Souffrance et angoisse liées à une sorte d'impuissance à agir pouvant conduire certains, dans les cas extrêmes, jusqu'au suicide.

DÉCONSTRUIRE LES BARRIÈRES CACHÉES? LA NÉCESSAIRE COOPÉRATION SYNDICATS — RECHERCHE

Tout ce qui précède soutenait l'idée que les barrières sont d'abord et surtout dans la tête des individus. Il est de notre devoir de scientifiques d'essayer de les déconstruire, mais il faut d'abord admettre que ce sont de vraies barrières. Peut-on les déconstruire? Comment passer outre?

Il s'agit là d'un sujet de discussion que l'on peut avoir entre chercheurs et syndicalistes; sur ce terrain-là, à mon avis, nous sommes vraiment dans le même combat, bien qu'à des places et avec des fonctions différentes. Dans mon laboratoire, en France, nous avons depuis longtemps considéré qu'en tant qu'ergonomes nous avions comme mission — comme les syndicalistes — de transformer le travail, et pour cela de chercher à *connaître pour agir*, c'est-à-dire d'allier les connaissances et l'action, mais que nous ne pouvions y parvenir tout seuls. En effet, les scientifiques n'ont pas le pouvoir de faire les transformations souhaitables ni de les imposer; en tout cas, dans notre domaine, qui touche à l'organisation sociale et économique, ils n'ont que celui de révéler, de *dire* les choses et, si possible, de permettre de les *comprendre*. Ce faisant, ils construisent des outils — outils symboliques, d'analyse, d'explicitation, de démonstration, d'argumentation — qui, en revanche, peuvent être utiles aux syndicalistes, dans leur action.

Le premier point évoqué ici était donc celui de voir comment l'analyse ergonomique pointue des situations de travail, de l'activité «réelle» des travailleurs pouvait amener à découvrir les exigences cachées du travail et les compétences «réelles» — mais elles aussi «masquées» — mises en oeuvre par les salariés; l'objectif étant de les faire reconnaître et prendre en compte dans l'organisation des systèmes de travail. Il s'agit bien d'une façon de déconstruire les barrières mentales en contribuant à transformer les points de vue stéréotypés et falsifiés sur le travail, la technique, les compétences des salariés, en s'attaquant au refus de voir la réalité, à la difficulté à voir les choses comme elles sont.

Le deuxième point sur lequel je voudrais insister avant d'ouvrir la discussion, concerne les possibilités de coopération entre les chercheurs et les organisations syndicales, en particulier, dans le domaine de la formation des syndicalistes à l'analyse du travail.

Pour les raisons mentionnées plus haut, il a toujours semblé absolument essentiel à un certain nombre d'ergonomes, dont je fais partie, que les travailleurs et leurs représentants puissent s'approprier non seulement les résultats des recherches — menées souvent avec leur collaboration — mais également une démarche fondée sur un ensemble de méthodes d'analyse, afin de pouvoir utiliser ces «outils» pour leur propre action (Teiger et Laville, 1991; Teiger et al., 1979). Un des moyens permettant cette appropriation est la formation.

La contribution des ergonomes à la formation syndicale appartient donc à une histoire déjà ancienne en France, qui remonte à une trentaine d'années (Teiger et Plaisantin, 1983). Dès le milieu des années 1960, certains syndicats ont demandé à ce que des chercheurs en conditions de travail les aident à comprendre ce qui se passait dans les situations de travail, et les conséquences de ces situations pour les salariés, en particulier sur leur santé. L'objet de la demande syndicale a évolué depuis cette période. Au départ, il s'agissait surtout de comprendre des points particuliers des conditions de travail, par exemple les problèmes du travail posté (travail en continu par équipes en alternance), qui étaient, à l'époque, posés surtout par les syndicats de la sidérurgie, de la métallurgie et du textile.

Ensuite, à la fin des années 1960, début des années 1970 — après les événements de 1968, pendant ces années de bagarres syndicales importantes dont D. Kergoat a parlé — on a commencé à pouvoir faire vraiment de l'analyse du travail et de ses conditions de réalisation dans les entreprises. En effet, certains syndicats ont pu alors obtenir, par l'intermédiaire, le plus souvent, des comités d'entreprise (structures paritaires internes aux entreprises), de faire entreprendre des recherches officielles sur des problèmes critiques. Les scientifiques ont pu ainsi sortir des laboratoires et avoir accès aux situations de travail, sur la demande de syndicalistes et en collaboration avec eux, en cherchant à mettre en évidence et à comprendre les liens inapparents entre travail et santé, santé physique certes, mais surtout santé mentale. On en parlait alors en termes de «charge de travail», physique et mentale, et aussi de «fatigue nerveuse»; une des grandes questions étant celle des cadences et de leurs conséquences à la fois dans le travail et hors du travail (Teiger, 1980).

Nous avons ainsi travaillé avec des syndicats de secteurs industriels composés surtout d'hommes et avec des syndicats de secteurs composés surtout de femmes. Deux types de problèmes sont apparus, qui sont précisément en rapport avec la question des «barrières cachées» à l'intégration sécuritaire des femmes au travail.

Nous avons, nous aussi, rencontré ce phénomène de croisement entre les rapports sociaux et les rapports de sexes — sur lequel travaille D. Kergoat et son équipe — dans les syndicats eux-mêmes, à propos de leur façon d'aborder les problèmes des conditions de travail des «secteurs de femmes» (montage d'appareils électroniques, confection, etc.). De ce fait, certaines situations ont été très difficiles à vivre, parce qu'il fallait presque mener une bataille, déjà, à l'intérieur des syndicats pour faire reconnaître les problèmes des conditions de travail des femmes. En effet, la plupart du temps, à cette époque, les responsables syndicaux étaient des hommes, même dans les secteurs industriels où la main-d'oeuvre est presque totalement féminine; ils avaient du mal à défendre les revendications des femmes concernant leurs conditions de travail, car ils ne les comprenaient pas. Ils avaient, en effet, comme tout le monde, une représentation extérieure et *a priori* des travaux exécutés par les femmes — travaux classés «légers» dans les grilles d'emplois industriels — comme étant répétitifs, donc simples, et pas vraiment fatigants puisque réalisés souvent en position assise, dans un environnement relativement propre et salubre par rapport aux situations de travail de l'industrie

sidérurgique ou mécanique. Certes, on reconnaissait le caractère monotone de ces travaux mais cette monotonie du travail permettait aux
femmes, qui comme chacun le sait (!) «aiment les travaux ennuyeux et
faciles» de penser tranquillement au menu du soir et autres préoccupations ménagères! Qui s'en plaindrait? Or, ces femmes se plaignaient de
fatigue et particulièrement de fatigue nerveuse. Un taux élevé d'absentéisme et de turnover venait d'ailleur concrétiser ces plaintes, sans comp-
ter les cas de «crises de nerfs» se produisant sur les lieux de travail. Les
résultats des premières recherches sur le terrain ont clairement montré,
alors, d'une part l'intensité de l'activité mentale mise en oeuvre, paradox-
alement, dans la réalisation de ces travaux prétendus répétifs qui n'en
perdaient pas pour autant leur caractère monotone et ennuyeux, ce qui
expliquait, au moins en partie, la «fatigue nerveuse» ressentie; ces résultats on démontré d'autre part, le degré de fatigue musculaire provoqué
par le maintien prolongé de la posture même dont l'immobilité est
accentuée par les exigences de précision et de vitesse associées (Teiger,
1977). Ainsi, la représentation de ce type de travail a pu se modifier et une
prise en compte plus efficace de ses exigences «réelles» dans les revendications syndicales a pu s'élaborer.

Le deuxième point évoqué ici découle du premier, tout en étant plus
général car il touche tous les travailleurs. Il est apparu qu'un des obstacles
les plus importants à l'action des syndicalistes sur les conditions de
travail, consistait, là encore, en l'existence d'une barrière cachée, formée
à partir de l'intériorisation que les travailleurs eux-mêmes faisaient de la
«non-valeur officielle» de leur travail, en termes de qualification — jugée
comme inexistante par l'organisation taylorienne — qui entraînait un
sentiment de dévalorisation de leurs propres connaissances acquises dans
le travail et même, parfois, de dévalorisation personnelle. En effet, dans
ces situations où le travail est supposé être objectivement «non qualifié»
— en réalité pas du tout objectivement mais uniquement salaire! —
alors qu'en réalité, comme je l'ai illustré tout à l'heure à propos des grèves
du zèle qui bloquaient rapidement la production, au contraire il est très
«qualifiées». Certains travailleurs peuvent finir par «croire» qu'ils font un
travail «non qualifié», et que par conséquent eux-mêmes sont «non
qualifiés» et sans valeur. Cette réaction s'observait chez les hommes, mais
davantage encore chez les femmes, affectées en plus grand nombre aux
tâches les plus taylorisées.

C'est pourquoi la formation des syndicalistes à l'analyse ergonomique
du travail est apparue comme un premier moyen de briser cette barrière
interne. En effet, l'apprentissage d'une démarche d'analyse, fondée sur la
réflexion sur sa propre activité, permet d'expliciter ce que l'on fait,

pourquoi et comment on le fait, et, en l'exprimant, elle permet de prendre conscience de toutes les compétences masquées — masquées parfois à soi-même, comme je l'ai dit tout à l'heure — mises en oeuvre dans le travail, et qui ont été principalement acquises par l'expérience directe du travail. La prise de conscience permet la prise de confiance et transforme le rapport au travail dont dépend, en partie, l'action (Teiger, 1987; 1993a). Ce type de formation contribue donc à redonner de la valeur à ce que les syndicalistes, en particulier, font, à ce qu'ils sont, à ce que font et sont les autres travailleurs qu'ils représentent; la formation devient bien un «outil pour l'action» (Teiger et Laville, 1991). L'on a pu observer que cette activité d'analyse et de prise de conscience était particulièrement importante pour les femmes, parce qu'elles étaient, en général, dans les situations de travail les plus dévalorisées et que même à l'intérieur des syndicats, elles occupaient bien souvent des positions subalternes (en France, du moins, au moment de l'étude).

CONCLUSION

Pour conclure, j'insiste à nouveau sur l'idée que pour transformer le travail, il faut vraiment arriver à changer la conception erronée que l'on s'en fait à tous les niveaux de la société. J'insiste aussi, encore une fois, sur la nécessité de briser ou de dissoudre ces barrières mentales qui sont, bien sûr, dans la tête des employeurs et des concepteurs des systèmes de travail, mais parfois aussi dans celle des salariés. Les scientifiques peuvent agir par les recherches et par la formation. Mais cela est insuffisant. Il faut agir ensemble, syndicalistes et chercheurs, de manière à lier les connaissances et l'action dans un projet de transformation, quel qu'il soit. La question de cette nécessaire articulation se pose à propos de la conduite des recherches sur le terrain, bien sûr, mais également à propos de la formation à l'analyse du travail. Celle-ci, en effet, peut être très déstabilisante pour les participants, car elle risque de remettre en question certaines pratiques syndicales, notamment dans le domaine de la prévention (comportements normatifs, par exemple). Si les découvertes faites au cours de la formation ne sont pas reprises, à un autre niveau dans le syndicat, dans une perspective d'action collective qui permette aux salariés de les réinvestir dans un projet, le résultat risque d'en être ou bien l'inefficacité pure et simple ou bien d'être assez dramatique sur le plan personnel (découragement, désinvestissement …). Pour toutes ces raisons il est donc tout à fait essentiel, de mon point de vue d'ergonome, de travailler en collaboration, chercheurs et syndicalistes, et de poursuivre un dialogue collectif tel que celui-ci.

BIBLIOGRAPHIE

Bernier, C. (en collaboration avec C. Teiger). *Le travail en mutation*. Montréal: Éd. St Martin, 1990.

Bernier, C., et C. Teiger. «Approches ergonomique et sociologique de la qualification du travail. Application à l'analyse des changements technologiques». *Cahiers de Recherche Sociologique* 3, 2 (1985a). pp. 81-97.

— «Les qualifications: un enjeu des nouvelles technologies» dans *Apprivoiser le changement*. CEQ (éd.). Québec: CEQ, 1985b. pp. 144-9.

— *Informatisation et qualifications*. Montréal: IRAT, 1985c. Rapport de synthèse accompagné de monographies:

- n°1: *Informatisation et qualifications, dans le bureau du registraire d'une université* (1985).

- n°2: *Informatisation et qualifications, dans une banque* (1986).

- n°3: *Informatisation et qualifications, dans une société de Fiducie* (1986).

— «Informatique et qualifications: les compétences masquées. Diffusion des nouvelles technologies». *Interventions économiques* (1987). pp. 225-67.

— *Nouvelles technologies: qualifications et formation*. Montréal: IRAT éd., 1988.

— «La contribution de l'analyse ergonomique du travail à l'étude sociologique des qualifications dans le tertiaire informatisé: une expérience de coopération interdisciplinaire», dans *Les analyses du travail: enjeux et formes*. M. Dadoy et al. (éd.). Paris: CEREQ éd., 1990a. pp. 183-92.

— *Nouvelles technologies, qualification et formation. Etude de l'évolution du travail de caissière et de commis dans une banque lors d'un changement de système informatique*. Montréal: IRAT éd., 1990b.

Boel, M., F. Daniellou, E. Desmares et C. Teiger. "Real Work Analysis and Workers' Involvement," dans *Ergonomics International 85, Proceedings of the 9th Congress of the International Ergonomics Association*. Bournemouth, septembre 1985. pp. 235-7.

Daniellou, F., A. Laville et C. Teiger. «Fiction et réalité du travail ouvrier». *Les Cahiers Français* 209 (1982). pp. 39-45.

Dejours, C. «Pathologie de la communication. Situation de travail et espace public: le cas du nucléaire». *Raisons Pratiques* 3 (1992). pp. 177-201.

— «Ergonomie, médecine du travail et santé des groupes de travailleurs», dans *Ergonomie et Santé. Actes du XXVIIIe Congrès de la SELF*. D. Ramaciotti et A. Bousquet, (éd.). Genève: M + H éd., 22-24 septembre, 1993. pp. XLIII-XLV.

Teiger, C. «Les modalités de régulation de l'activité comme instrument d'analyse de la charge de travail dans les tâches perceptivo-motrices. Modes opératoires et postures». *Le Travail Humain* 40, 2 (1977). pp. 257-72.

— «Les empreintes du travail», dans *Equilibre ou fatigue par le travail*. Paris: Entreprise Moderne d'Édition, 1980. pp. 25-44.

— «Travail théorique et travail réel. Contribution ergonomique à la discussion de travaux d'économistes du travail», dans *Formation et Emploi*. Paris: Éd. du CNRS, 1982. pp. 43-8.

— «Ce qui se passe dans les sessions de formation» dans *Souffrance et plaisir dans le travail*. C. Dejours (éd.). Paris: Éd. du CNRS, 1987. pp. 89-94.

— «Représentation du travail, travail de la Représentation», dans *Représentations pour l'action*. A. Weill-Fassina et al. (éd.). Toulouse: Octarès éd., 1993a. pp. 311-44.

— «L' approche ergonomique: du travail humain à l' activité des hommes et des femmes au travail». *Education Permanente* 166 (1993b). pp. 71-96.

Teiger, C., et C. Bernier. «Intérêt de l'analyse ergonomique du travail pour la mise en évidence des compétences méconnues: le cas des tâches de saisie dans le tertiaire informatisé au Québec», dans *Sexe faible ou travail ardu?* C. Brabant et K. Messing (éd.). Montréal: Les cahiers scientifiques de l'ACFAS, n°70, 1990. pp. 61-70.

— «Polyvalence et informatisation: tâches ajoutées ou fonction élargie? Le cas du secteur bancaire au Québec». *Performances* (1991).

— "Ergonomic Analysis of Work Activity of Data Entry Clerks in the Computerized Service Sector can Reveal Unrecognized Skills." *Women and Health* 18, 3 (1992). pp. 67-77.

Teiger, C., et F. Daniellou. «Formation à l'analyse de l'activité et rapport au travail» dans *Souffrance et plaisir dans le travail*. C. Dejours (éd.). Paris: Éd. du CNRS, 1987. pp. 75-95.

Teiger, C., et A. Laville. «Nature et variations de l'activité mentale dans des tâches répétitives». *Travail Humain* 35, 1-2 (1972). pp. 99-116.

— «L'apprentissage de l'analyse ergonomique du travail, outil d'une formation pour l'action». *Travail et Emploi* 1, 47 (1991). pp. 53-62.

Teiger, C., A. Laville, D. Dessors et R. Toutain. "Trade Union Participation in Research and Training in Ergonomics." Présentation au conférence annuelle du Ergonomics Research Society, Oxford, 2-5 avril, 1979.

Teiger, C., et M.C. Plaisantin. «Quelle coopération possible entre syndicalistes, travailleurs et chercheurs pour une action sur les conditions de travail? Questions et propositions à partir de quelques expériences», dans *Les effets des conditions de travail sur la santé des travailleuses*. J.A. Bouchard (éd.). Montréal: CSN éd., Actes du Colloque International, mai 1983.

Lucie Dumais

Des variables sociologiques dans la recherche en santé-sécurité du travail

Within sociology, considerable progress has been made in addressing the question of the social regulation of prevention. Sociological indicators remain vague, however, about the social sources of risk. The clients of this research have been somewhat discontented with these results. By drawing on the research experiences of a sociologist working with an interdisciplinary research team to study women's occupational health problems, this paper examines some possible reasons for this discontent and for the limited effectiveness of sociological research into the social sources of risk. There is a gap between the expectations of clients and what sociologists feel they can offer. This results from an inability to clearly explain areas of competence within sociology, a tendency to reformulate the demands of clients to fit sociologists' skills, and clients' tendencies to bring sociologists into occupational health research in order to explain what cannot be explained by other disciplines. The limited usefulness of sociological research into occupational health risks is linked to the problems of imperfect knowledge in science and the limits of both methodological individualism and the usefulness of representations as tools for intervention. Conflicts may also arise between the pursuit of sociologically interesting questions and the risks such research might pose for workers. Yet sociologists can make valuable, if imperfect, contributions to research on occupational health by studying social indicators in greater depth or by documenting conflicts between different social groups precipitated by the social stakes related to occupational health.

Les sociologues ont fait développé considérablement la question de la régulation sociale de la prévention. En revanche, en ce qui a trait aux origines sociales des risques, les indicateurs sociologiques demeurent imprécis. La clientèle de recherche des sociologues a été plutôt insatisfaite de ces derniers résultats. Cet article examine certaines raisons qui ont pu causé l'insatisfaction de la clientèle et les limites de la recherche sociologique sur les origines sociales des risques. Le tout, à partir de recherches sur la santé au travail des femmes d'une sociologue travaillant dans une équipe interdisciplinaire. Il y a un écart entre les attentes de la clientèle et ce que les sociologues peuvent offrir. Cet écart résulte d'une difficulté à expliquer clairement le domaine de compétence de la sociologie, une tendance à reformuler les demandes de la clientèle en fonction de ces compétences, et la tendance de la clientèle à inviter les sociologues à répondre aux questions laissées en suspens par d'autres disciplines. L'utilité limitée de la recherche sociologique est liée au problème de la connaissance imparfaite en science et de l'individualisme méthodologique, ainsi qu'aux lacunes de l'approche des représentations comme outil d'intervention. Des conflits peuvent aussi exister entre la poursuite de questions sociologiques pertinentes et la menace que cela peut poser aux travailleuses. Du reste, les sociologues peuvent contribuer, quoiqu'imparfaitement, à la santé du travail en documentant davantage les indicateurs sociaux ou en documentant les différents groupes sociaux sur les enjeux sociaux de la santé.

INTRODUCTION

La sociologie (et d'autres disciplines des sciences sociales telle l'anthropologie) s'est distinguée comme discipline pertinente dans le domaine de la recherche en santé.

Plusieurs variables et indicateurs sociologiques sont très évocateurs des variations de la santé dans la société, ou même des facteurs déterminant les variations dans la santé d'une société. Par exemple, l'éducation des femmes est associée à un meilleur contrôle des naissances et une baisse de la mortalité infantile; les antécédents familiaux comptent beaucoup dans la prévalence de comportements de violence familiale et d'alcoolisme; le revenu est inversement proportionnel à la consommation de tabac; la pauvreté et la mauvaise santé sont des phénomènes corrélés; les femmes consomment plus de médicaments et de soins, mais ne sont pas davantage en santé que les hommes (voir, par exemple, Guyon, 1990; Quéniart, 1991; Gervais, 1992; Ferland et Paquet, 1994; Pompalon, 1994.)

Bref, les sociologues peuvent être satisfaits du travail sociologique dans le domaine de la recherche en santé en général. Car n'est-il pas entré dans les mœurs de nos institutions publiques et des citoyens que la santé est autant une affaire de prédispositions génétiques et de mesures d'hygiène que de conditions économiques et d'éducation? Du reste, il faut admettre que les connaissances générées sur les déterminants sociaux de la santé n'ont pas nécessairement entraîné des progrès sociosanitaires pour toutes les catégories sociales (Colin et al.; 1992; Québec, 1992). Les «clientèles» potentielles des sociologues de la santé (comme le Ministère de la Santé, le réseau public des services et des soins, les intervenants en santé, les diverses classes de la population, les hommes, les femmes) n'ont donc peut-être pas été aussi satisfaites — ou optimistes — que les sociologues mêmes.

Que peut-on espérer de la sociologie dans le domaine de la recherche en santé au travail?

Disons d'emblée que le domaine de la santé au travail est relativement jeune, et d'autant plus en sociologie puisqu'il ne constitue pas un champ propre, se situant à l'entre-deux des champs de la sociologie du travail et de la sociologie de la santé (Renaud et Simard, 1986). Deux avenues prometteuses se profilaient déjà voilà 10 ans: l'établissement des risques d'origine sociale (c'est-à-dire le lien entre les accidents et maladies et l'organisation du travail) et les mécanismes sociaux de prévention et de régulation des risques de tous genres (*ibid.*). Par rapport au second axe, je pense qu'on peut aujourd'hui répondre positivement à la question de savoir si la sociologie a réussi à légitimer les questions d'ordre politique qu'elle pose devant les limites de la médecine, du système public de santé et de la gestion de la main d'oeuvre dans les entreprises. L'analyse sociologique a bien démontré dans divers contextes que la prévention des risques et l'accès aux soins de santé ne sont pas une simple question médicale ou biologique; qu'en fait, la médecine et la santé au travail sont des systèmes sociaux publics, dans lesquels la prévention et les soins sont des enjeux politiques, économiques et de relations industrielles, autant que médicaux et techniques (voir, parmi d'autres, Berthelette, 1981; Chavkin et al., 1984; White, 1988; Harrisson, 1991; Hall, 1993; Malenfant, 1993; Lemieux et al., 1994).

Mais c'est par rapport au premier axe que je me situerai dans ce texte. Sur ce point, je pense humblement que les variables sociologiques restent encore aujourd'hui plutôt nébuleuses, imprécises dans leur contenu et leurs effets. Elles possèdent un pouvoir évocateur certain, mais elles sont encore peu documentées (voir Simard et al., 1988; Chanlat, 1992; Lowe, 1989; Dwyer et Raftery, 1991).

Cela est-il dû au fait que la sociologie est par nature impropre à répondre aux questions pointues posées dans le domaine de la santé au travail? Ou est-ce une affaire de temps avant qu'elle ne polisse ses concepts et teste ses variables de façon satisfaisante?

Incidemment, la fonction de la sociologie dans le domaine de la santé au travail est-elle claire aux yeux des non-sociologues, qu'ils soient chercheurs, intervenants en santé ou acteurs du marché du travail? Les sociologues et leurs clientèles (par exemple les syndicats, les employeurs, les professionnels de la santé, les chercheurs en médecine et en santé au travail) partagent-ils la même vision de ce que peut apporter la sociologie à leur questionnement? C'est à ces interrogations que je tenterai de répondre dans cet essai. J'y montrerez ma vision de ce que la sociologie peut apporter, dans la perspective de mes expériences pratiques avec des syndicats de travailleuses de l'industrie et des services et avec des chercheurs en sciences appliquées à la santé. Je crois que le forum constitué pour ce colloque est particulièrement approprié pour réagir à mes propos, puisque nous avons été témoins de demandes diverses envers la recherche sociale provenant à la fois des intervenantes syndicales et des chercheures des sciences de la santé (médecins, biologistes, ergonomes, épidémiologistes). Je débuterai d'abord par une réflexion d'ensemble sur la discipline sociologique, et procéderai ensuite par des illustrations d'indicateurs utilisés en recherche en santé au travail.

CE QU'ONT DIT LES SOCIOLOGUES SUR LEUR PROPRE DISCIPLINE

Peu d'entre nous, sociologues, peuvent dire de façon claire et certaine quelle est la «fonctionnalité» de la sociologie. Car il n'y a pas question plus épineuse (voir par exemple, Brodbeck, 1968; Dumas, 1992; Légaré, 1994). Durant tout ce siècle, la sociologie a tenté de s'expliquer à elle-même comment elle peut bien étudier les faits sociaux (comme la culture, les structures sociales, les organisations) alors que, en règle générale, les données qu'elle va aller chercher sont des données individuelles (comme les perceptions, les dispositions, les comportements, les attitudes, les discours, les textes écrits). La sociologie fait beaucoup d'effort pour établir les traits distinctifs ou les points communs entre les groupes, les régions, les sexes, les classes, les ethnies, en se donnant comme but de trouver les déterminismes sociaux et l'influence des structures sociales sur l'action humaine. Mais en même temps, elle a toujours eu à composer avec cette part de liberté qu'a l'être humain dans sa façon de penser et d'agir, et à vouloir comprendre comment les mouvements sociaux arrivent à changer les structures sociales. Les sociologues, en visant à analyser l'action et le discours de ces mouvements sociaux, ont dû se démarquer scientifiquement de ces mêmes mouvements sociaux par l'élaboration de théories et par des méthodes critiques. Mais depuis des décennies, ils se demandent jusqu'à quel point l'on peut, comme intellectuels, se distancier soi-même des idéologies, des groupes d'intérêt, des normes sociales pour arriver à faire de telles analyses.

Comme l'a exprimé N. Mouzelis (1993), la sociologie avait jusqu'aux années 1970 privilégié le macrosocial comme substance de ses analyses.

Mais elle a depuis été contrainte à remettre en question la valeur de ses théories générales. Or, depuis qu'il n'y a plus de fondement universel qui tienne — ni de point de vue purement objectif — c'est toute la théorie sociologique qui en a pris pour son rhume. Avec les méthodes qualitatives, c'est le microsocial qui devient la substance même de la sociologie, et qui semble, par conséquent, nous amener à «ratatiner» la théorie générale.

Les courants nouveaux de la sociologie, et notamment les études féministes, se rapprochent de plus en plus de l'expérience vécue telle que racontée par les acteurs, actrices sociaux eux-mêmes. Mais là où le bât blesse, maintenant, c'est qu'en même temps que l'on privilégie le microsocial et le discours des acteurs, on ne dit pas que le sens commun doit remplacer la théorie sociologique (voir par exemple Harding, 1991). Au contraire, on réaffirme la puissance critique de la théorie sociologique par rapport aux opinions reçues, «de rendre visibles les problèmes occultés, de désamorcer les préjugés et les conceptions toutes faites», diront Renaud et Simard (1986:6) à propos de la sociologie appliquée à la santé au travail. Il n'y a à peu près pas de nouveaux textes de sociologie qui ne précisent d'emblée que leur analyse est «critique».

Ce nouveau contexte de recherche place la sociologie devant le problème suivant: d'un côté elle se rapproche des acteurs sociaux, des individus, de leur subjectivité, elle écoute leurs malaises. De l'autre, elle tient à garder sa distance du sens commun et à parler un autre langage: le langage de la critique, critique des institutions, du poids de l'histoire, de la culture et des représentations, du pouvoir et de la subjugation. Or ce langage peut, à raison, paraître éloigné des préoccupations directes des gens et des milieux de travail, ou alors ne pas répondre à ces préoccupations par des solutions immédiates.

Le domaine de recherche en santé au travail m'a continuellement confrontée à cette contradiction de principe: me rapprocher des gens et de leurs problèmes, mais me questionner continuellement sur ma spécificité comme intellectuelle — alignée ou non? engagée ou non? critique ou non?[1] Cette ambivalence qui, selon moi, vient à la fois de la position personnelle de chaque chercheur et de la profession de sociologue elle-même, affecte ultimement les rapports des chercheurs avec leurs clientèles en santé au travail.

QUELQUES PROBLÈMES À SURMONTER POUR UN RAPPROCHEMENT ENTRE SOCIOLOGUES ET CLIENTS POTENTIELS POUR LA RECHERCHE

Les intervenants en santé au travail et les autres chercheurs des sciences de la santé qui ne sont pas sociologues à proprement parler, forment, en quelque sorte, une partie de notre clientèle de recherche. Or, j'ai l'impression que les rapports entre sociologues et clientèles en santé au travail ne sont pas des plus limpides.

À maintes reprises, au long de ma pratique dans le domaine, j'ai ressenti que nos clientèles ne savent pas souvent très bien quoi nous demander. Au cours du colloque, j'ai en fait eu la chance de répertorier divers types de demandes. Certaines m'ont choquée: par exemple, des intervenantes ont affirmé ne pas avoir besoin d'aide pour détecter les problèmes de terrain, mais plutôt pour trouver des solutions. Je pense, au contraire, que la sociologie a une capacité d'analyse utile à partager, alors que loin de moi l'idée de trouver la solution à un problème concret. D'autres demandes sont venues me rassurer: par exemple une intervenante et une chercheure ont dit qu'elles espéraient tirer une meilleure compréhension des problèmes de terrain, et peut-être aussi recevoir des propositions de solution.

Je pense que nos clientèles en santé au travail nous font des demandes légitimes. Mais nous ne sommes pas habitués à les remplir. Avec la double conséquence suivante: ou bien on fait à peu près ce qu'on nous a demandé, ou bien on fait carrément autre chose parce que c'est ça qu'on sait faire le mieux. J'ai toujours eu un malaise face à cet état de choses et j'aimerais aujourd'hui commencer à mettre cartes sur table. D'abord en essayant de mettre au jour les raisons de l'écart entre demandes et offres. Puis, en commençant à expliquer le mieux possible ce que, selon moi, la sociologie *peut faire* et ce qu'elle *ne peut pas faire* dans les cirsconstances.

Je présume d'au moins trois raisons de l'opacité des rapports entre sociologues et clientèle de recherche. *Primo*, beaucoup de sociologues ont du mal à énoncer clairement leurs compétences et notamment à décrire «de quoi a l'air» leur produit fini. Cela n'aide donc pas à approcher la clientèle. Je pense que c'est autant une question de «mauvaise habitude» qui pourrait être résolue avec le temps et la pratique, qu'une question de concepts et de langage scientifique. N'oublions pas que la sociologie a par tradition tenté de se distancer des explications de sens commun, du «bon sens» quotidien, car elle visait précisément à expliquer la société et son bon sens à l'aide de concepts plus généraux (Schutz, 1962), et cette tendance n'a fait que s'intensifier dans le contexte du post-modernisme — avec la déconstruction des idéologies et des discours (Foucault, 1969; Spivak, 1988). D'où que ses théories, bien qu'elles visent véritablement un enrichissement de notre compréhension de la société, ont toutes tendance à utiliser des mots «hors du commun» et donc à rester à un niveau de langage hermétique.

Secundo, à l'instar d'autres chercheurs, les sociologues pourraient avoir tendance à reformuler les demandes de clientèle potentielle à leur convenance, c'est-à-dire selon leurs intérêts ou selon leurs spécialités de recherche. Cette tendance semble s'accentuer encore une fois, si l'on en juge par les «essais» de plus en plus nombreux de recherches interdisciplinaires et les recherches cliniques, notamment dans le domaine de la santé où sciences sociales, sciences de la santé, et médecins — avec leurs «clients» — se côtoient (ACSALF, 1994). Bien que je croie cela légitime, parce que les sociologues doivent garder une certaine autonomie de pensée et une certaine distanciation, je crois aussi qu'il faut savoir où arrêter cette tendance dans les cas où nous nous engagerions en même temps à être au service d'une clientèle (ou à être collaborateur, si l'on parle de recherche en partenariat ou de recherche-action, par exemple). Dans ces derniers cas, il faut d'une part assurer nos clientèles de notre flexibilité et de notre capacité à faire des compromis; et d'autre part, faire un effort pour expliciter ce que la sociologie peut faire concrètement. Par exemple, il faut une bonne dose de transparence et de confiance mutuelle entre partenaires pour laisser le (la) sociologue faire une analyse des conflits et parler de théorie critique quand le (la) partenaire est lui (elle)-même partie prenante du conflit sur le terrain. (Voir, par analogie avec l'ergonomie, le texte de Teiger dans ce livre.) Or cela n'est pas facile, car une telle tradition de partenariat est presque inexistante dans notre discipline. De plus, les groupes interdisciplinaires en santé n'ont pas nécessairement fait le choix entre l'intégration et la cohabitation: les chercheurs de diverses disciplines ne travaillent pas nécessairement «ensemble», car il est difficile de s'entendre sur l'endroit où les disciplines doivent fusionner leurs problématiques et là où elles doivent éviter à tout prix de diluer leur force explicative traditionnelle (Dejours, 1993; Dumais, 1994).

Tertio, il m'apparaît que le rôle qu'on donne aux sociologues de la santé au travail leur a été dévolu un peu par défaut, et moins parce qu'ils auraient fait une démonstration «pro-active» du potentiel de la discipline pour le domaine de la santé au travail. Comme si, après avoir été témoin des limites des sciences médicales dans le domaine de la santé, nos clients s'étaient tournés vers les sciences sociales et y avaient mis toutes leurs espérances afin «d'expliquer le non-expliqué», diront Renaud et Bouchard (1994). Or la grande vertu de la sociologie actuellement, du moins en ce qui concerne l'établissement des risques à la santé, c'est de démontrer qu'il y a des variations de la santé selon certains axes sociaux, mais sans avoir apporté réellement une compréhension approfondie des mécanismes précis qui sont en jeu dans la santé d'un milieu de travail. Je pense que les sociologues ont beaucoup à faire pour approfondir les facteurs explicatifs des variations de la santé, tels que l'organisation du travail, le style de gestion en santé, la démocratisation du milieu, la culture d'entreprise; ou même des indicateurs plus tangibles, tels que l'absentéisme, la satisfaction au travail, l'autonomie et le contrôle sur le travail, les comportements de prévention. L'état actuel de la recherche démontre que l'apport des variables sociologiques à la valeur du R^2 dans les analyses de type épidémiologique fait l'objet de querelles d'interprétation (voir par exemple dans Hall, 1990; Gervais, 1992).

Je viens donc de relever certains angles sous lesquels on peut examiner de façon critique l'utilité des variables sociologiques en santé au travail. Il s'agit: (1) de la nature hybride des faits sociaux, c'est-à-dire qu'ils peuvent être des agrégats de faits individuels ou des entités sociales *per se* qui influencent les individus; (2) le niveau de langage «distinct» de la sociologie par rapport aux verbalisations de sens commun; (3) la re-définition en termes sociologiques traditionnellement reconnus d'un problème soulevé «par nos clients»; et (4) l'approfondissement d'indicateurs décrivant les mécanismes précis des variations de la santé en milieu de travail. Je crois que de ces quatre angles de vision, on pourra saisir un peu mieux ce que la sociologie *peut faire* et ce qu'elle *ne peut pas faire* dans le domaine de la santé au travail.

NATURE HYBRIDE DE LA SOCIOLOGIE ET TYPES DE VARIABLES EXPLICATIVES EN SANTÉ AU TRAVAIL

Commençons par la nature hybride de la sociologie et du niveau de langage qu'elle peut employer pour expliciter les aspects sociaux de la santé. Un détour par trois notions importantes en philosophie des sciences sociales sera utile à cette fin. Ces notions sont celles de la connaissance imparfaite, de l'individualisme méthodologique et de l'interprétation.

A. Connaissance imparfaite et individualisme méthodologique

La science cherche à découvrir les facteurs qui déterminent les faits de la nature et les faits sociaux. Vu sous cet angle, la sociologie produit des connaissances imparfaites. Mais personne n'en sera étonné, ni choqué. Car on peut faire un grand bout de chemin, et fort utile, même avec une connaissance imparfaite (on n'a qu'à regarder la médecine pour s'en convaincre).

Ce qui est plus embêtant c'est qu'elle ne produit que des connaissances imparfaites.[2] Ainsi elle n'a pas de pouvoir de prédiction comme tel, du moins au sens où on l'entend avec les théories en physique, en chimie, ou même en biologie. Ces dernières seraient plus aptes à prédire l'occurence d'un événement de la nature en fonction de la présence de certains facteurs explicatifs.[3]

La sociologie ne produit donc que des connaissances imparfaites, au sens où, même en connaissant les facteurs explicatifs (ou conditions d'occurence), elle ne peut jamais prédire que tel événement individuel se produira. Pourquoi? Simplement parce qu'en général, c'est une *question de probabilité*, de statistiques, et non de certitude: en effet, quand on fait de la recherche avec des facteurs sociologiques (variables, indicateurs), la seule chose qu'on peut savoir c'est que dans telles conditions il y a x chances sur 100, ou y chances sur 20 que le fait social z arrive. On ne peut pas prédire un phénomène social *singulier*; on peut seulement dire que, dans l'ensemble il y a de fortes chances que ce phénomène arrive. Prenons l'exemple classique des dés. À chaque coup de dés, je ne peux pas prédire quel chiffre sortira, mais sur 1000 coups de dés, je peux prédire que dans l'ensemble, tel chiffre sortira tant de fois. En somme, je n'ai pas de théorie parfaite d'un coup de dé; je n'ai qu'une connaissance imparfaite de l'ensemble des coups de dés. C'est la même chose en sociologie. En fait, ce serait aussi le cas de la biologie (et même de la physique et de la chimie), au sens où même les sciences naturelles ne font que «tendre vers» des connaissances «parfaites» sans les atteindre.

L'analogie avec une question en santé au travail est maintenant facile à démontrer. Supposons que nous allions dans un atelier de couture. Il y a de fortes chances que dans cet atelier, en dedans de cinq ans, un grand pourcentage de femmes (puisque ce sont surtout des couturières) développeront le syndrome du tunnel carpien. C'est une connaissance très valable, même si elle est imparfaite. On ne pourra jamais dire que Madame Unetelle va dans les cinq prochaines années développer un syndrome du tunnel carpien. Mais on sait que les conditions de travail des ateliers de couture sont dommageables pour un grand nombre de femmes dans l'ensemble. Ce n'est pas à négliger comme connaissance.[4]

L'individualisme méthodologique est indissociable de cette manière de concevoir la science (en termes de connaissance parfaite/imparfaite ou en termes de prédiction statistique). Cependant la notion d'individualisme méthodologique est limitative par rapport à notre «manière de concevoir les faits sociaux et l'être humain». Par exemple, un grand nombre de sociologues refusent totalement l'idée de pouvoir prédire — même de façon imparfaite — des faits sociaux ou des comportements. D. Kergoat (voir autre texte dans ce livre) suggère que le substrat de la sociologie, n'est pas fait de *patterns* de comportements communs, mais bien des formes sociales en constante transformation. En fait, elle propose que l'idée même de prédiction n'est ni pertinente ni même éthique[5].

B. Limite de l'individualisme méthodologique: interprétation, contexte et langage distinct du sens commun

Comme je l'ai mentionné précédemment, l'individualisme méthodologique est une position philosophique qui suppose que les faits sociaux sont ni plus ni moins des «agrégats» de dispositions, attitudes, comportements, discours individuels. Prenons un exemple. Qu'est-ce qu'une «foule en délire»? Au moins 50 p.100 + 1 personnes en délire dans un groupe de personnes? On peut dire que oui; enfin, à peu près. Ce serait la somme, la synthèse des dispositions de chaque personne.

Mais est-ce *seulement* cela? Cette fois, je crois qu'on doit dire non. Car une foule en délire, c'est d'abord et avant tout davantage que la somme des individus. Une foule en délire, c'est aussi la représentation sociale qu'on a de l'agrégat des personnes, et en même temps l'effet psychologique (sur leur niveau d'excitation ou sur leur niveau d'angoisse) que cette représentation a sur ces mêmes personnes. La foule en délire est donc une entité indépendante des dispositions des individus qui la composent, car c'est elle qui va en quelque sorte influencer les individus et non l'inverse. C'est une entité sociale (ici la représentation qu'on a de la «foule en délire») qui a le pouvoir d'influencer les dispositions individuelles des gens qui en font partie — et même des gens qui l'observent. Donc, bien que l'entité sociale elle-même n'ait pas de dispositions psychologiques au même titre qu'un individu (ça, c'est carrément fou de le supposer, et pire, de l'argumenter), elle a quand même des effets indéniables sur la psychologie des individus.

La limite de l'individualisme méthodologique ne sera donc pas solutionnée grâce à plus d'enquêtes de terrain pour documenter ses théories explicatives. Sa limite est aussi liée au fait que les facteurs explicatifs que nous cherchons à découvrir en sociologie ne sont pas seulement de l'ordre des agrégats de dispositions individuelles, mais aussi de l'ordre des représentations sociales (culturelles, politiques ou économiques), c'est-à-dire des valeurs, des modes de pensée, des institutions influant sur les dispositions et comportements des individus[6].

Je vais maintenant donner deux exemples d'études propres au domaine de la santé au travail pour illustrer les découvertes de l'ordre des représentations, et aussi pour réfléchir à leur utilité en santé au travail.

DEUX EXEMPLES DE REPRÉSENTATIONS EN SANTÉ AU TRAVAIL DES FEMMES

Dans une étude d'un milieu col bleu non traditionnel à laquelle j'ai participé, nous cherchions à savoir si les équipements de sécurité et l'organisation du travail étaient mésadaptés pour les femmes dans des postes de concierge, de jardiniers et d'entretien de la voirie. Dans chacun de ces groupes d'emplois, nous avons d'abord trouvé que plus de femmes que d'hommes rapportaient des problèmes physiques avec des charges similaires (vadrouilles, polisseuse; charettes, pelles; barrières en fer, marteau piqueur). À cette étape de notre étude, notre méthode était tout à fait inspirée de l'individualisme méthodologique. Car nous avons fait un décompte des dispositions et des perceptions de chaque individu et nous avons conclu que l'appartenance dans le groupe des femmes «prédisposait» davantage à certains problèmes (comme la difficulté de soulever des poids lourds ou d'avoir mal aux poignets) alors que l'appartenance dans le groupe des hommes «prédisposait» davantage à d'autres types de problèmes (se pencher fréquemment et souffrir de maux de dos, par exemple) (Messing et al., 1994).

Nous avons ensuite remarqué que les postes de concierges étaient subdivisés entre les sexes selon des aptitudes qu'on disait non seulement propres à chacun des sexes (selon l'opinion de leur superviseur et de plusieurs d'entre eux et d'entre elles), mais réellement plus présentes chez les femmes (minutie, nettoyage à fond) ou chez les hommes (force musculaire, intérêt pour les machines) (selon nos observations et nos questionnaires individuels). Il en allait de même dans le jardinage: la plantation et le désherbage étaient alloués aux femmes, la motoculture (culture à l'aide d'un rotoculteur motorisé) et l'épandage de pesticides, aux hommes. Nonobstant l'existence d'obstacles physiques réels pour plusieurs femmes, il nous est apparu évident que les représentations de ce que chacune et chacun doivent faire étaient assez fortes pour empêcher une situation où la majorité des femmes (qui n'avaient pas de problèmes physiques majeurs) feraient des «jobs d'hommes», et où plus d'hommes que de femmes feraient des «jobs de femmes».

Les représentations sociales nous aidaient donc à comprendre le sens implicite de certaines situations de travail. Mais elles restaient intangibles au sens où elles ne sont pas des variables comme telles, car elles ne discriminent pas les individus entre eux (sur une échelle de perceptions, de douleurs, ou de dispositions par exemple); ensuite, leur effet n'est pas mesurable par rapport à des problèmes physiques observables; enfin, leur valeur de vérité n'est donc testable que par la discussion (et non par groupe-contrôle ou significativité statistique). Leur fonction explicative restait, à ce moment du moins, accessoire, mais c'était une fonction non négligeable pour comprendre certains problèmes de santé au travail.

Finalement, la «découverte» de représentations sociales laissait bien peu de prise à une intervention pour la désexisation, car elle ne disait en rien comment réconcilier les représentations conflictuelles entre les femmes et les hommes. Car si la sociologie s'est donné le pouvoir d'expliquer les obstacles à l'entrée des femmes dans des emplois non traditionnels en termes de résistances culturelles, et peut s'en servir pour aviser les intervenants sur les conséquences possibles de leur décision; en revanche, elle n'a ni le pouvoir, ni le mandat, ni la compétence pour imposer un changement dans les représentations; ni non plus l'autorité intellectuelle pour décider arbitrairement quelles représentations sont les plus «saines» pour la société.

Passons au second exemple. Dans une usine pâtissière, la «désexisation» des postes était à peine tolérée. Les hommes nous disaient n'être aucunement intéressés à faire les «jobs» des femmes à la chaîne, et les femmes répondaient «c't'une job d'homme» quand nous leur présentions l'éventualité de faire les «jobs» des hommes. Encore là, il était apparent que les difficultés physiques rapportées par les femmes ou leur crainte d'essayer les machines faisaient autant référence à leur incapacité physique à soulever des sacs de farine de 40 kilograms qu'à leur représentation sociale de leur place dans l'usine (elles se disaient craintives d'avoir à ajuster la machine d'assemblage de boîtes de biscuits, ou d'avoir à subir les remarques ironiques des hommes). Cette interprétation de la situation ne correspondait pas nécessairement à ce qui nous avait été rapporté par questionnaire, mais à une explication, à un déterminant plus implicite, suggéré par une théorie sociologique des représentations, et contribuant en quelque sorte à notre compréhension de la santé au travail (Dumais et al., 1993; Dumais, 1995). Car elle expliquait en partie pourquoi les hommes avaient trois fois plus d'accidents que les femmes (et pourquoi ils acceptaient cet état de choses, même pour un salaire un peu plus élevé), alors que les femmes rapportaient plus qu'eux des problèmes chroniques aux épaules et au cou (et pourquoi elles préféraient cet état de choses, et aussi s'accommodaient d'un salaire un peu plus faible). Bref, la sociologie nous apportait une connaissance qui enrichissait notre compréhension de ce milieu de travail, sans toutefois nous indiquer comment instaurer un changement. Comme le dit la maxime philosophique en science: «*an is is not an ought*»: une description de l'*état* des choses n'équivaut pas à une prescription des choses *à faire*.

En résumé, nous avons vu que certaines questions qui nous sont posées en santé au travail amènent les sociologues à des conclusions de recherche valables, mais pas toujours «utilisables» en pratique. Nous en avons vu au moins deux sortes, que je reprends ici en passant de celle que je considère la «moins» surprenante à la «plus surprenante». Les conclusions des sociologues n'aident pas à prédire des phénomènes individuels (dispositions à la maladie, à certains comportements, à certaines attitudes), mais seulement des probabilités (ou pourcentages) d'occurence propres à un ensemble de personnes et de conditions environnementales. Les représentations sociales que les sociologues suggèrent sont de l'ordre du sens, et il est à peu près impossible de quantifier (même de façon probabiliste) leur force d'impact sur la santé mentale ou physique des individus. Les interprétations des sociologues nous mettent devant des situations conflictuelles et contradictoires, sans nous donner aucun critère pour décider quelle partie du conflit ou de la contradiction privilégier pour l'intervention.

REDÉFINITION DES QUESTIONS EN SANTÉ AU TRAVAIL ET INDÉPENDANCE DES SOCIOLOGUES

Il y a d'autres genres de questions que les sociologues aiment approfondir, mais qui n'ont pas de pertinence directe avec la santé au travail, ou alors qui sont préjudiciables à un équilibre social garant d'un niveau de santé durement acquis. À partir de cet angle de réflexion sur ma discipline, je pose donc la question suivante: est-ce que dans une recherche commanditée, en collaboration, ou en partenariat, les commanditaires, collaborateurs et collaboratrices ou partenaires peuvent imposer des limites au genre de questionnement que les sociologues sont habitués à se poser?

Ma position est que seuls le pragmatisme et l'expérience de recherche peuvent nous aider à faire de la recherche tout en tenant compte de cette interrogation. Je vais me contenter d'un exemple pour illustrer ce dernier point.

Il s'agit d'un questionnement fort intéressant du point de vue sociologique, mais qui risque d'être préjudiciable pour certains acteurs du milieu de travail. Dans trois milieux de travail où nous avons étudié des postes considérés comme «désexisés» (Dumais, 1995), les femmes ont rapporté en plus grande proportion certains problèmes musculo-squelettiques. Nous voulions savoir «pourquoi», et nous avons donc considéré trois façons de répondre à cette question.

En premier, nous avons contrôlé si les deux sexes faisaient les mêmes tâches. Il s'est avéré que la division sexuelle était présente dans la moitié des emplois. Car dans ceux-ci, pour une même titre d'emploi, les femmes ne faisaient pas les même tâches que les hommes.

En second, nous avons, dans les emplois réellement «désexisés», examiné l'aménagement des postes et les mouvements exigés des personnes de différentes taille et force. L'aménagement des postes nous paraissait passablement défavoriser les personnes de petite taille, mais encore plus les femmes que les hommes. Cette question typiquement ergonomique nous poussait à conclure que le fait que les femmes rapportaient plus de problèmes musculo-squelettiques était dû aux conditions physiques des postes, sans préjuger des dispositions individuelles de femmes en particulier.

En troisième lieu, nous avons considéré les antécédents d'emplois, parce qu'ils pouvaient indiquer à la fois l'acquisition de trucs de métier et d'expériences utiles dans l'accomplissement des dites tâches, mais aussi indiquer le genre d'usure physique et mentale en général accumulé par les femmes et par les hommes. Cette troisième question est une question typique de la sociologie de la mobilité occupationnelle, une spécialité de la sociologie extrêmement bien documentée. Or, cette question est aussi extrêmement litigieuse. Car dans un milieu de travail, l'enjeu pour les syndicats, c'est de se tenir dans les limites des conditions collectives de travail, alors que l'enjeu pour l'employeur, c'est d'en faire un enjeu pour l'embauche du personnel, et donc d'ordre plutôt individuel. Or, la théorie de la mobilité occupationnelle est fortement associée à l'individualisme méthodologique, en ce sens que c'est par une quantification probabiliste qu'elle jette les bases de sa théorie: savoir à la base combien de personnes passent d'une classe à l'autre en dedans de deux générations, ou d'une occupation à l'autre au cours de leur carrière. Cette théorie peut servir la connaissance en santé au travail à son tour, au sens où sachant que les antécédents des femmes en emploi peuvent en grande partie affecter leur disposition «physique», et que la plupart des femmes en emploi non traditionnel en usine ont des antédécents d'emplois caractérisés par le travail répétitif, il est important de les considérer dans le contexte d'un programme d'accès sécuritaire aux métiers non traditionnels. Or, par pragmatisme, cette question n'a pas fait l'objet de nos analyses approfondies, à cause de la menace qui aurait pesé sur les femmes dans l'hypothèse d'une résultat positif, c'est-à-dire si leurs antécédents d'emplois les avaient rendues effectivement plus «usées» que les hommes pour certaines tâches.

Je pense donc que si l'on menace de limiter la sociologie dans son questionnement en santé au travail, il y a de bonnes raisons pour le faire. C'est aux sociologues de prouver à leurs partenaires que, par un effort pragmatique, ils et elles vont s'assurer de poser leurs questions de manière à ne pas menacer, par exemple, l'emploi des femmes ou les programmes d'accès à l'égalité.

CONCLUSION: DE LA PRÉCISION ET DE LA VALIDATION DES INDICATEURS SOCIOLOGIQUES

En résumé, les sociologues, selon leur préférence, choisissent de suivre l'un des deux principaux paradigmes (individualisme méthodologique ou interprétation), chacun de ces paradigmes conduisant à des connaissances valables, quoique imparfaites. Pour chacun de ces paradigmes, les sociologues délimitent à des degrés divers, le poids des structures sociales par rapport au principe du libre choix et de la subjectivité sur la pensée et l'action des individus. Chacun de ces paradigmes a finalement montré son incapacité légendaire à faire de l'intervention dans la mesure où ses méthodes et ses théories ne donnent aux sociologues ni la certitude de prédire quoi que ce soit, ni le mandat de décider de ce qui est bon ou mauvais, de ce qui est sain ou malsain d'un point de vue social.

Mais force est de constater que la sociologie est devenue partie prenante du pari de la santé au travail, tant auprès de l'Institut de recherche en santé-sécurité du travail (IRSST) que des syndicats (et de mes collègues biologistes), notamment parce qu'elle s'avère utile pour aviser les intervenants des impacts possibles de leurs décisions.

Or si les sociologues en santé au travail ont fait un bout de chemin, ils et elles n'ont pas, à mon avis, vraiment amorcé le boum du développement du champ de la santé au travail en termes de déterminants des risques d'origine sociale. Il y a certes des variables sociologiques intéressantes dans le champ telles que l'absentéisme, l'autonomie et le contrôle sur le travail, les modes de gestion des ressources humaines, la satisfaction au travail. Mais je ne constate pas l'existence de modèles théoriques encore suffisamment documentés (je pense aux «modèles de gestion» qui sont trop généraux pour être vraiment testables), sinon très peu de modèles qui font un brin d'unanimité (je pense au modèle psychosociologique de Karasek sur la charge mentale du travail qui, même en étant populaire, reste fort controversé dans le milieu sociologique).

Par contre, je crois qu'il y a beaucoup de variables et d'indicateurs courants qui méritent d'être approfondis. En vertu des méthodes d'analyse propres à l'individualisme méthodologique, notamment. Si bien que même si nombre de sociologues sont ambivalents à l'idée de n'employer que cette conception de la sociologie[7], ils et elles l'utilisent la plupart du temps, faute de mieux. Je fais ainsi mienne la position à l'effet que l'individualisme méthodologique n'est ni inutile au plan de la connaissance, ni une conspiration au profit des plus puissants. Au contraire, il nous sert beaucoup dans notre compréhension du monde, et dans notre volonté d'orienter le plus sagement possible l'action de l'État au profit des plus démunis, des plus nécessiteux, bref du plus grand nombre. Mais gardons-nous d'en faire la caution ultime pour l'intervention.

Je crois que la place des sociologues en tant qu'interprètes du sens et des représentations est valable dans le monde du travail, même si c'est un rôle peu fonctionnel, voire ingrat. Car d'expliciter la disparité des points de vue et des rationalisations des divers acteurs sociaux fait, à juste titre, sonner les cloches là où il y a doute, incertitude, questionnement, interprétation à «double sens», conflits. C'est dire, en revanche, que ce rôle nous fera prendre en compte que la résolution des problèmes de relations de travail ou dans le système de santé n'est pas nécessairement fournie par une technique, par une formule choc, ou par une recherche, mais bien plus souvent en fonction de négociations entre les acteurs politiques du système de santé.

NOTES

1. Une autre contradiction de principe est celle-ci: la sociologie se rapproche des malaises des individus, mais la plupart des sociologues tiennent à rester idéologiquement indépendants des groupes d'intérêts qui ont le pouvoir de transformer les conditions sociales qui affectent ces malaises. En ce sens, si la plupart affichent leur préjugé favorable envers certaines catégories sociales, comme les féministes, comme les socio-démocrates, comme les libéraux, les sociologues, surtout universitaires, restent en bon nombre non engagés politiquement. Les présents actes de colloque reflètent assez bien la diversité de ces tendances chez les chercheures (bien qu'elles ne soient pas toutes sociologues): la plupart féministes, certaines ne sont pas engagées dans l'action sociale ni dans le partenariat avec des groupes d'action, alors qu'au contraire, d'autres ne séparent pas la recherche de l'action.

2. Je tiens à mettre au clair que je ne serais pas d'accord avec ceux qui utiliseraient ce «défaut» de la sociologie pour la discréditer en tant que discipline de rigueur scientifique. Ce que je reprocherais à la sociologie en revanche, c'est l'imprécision des facteurs explicatifs qu'elle mettrait de l'avant. Car lorsqu'on manque de précision, on peut alors faire dire n'importe quoi à une explication, sans jamais être en position pour la tester. Et c'est là je pense qu'à moyen terme le discrédit de la sociologie peut surgir dans le domaine de la santé au travail.

3. Cette distinction entre connaissances parfaite et imparfaite, bien qu'elle-même idéale et point réelle, demeure une des meilleures analogies pour exprimer les différences entre les sciences sociales (ou humaines) et les sciences naturelles, et pour aider à expliciter la nature hybride de la sociologie. Car il ne fait pas de doute que la sociologie est plus éloignée du modèle des connaissances parfaites que ne l'est la chimie, et *vice versa*.

4. Remarquer bien que je n'ai pas dit science, mais bien connaissance. Pourquoi? Parce qu'il est possible que cette imperfection soit due au stade d'évolution de nos connaissances, et non pas à la nature même de notre science. Parce qu'il est possible que notre recours à la statistique devienne inutile le jour où nous connaîtrons tous les facteurs explicatifs du canal carpien, des conditions environnementales aux dispositions individuelles. Alors, sachant parfaitement quels sont ces facteurs, on pourra expliquer des phénomènes individuels de façon parfaite.

5. Je tiens à suggérer la lecture de Gellner (1974) pour la nuancer avec celle de Kergoat. Gellner n'est pas en total désaccord avec Kergoat sur le fait que le substrat (ontologique) de la sociologie n'est pas constitué nécessairement des *patterns* communs, de

comportments ou d'attitudes. Mais il suggère que cela n'empêche pas que la théorie sociologique peut, elle, être basée sur l'idée de prédiction, de structures et de déterminismes de comportements ou attitudes. Car le substrat ontologique est du domaine de l'expérience, alors que la théroie est du domaine de la cognition. Dans la logique de Gellner, le problème éthique ne résiderait donc pas dans la théorie mais plutôt dans ce qu'on veut la concevoir comme étant le reflet exact de la réalité, de l'expérience vécue, plutôt que comme étant une idée, une représentation.

6. Ce à quoi se réfère d'une part la notion même d'individualisme méthodologique, mais aussi la théorie de l'action ou du paradigme de l'*agency*; et d'autre part ce à quoi se réfère la théorie des entités sociales, mais aussi de la théorie du sens et de l'interprétation ou du paradigme des *structures*.

7. Or l'individualisme méthodologique prétend justement qu'il n'y a pas d'entité sociale hormis des agrégats de dispositions ou attitudes individuelles. L'individualisme méthodologique correspond bien à l'argument des 50 p.100% personnes en délire pour décrire une foule en délire; ou encore à l'explication 'par agrégats' d'une institution bureaucratique; ou encore du marché du travail; ou encore du mileu de travail délétère. Bref, l'individualisme méthodologique et son pendant, la connaissance imparfaite, constituent, je le pense, la conception de la sociologie la plus analogique à faire en fonction des questions que nous pose à l'heure actuelle le domaine de la santé au travail.

RÉFÉRENCES

Association canadienne de sociologie et d'anthropologie de langue française (AC-SALF). *Bulletin d'information de l'ACSALF* (no. spécial sur «La sociologie clinique en question») 16, 1 (1994).

Brodbeck, M. *Readings in the Philosophy of the Social Sciences.* Londres: MacMillan, 1986.

Berthelette, D. *La rémunération au rendement et la santé au travail.* Montréal: IRSST, 1981.

Chanlat, J.F. «Vers une anthropologie de l'organisation». *Interface* 13, 1 (janvier 1992). pp.17-21.

Chavkin, W., et al. *Double Exposure: Women's Health Hazards on the Job and at Home.* New York: Monthly Review Press, 1984.

Colin, C., et al. *Extrême pauvreté, maternité et santé.* Montréal: Saint-Martin, 1992.

Dejours, C. «Problématiser la santé en ergonomie et en médecine du travail». *Communication au Congrès de la Société d'ergonomie de la gue française*(octobre 1993).

Dumais, L. «L'interdisciplinarité entre la sociologie et l'ergonomie: sur les ailes du désir». *Bulletin d'information de l'ACSALF* 16, 1 (mars 1994). pp. 9-10.

— «Organisation d'emplois non-traditionnels cols bleus et facteurs facilitant l'intégration des femmes», dans *Plaisir et souffrance* (les cahiers scientifiques de l'Association Canadienne Française pour l'avancement des sciences [ACFAS], 81). Montréal: ACFAS, 1995, pp. 104-40.

Dumais, L., K. Messing, A.M. Seifert, J. Courville et N. Vézina. "Make Me a Cake as

Fast as You Can." *Work, Employment and Society* 7, 3 (1993). pp. 363-82.

Dumas, B. «Positivité et normativité en sciences humaines», dans *La culture en mouvement: Nouvelles valeurs et organisations*. D. Mecure (éd.). Sainte-Foy, Québec: Presses de l'Université Laval, 1992. pp. 273-83.

Dwyer, T., et A.E. Raftery. «Industrial Accidents are Produced by Social Relations of Work: A Sociological Theory of Industrial Accidents». *Applied Ergonomics* (June 1991). pp. 167-78.

Ferland, M., et G. Paquet. «L'influence des facteurs sociaux sur la santé et le bien-être», dans *Le système de santé au Québec*. V. Lemieux et al. (éd.). Sainte-Foy, Québec: Presses de l'Université Laval, 1994. pp. 53-72.

Foucault, M. *L'archéologie du savoir*. Paris: Gallimard, 1969.

Gellner, E. *Legitimation of Belief*. Londres: Basil Blackwell, 1974.

Gervais, M. *Interprétation des enquêtes de santé*. Montréal: IRSST, 1992.

Guyon, L. *Quand les femmes parlent de leur santé*. Québec: Publications du Québec, 1990.

Hall, A. «The Corporate Construction of Occupational Health and Safety: A Labour Process Analysis». *Canadian Journal of Sociology* 18, 199 (1993). pp. 1-20.

Hall, E.M. *Women's Work: An Inquiry into the Health Effects of Invisible and Visible Labor*. Stockholm: Kingl Carolinska Medico Chirurgiska Institutet, 1990.

Harding, S. *Whose Science? Whose Knowledge? Thinking from Women's Lives*. Ithaca: Cornell University Press, 1991.

Harrisson, D. «La santé et la sécurité du travail: de nouveaux rapports à la lumière des mutations de la décennie 1990». *Revue internationale d'action communautaire* 25, 65 (1991). pp. 53-63.

Légaré, J. «Les relations formation-travail en sociologie et en anthropologie». *Bulletin d'information de l'ACSALF spécial «Quel(s) métier(s) pour les sociologues et anthropologues»* (août 1994). pp. 18-9.

Lemieux, V., et al. *Le système de santé au Québec. Organisations, acteurs et enjeux.* Sainte-Foy, Québec: Presses de l'Université Laval, 1994.

Lowe, G. *Le travail des femmes et le stress: Nouvelles pistes de recherche*. Ottawa: Conseil consultatif sur la situation de la femme, mars 1989.

Malenfant, R. «Le droit au retrait préventif de la femme enceinte ou qui allaite: à la recherche d'un consensus». *Sociologie et sociétés* XXV, 1 (1993). pp. 61-76.

Messing, K., L. Dumais, J. Courville, A.M. Seifert et M. Boucher. "Comparing Accident Rates for Women and Men in Jobs Traditionally Held by Men." *Actes du congrès de l'Association Internationale d'Ergonomie* 5 (août 1994). pp. 156-8.

Mouzelis, N. «The Poverty of Sociological Theory». *Sociology* 27, 4 (1993). pp. 675-95.

Pompalon, R. «La santé des Québécois et des Québécoises», dans *Le système de santé au Québec*. V. Lemieux, et al. (éd.). Sainte-Foy, Québec: Presses de l'Université Laval, 1994. pp. 33-52.

Renaud, M., et L. Bouchard. «Expliquer l'inexpliqué: l'environnement social comme facteur clé de la santé». *Interface* 15, 2 (mars-avril 1994). pp. 14-25.

Renaud, M., et M. Simard. «Présentation: Travail, santé, prévention: la place de la

sociologie». *Sociologie et sociétés* (numéro spécial sur «Travail, santé, prévention»)
XVIII, 2 (1986). pp. 3-10.

Québec. *La politique de santé et de bien-être.* Québec: Ministère de la santé et des
services sociaux, 1992.

Quéniart, A. (éd.) *Femmes et santé. Aspects psychosociaux.* Boucherville, Québec:
Gaetan Morin, 1991.

Schutz, A. *The Problems of Social Reality.* The Hague: Martinus Nijhoff, 1962.

Simard, M., C. Levesque et D. Bouteiller. *L'efficacité en gestion de la sécurité du travail:
Principaux résultats d'une recherche dans l'industrie manufacturière.* Montréal:
GRASP (Groupe de recherche sur les aspects sociaux de la prévention), Univer-
sité de Montréal, 1988.

Spivak, G.C. *In Other Worlds. Essays in Cultural Politics.* New York: Routledge, 1988.

White, D. *Social Policy and Social Change. Reproduction and Transformation in the
Field of Occupational Health in Québec.* Thèse de doctorat. Montréal: Département de sociologie, Université de Montréal, 1988.

Donna Mergler

Adjusting for Gender Differences in Occupational Health Studies

Le type d'analyses statistiques que l'on applique à des données de recherche détermine en grande partie les résultats que l'on obtient. Il est donc important de connaître des prémisses qui sous-tendent les procédures mathématiques que l'on emploie. En santé au travail, des conclusions fausses, tirées d'analyses partielles ou inexactes, peuvent entraîner des mesures discriminatoires au niveau de l'embauche, des soins de santé inadéquats ou des actions préventives déficientes. Cet article traite des hypothèses sous-jacentes à la procédure d'ajustement utilisée pour tenir compte des différences observées au niveau de la santé mentale entre les travailleuses et les travailleurs. Les données que nous utilisons proviennent de l'Enquête Santé-Québec de 1987, réanalysées à l'égard du travail par un comité provincial sur la santé mentale au travail. Elles indiquent qu'une proportion significative de travailleuses (17.8 p.100) présentent un indice élevé de détresse psychologique en comparaison avec les travailleurs (9.1 p.100). Si l'on ajuste les statistiques pour cette différence entre femmes et hommes, lors de l'analyse de la distribution de la détresse psychologique par rapport au secteur et catégorie d'emploi, on tient pour acquis que cette différence relève de facteurs autres que le milieu de travail. Par contre, si cette différence n'est pas prise en compte lors des analyses, cela suppose que les femmes et les hommes devraient manifester des niveaux de détresse psychologique similaires lorsqu'ils effectuent le même travail. Pour les emplois où la majorité de la main-d'oeuvre est composée de femmes, le degré de risque varie en fonction de la procédure utilisée, avec des conséquences en termes d'interventions préventives ou curatives. Des modèles alternatifs pour étudier la relation entre la santé des femmes et des hommes par rapport à leur travail sont abordés en conclusion.

Since statistical analyses determine the findings of many studies, it is important to examine the underlying premises of the procedures that are applied to research data. In occupational health, false conclusions drawn from partial or inaccurate analyses can lead to discriminatory hiring policies, inadequate health treatment and deficient preventive action. The present article examines some of the assumptions in mathematically adjusting for sex differences in health studies, using data from the 1987 Quebec Health Survey, which was re-analyzed by a committee on mental health and the workplace. The results of the survey indicate that significantly more women workers (17.8 percent) as compared to men workers (9.1 percent) present a high index of symptoms of psychological distress. When analyzing the distribution of high psychological distress with respect to work sector and/or job, statistical adjustment for the sex difference carries the assumption that the difference is due to factors inherent to each sex. On the other hand, not adjusting for these differences carries the assumption that women and men should have similar levels of psychological distress if they perform the same work. Attributing risk of psychological distress to specific jobs in which women make up the majority of the workforce varies depending upon which procedure is used. This can affect the focus of preventive or curative intervention. Alternative models for examining women's and men's health in relation to work are discussed.

INTRODUCTION

When doing statistical analyses, it is important to examine the underlying premises of the procedures researchers apply to their data. In occupational health, not doing so may have important (and possibly dire) consequences, since false conclusions drawn from partial or inaccurate analyses can lead to discriminatory hiring policies, inadequate health treatment, and deficient preventive action. The way in which data are treated determines the conclusions; numbers or statistics, often quoted out of context as "truths," form the basis of policy decisions. Although most occupational health researchers would adamantly deny that they employ discriminatory practices, their failure to question some accepted methodological techniques that have evolved in a sexist and classist context can make them unwilling and unknowing participants in the dissemination of distorted or imprecise findings.

Most studies comparing the health of female and male workers have shown that women workers report more symptoms of poor physical or mental health than their male counterparts (McIntosh et al., 1994; Cox et al., 1984; Courville et al., 1991; Mergler et al., 1987; Messing and Reveret, 1983). Although some authors have suggested that this may be due to differences in working and/or living conditions (Courville et al., 1991;

Mergler et al., 1987; Messing and Reveret, 1983; Skov et al., 1989) — and in spite of some evidence that there is no difference in the proportion of health problems when women and men do work in similar conditions (Cox et al., 1984; Mergler et al., 1987; Loscocco and Spitze, 1990) — most researchers will automatically "adjust" or "control" for observed gender differences when examining the relation between work and health.

Adjusting is a statistical procedure that corrects for the effect of factors not related to the hypothesis being tested. This is done in order to isolate, as much as possible, the relation between factors under scrutiny and health. For example, when examining the relation between workplace exposure and lung damage, one would adjust for smoking status since it has been repeatedly shown that smoking affects the lungs; by adjusting, the contribution of smoking to lung damage is mathematically estimated and removed from the equation. In the same way, when adjusting for differences in health outcomes between women and men workers, the differences attributed to gender are removed from the relation between work and health. In other words, one makes the assumption that female/male differences in health outcomes are due to something (for the most part, unnamed) other than possible differences in working conditions.

Analysis of the relation between work and health is further complicated by the fact that women work in fewer job categories than men (Messing, 1991; Bradley, 1989; Lacroix and Haynes, 1987). This results in a "dilution" effect, since women whose working conditions may differ greatly are grouped together in the same job category. Moreover, even when women and men have the same job title, they often do different types of work with different patterns of exposure to health risks (Messing et al., 1994).

In the course of producing a document on mental health and the workplace for the Quebec Mental Health Advisory Council, a government appointed committee (including the author) had to deal with the question of adjusting for gender differences. The committee was mandated to review current knowledge on the effects of working conditions on mental health, and make recommendations for preventive intervention. The resulting book (Vézina et al., 1992) reviewed an extensive literature on workplace factors that can contribute to mental health problems. When the book was being written, however, the only available data on the mental health of the Quebec workforce were contained in the 1987 Quebec Health Survey (QHS-87), which had been conducted in order to provide a portrait of the health status of the Quebec population

(Enquête Santé Québec, 1988). Although the authors of *Pour donner un sens au travail* were aware of the methodological limits of using data from a survey that was not designed to examine workplace effects on mental health (Vézina et al., 1992), we felt that the paucity of material on the situation in Quebec justified its use. Indicators of mental health status were gleaned from data gathered for the QHS-87 and analyzed for active workers, with respect to job and work sector.

This articles relates some of the methodological issues raised in the analysis and gives an interpretation of the association between women's and men's mental health outcomes and work. Using the data available from QHS-87, I will examine some of the assumptions and methodological choices that have been unquestioningly made in studies of occupational health. I will also examine the consequences of making such assumptions about women's health and well-being.

MENTAL HEALTH AND THE WORKPLACE

The Quebec Health Survey of 1987 covered 13,700 households. One of the indicators of mental health used in the survey was the Psychiatric Symptom Index (PSI) developed by Ilfeld (1976). It is composed of 29 questions which examine the symptomatology of depression, anxiety, agression and cognitive difficulty. The questions refer to the previous week, with a four-category response scale. The responses are scored on a scale from 0-100.

The analyses performed by Vézina et al. (1992:79-91) included 10,499 active workers (3,353 women [38.6 percent] and 6,646 men [61.4 percent]). Active workers were defined as those aged 18-64 who had been in the workforce for more than one year. Persons who worked part-time were included, as were the currently unemployed. Jobs were classified from responses of workers or their families, according to sectors of economic activity developed by the Quebec Bureau of Statistics (1984), or by profession, using the classification system of the Canadian Code of Professions (1987). The workers' PSI scores were dichotomized: a score in the upper 15 percent of the entire population (scale score 26.2) was considered a high PSI. In the total working population, 12.5 percent were in this category; thus, workers in general suffered less psychological distress than those who reported not working.

Prior to analyzing the relationship between work and high PSI scores, the relation of non-workplace factors to high PSI scores was examined in order to adequately adjust for those factors. The table below lists the variables that were significantly associated with high PSI scores among the working population and that were initially considered in the analyses as "control" variables.

Table 1   Distribution of Elevated Psychiatric Symptom Index with Respect to Sex, Stressful Events, Health Problems and Social Support

Variable		% High PSI
Sex	men	9.1
	women	17.8
Stressful extra-professional life events in the past 12 months	few	11.4
	many	29.0
Social support	presence	11.2
	absence	20.0
Health problems	minor	9.1
	major	17.2

From *Pour donner un sens au travail*, Vézina et al., 1992, p. 142.

Twice as many women workers (17.8 percent) as men workers (9.1 percent) had high PSI scores. This highly significant difference between the sexes led to a heated debate among the committee members on the meaning of the variable "sex" and how it should be treated statistically. One of the points raised was that the four categories examined were not of the same order. "Stressful extra-professional life events," "health problems" and "lack of social support" refer to well-defined, specific events or conditions, while "sex" refers to normal population characteristics.

In the Quebec Health Survey (Enquête Santé Québec, 1988), stressful life events were determined according to an accepted, or validated, scale (Holmes and Rahe, 1967), which ranks identified occurrences such as death in the family, divorce, losing one's job, etc., according to the degree of psychological stress that they generate. A large number of studies have reproduced these results (Yodfat et al., 1993; Harmon et al., 1970; Kohn and Frazer, 1986). Health status was also rated on a validated scale (Belloc et al., 1971) which included the presence or absence of incapacities, health problems or chronic symptoms. The relative weight of these factors was ascertained by interview. Social support, although not a scaled score, was defined dichotomously as the presence or absence of a person or persons within the subject's family or entourage, to whom the subject could freely talk and in whom he or she could confide problems. Previous studies have shown the association between these specific variables and indicators of psychological distress (Schutt et al., 1994; Cohen and Williamson, 1991;

Tafari et al., 1991; Norfleet and Burnell, 1990; Nations et al., 1988; Kaplan et al., 1987; Roberts, 1980; Rousseau and Jenicek, 1977; Berkman, 1971).

But what is the definition of "sex"? What are we measuring when we say that there is a difference in PSI scores between men and women? The difference between a penis and a vagina? Or are we examining genetic, physiological, social, economic and cultural differences? And, most important in the context of the present analysis, what is the bearing of these differences on the relation between working conditions and high PSI scores?

The initial analysis of high PSI scores with respect to job category was "adjusted" mathematically for the four factors listed in Table 1, thereby implicitly attributing these differences in high PSI scores to factors other than the workplace. An "odds ratio" (OR), which provides an estimate of the risk of a high PSI score, was calculated for the different sectors and jobs for which the sample was sufficiently large (Vézina et al., 1992:137-43). A simplified definition of an odds ratio is given below.

Odds Ratio (OR) = $\dfrac{\text{risk in part of the group under study}}{\text{risk in the rest of the group}}$

If the risk in part of the group under study = risk in the rest of the group, then OR = 1

If the risk in part of the group is greater than the risk in the rest of the group, then OR is greater than 1.

If the risk in part of the group is less than the risk in the rest of the group, then OR is less than 1.

The results indicated that the highest PSI scores were mainly associated with jobs and/or sectors of activity where the majority of workers are men. Few workplaces where the majority of workers are women showed significantly high PSI rates, despite the fact that many of the work characteristics identified as especially detrimental to mental health, such as repetitive and/or monotonous tasks, deficient communications, ambiguity and role conflict, lack of autonomy, overwork and employment in helping professions (Vézina et al., 1992:61) are commonly found in workplaces where the majority of the workforce are women (Mergler et al., 1987; Messing, 1991; Lacroix and Haynes, 1987; Doyal, 1991; Billette and Piché, 1987; Lowe, 1989).

After much discussion among committee members, a compromise position was reached wherein gender would not be adjusted for sectors or jobs where either women alone or men alone made up over 80 percent of the workforce. Subsequent reanalysis of the data revealed that job categories such as cashier, teller, stenographer, typist and secretary, which had previously not been associated with high PSI scores, were now identified with high levels of psychiatric symptoms (Vézina et al., 1992:85-86). Note that this "solution" does not entirely solve the problem since men and women with the same job title in "mixed" professions may not in fact be assigned the same tasks (Messing et al., 1994).

THE IMPACT OF ADUSTING FOR SEX: FURTHER ANALYSES

Adjusting or not adjusting for sex is not merely a mathematical exercise, since the use of this procedure can substantially modify the results. Further analyses of the data illustrate the consequences of adusting for sex. Table 2 shows the difference in an OR adjusted for sex ("adjusted OR") and not adjusted for sex ("OR not adjusted") for the jobs listed in *Pour donner un sens au travail* where women constitute the majority of the workforce.

When the OR is adjusted for sex, only three jobs yield figures that are significantly different from those in Table 1: cashier and teller; nursing aide; and food services worker. However, when the OR is not adjusted for sex, six of the seven jobs examined here are significantly different from their equivalents in Table 1.

Table 2   Comparison of Odds Ratio (OR) for High PSI, Adjusted and Not Adjusted for Sex for Job Categories Where Women are in the Majority

Job	n	% Women	OR Not Adjusted	Adjusted OR
Stenographers, typists, secretaries	484	99.4	1.45*	0.95
Cashiers, tellers	2174	93.0	1.94**	1.32*
Nursing aides	71	88.7	2.19*	1.63*
Food services	120	83.3	4.05***	3.13**
Data entry personnel	52	82.7	2.27*	1.73
Garment and leather workers	212	75.0	1.39	1.07
Nursing personnel	43	69.8	2.54*	2.11

*p<0.05; **p<0.0.01; ***p<0.001

(All of these values are adjusted for social support, health problems and stressful life events.)

Job categories listed in *Pour donner un sens au travail*, op. cit.

As the percentage of women in a particular sector or job increases, so does the difference between the adjusted OR and non-adjusted OR. If the job is carried out entirely (100 percent) by women, adjustment for sex compares the percentage of workers in that job with high PSI scores to the percentage of women in general with high PSI scores (17.8 percent), rather than to the overall mean of workers with high PSI scores (12.5 percent). The comparison percentage decreases in proportion to the ratio of men and women. At the other extreme, if there are no women in the job, the percentage of men with high PSI scores is compared to the proportion of all men with high PSI scores (9.1 percent).

For women, the non-adjusted ORs are proportionally higher then the adjusted ORs as the percentage of women workers in the job increases. In other words, the greater the proportion of women in the job, the more that adjustment minimizes the results.[1] Using the data from Table 2, the percent decrease in OR from the non-adjusted value to the adjusted value was calculated. For example, for cashiers whose non-adjusted OR = 1.94 and adjusted OR = 1.32, there is an decrease of 32 percent (OR non-adjusted - OR adjusted/OR non-adjusted). In Figure 1, the percent decrease in OR at each job is plotted against the percentage of women in the particular job. For the group classified as stenographers, typists and secretaries, where women constitute 99.4 percent of the workforce, the OR decreases by 34 percent after adjustment, whereas for nursing personnel, where women constitute 70 percent of the sample, the decrease after the adjustment is of the order of 17 percent.

It is clear, then, that whatever causes the PSI results of men and women to differ, adjusting for sex as if it were a single well-defined entity changes the results and therefore changes the conclusions that are drawn about the relation between women's work and health.

A further difficulty arises from the fact that women occupy fewer job titles than men; as well, those jobs women do hold are often poorly defined (Messing et al., 1994; Messing, 1991; Lacroix and Haynes, 1987; Strang and Baron, 1990). In the example given above, secretaries, typists and stenographers are all grouped together despite the fact that their jobs and their working conditions may be quite different. If, for example, a subgroup of these workers has particularly difficult working conditions, this would remain undetected if they are part of a larger group with better working conditions. It is quite possible that such an oversight might occur, since the subsector classification of "secretaries, typists and stenographers" includes 484 persons, of whom 481 are women, and represents 27.3 percent of all office workers surveyed. Proportionally, this is the largest subgroup of all the sectors surveyed.

Figure 1   The Percentage Decrease in OR for High PSI Following Adjustment with Respect to the Percentage of Women in a Particular Job or Sector

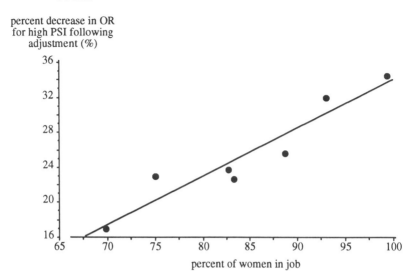

percent decrease in OR
for high PSI following
adjustment (%)

percent of women in job

DO THE STATISTICAL MODELS REFLECT REALITY?

Variables that need to be "adjusted for" are those that are unrelated to the studied exposures but can independently produce the outcome under study. The model that is traditionally used in epidemiological investigations, shown here as Model 1, is that sex, like smoking, drinking and poor dietary habits, affects health independently of work, making it an independent variable that must be adjusted for if one wants to examine the relation between work and health.

Model 1

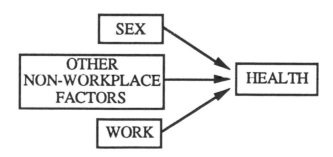

For example, in the analyses performed by Vézina et al. (1992:79-91), the effects on PSI scores of high scores in the stressful extraprofessional life events, major health problems and social support scales were statistically accounted for when analyzing the relationship between work and mental health. When sex is included as an independent variable in the analysis, differences in the scores of men and women are likewise eliminated. Thus we are, in effect, presuming that differences in PSI scores between the sexes are not due to possible differences in working conditions. In fact, if women's working conditions are particularly stressful, adjustment for sex differences may remove the very relation that we are trying to examine.

There is an extensive literature on the sexual division of labour (Hartmann and Reskin, 1986; Cockburn, 1988; Bradley, 1989), and a growing literature on women's occupational health, that shows that men and women's working conditions and resulting health problems are often different (Bureau of National Affairs, 1989; Stellman, 1977; Bradley, 1989; Dumais et al., 1993). Since women are "ghettoized" in a certain number and type of jobs, and the particular working conditions of these jobs affect both physical and mental health, an alternative model (Model 2) might better describe the situation. In this model, sex is a determinant of the type of work available and of working conditions, which are in turn a determinant of health. A still more complex model would include sex as a determinant of certain non-workplace factors (Model 3), which

Model 2

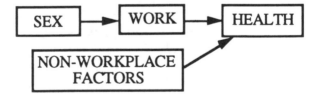

Model 3

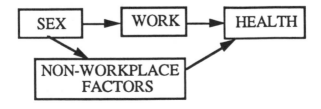

could, in turn, affect health outcomes. We could likewise hypothesize interactive models where work would affect *non-workplace* factors, and vice versa, and health could affect both workplace and nonworkplace factors. These models would require very different analytical approaches.

CONCLUSION

Whether we postulate that the prevalence of psychiatric symptoms is higher among women workers than men for reasons of biology, socio-economic status or working conditions, relegating this difference to "sex" and adjusting through statistical analysis is like sweeping the problem under the rug. It is interesting to note that epidemiology — a discipline that prides itself on its rigour and methodology — continues to accept a gross classification such as "sex" in examining the relation between work and health, without questioning which aspects of "sex" account for this difference and without asking if the sex of the person is related to the type of work that is performed. A similar logic has been questioned in epidemiological studies which control for "race" (Strang and Baron, 1990) or for "socioeconomic status" as if they were separate from work (Brisson et al., 1987; Semiatycki et al., 1988). Race, like sex, is a determinate of the type of job one is likely to do, and socioeconomic status reflects the job that one does and the conditions in which the job is performed (Messing and Mergler, 1995).

Margrit Eichler (1992) suggests that the appropriate procedure is to analyze data separately for both sexes, considering them together only if the same relationships appear to be operating in both sexes. In the study of women's occupational health, this could be possible if there were more precision in describing women's jobs. Ironically, with the limited infor-mation available for job classification in surveys such as *Pour donner un sens au travail* separate analysis of the data by sex would reveal that very few women's jobs are associated with high PSI scores. The lack of knowledge about (and lack of interest in) women's working conditions may also form the basis of inappropriate diagnoses. For example, in a review of the literature on mass hysteria in occupational settings, Brabant and coauthors (1990), demonstrate that physical, chemical and organiza-tional hazards, rather than unknown psychogenic factors particularly present in women, probably account for the psychological symptomat-ology.

If we want to know more about the relation between work and health, professional exposures should be treated with the same precision as extraprofessional exposures. In many epidemiological studies, and in national health surveys like the Quebec Health Survey or the Canada Health Survey (The Health of Canadians, 1981), emphasis is placed on individual factors such as smoking, drinking, exercise and dietary habits, while work is limited to job title, which has been shown to be a highly inaccurate means of job classification (Messing et al., 1994; Messing and Reveret, 1983; Skov et al., 1989; Murgatroya, 1984; Hunter and Manley, 1986; Jessell and Beymer, 1992; Bielby and Baron, 1986), particularly for women's jobs (Messing, 1991; Lacroix and Haynes, 1987; Messing et al., 1991). Indeed, different conditions of exposure can be present within the same job title. Moreover, in many workplaces, men and women may have very different exposures even though their job titles are similar (Messing et al., 1994; 1991). The overall effect of using job title to examine the relation between work and health is akin to misclassification. Persons with very different exposures are grouped together. The overall effect is to tend toward the mean prevalence of the health problem. For example, workplace studies have shown that office workers who use computers are more tense than those who don't use computers (Steffey and Jones, 1989) and that video dispay users with restrictive and less stimulating tasks report more psychological and physical symptoms than those whose work involves active dialogue with the computer (Elias and Cail, 1986). However, when the job categories of secretaries, stenographers and typists are grouped together — so that they include computer users of different categories as well as women who do not use video display terminals at all — as in the data used in the Quebec Health Survey analyses, the overall risk for high PSI scores is 0.95 (just about the mean for all workers). Had the type of work with computers been used as a measure of exposure to risk, the effect of work on mental health for secretaries, stenographers and typists might have become more evident.

The imprecise treatment of working conditions, and particularly of women's working conditions, minimizes, in a mathematical way, the effects of work on health. This has important consequences for health promotion. Government policies and campaigns for health improvement focus on individual lifestyle (eat better, exercise more, stop smoking and drink less), for which precise information is available, and ignore the contribution of poor working conditions to poor health. The irony of this approach was all too evident in one plant we visited during our research, where government agency posters on the wall attested to and praised the company's contribution to workers' good health through organizing midday exercise programs. No consideration was given to the fact that the level of exposure to toxic substances in the plant was sufficient to make the workers feel giddy and dizzy, and to give them pounding headaches. Workers also suffered from memory loss and dermatological problems. One woman told us that she could no longer do the dishes because her hands broke out in a terrible rash, and that no ointment or cream seemed to help.

There is a clear need for better characterization and classification of women's jobs, and new methodologies must be applied in examining the relation between women's work and health. The old concepts, which are not necessarily accurate for men's work, must be rethought in light of the various interactions between sex, work, working conditions, living conditions and health (Messing and Mergler, 1995). We should be looking at women's working conditions (as opposed to job titles), differences in socioeconomic situations (a woman worker who is the sole supporter of her family is not in the same situation as a working couple or a man who is the sole supporter of his family, with a spouse to look after the home and children).

Alice Hamilton, an American pioneer in occupational health, reanalyzed data from other scientists that showed women to be more sensitive to lead intoxication than men. By examining the tasks and socioeconomic status of the workers and reanalyzing the data she explained the male/female differences in blood lead levels: the women were in poorer paying jobs with higher exposures. When unexplained differences between men and women are observed in occupational health studies, we, like Alice Hamilton, must delve into the problem until we understand the underlying causes.

ACKNOWLEDGMENTS

The author wishes to thank Louise St-Arnaud and Dala Bortolussi for their invaluable help, and Suzanne Gingras, who carried out the analyses. This work was supported by the Conseil québécois de recherche sociale.

NOTES

1. For men, the differences between adjusted and non-adjusted ORs likewise increases with the percentage of men, except in the opposite direction — the more men there are on the job, the more the results on the risk of PSI are maximized.

REFERENCES

Belloc, N.B., L. Breslow and J.R. Hochstim. "Measurement of Physical Health in a General Population Survey." *American Journal of Epidemiology* 93 (1971). pp. 328-36.

Berkman, P.L. "Measurement of Mental Health in a General Population Survey."

American Journal of Epidemiology 94 (1971). pp. 105-11.

Bielby, W.T., and J.N. Baron. "Occupations and Labor Markers: A Critical Evaluation." *American Economic Review* 76 (1986). pp. 43-7.

Billette, A., and J. Piché. "Health Problems of Data Entry Clerks and Related Job Stressors." *Journal of Occupational Medicine* 29 (1987). pp. 942-8.

Brabant, C., D. Mergler and K. Messing. "Va te faire soigner, ton usine est malade: la place de l'hystérie de masse dans la problématique de la santé des femmes au travail." *Santé mentale au Québec* 15 (1990). pp. 181-204.

Bradley, H. *Men's Work, Women's Work. A Sociological History of the Sexual Division of Labour in Employment.* Minneapolis: University of Minnesota Press, 1989.

Brisson, C., D. Loomis and N. Pearce. "Is Social Class Standardization Appropriate in Occupational Studies?" *Journal of Epidemiology and Community Health* 41 (1987). pp. 290-4.

Bureau of National Affairs. *Working Women's Health Concerns: A Gender at Risk? A BNA Special Report.* Washington, DC: Bureau of National Affairs, 1989.

Cockburn, C. *Machinery of Dominance.* London: Pluto Press, 1988.

Cohen, S., and G.M. Williamson. "Stress and Infectious Disease in Humans." *Psychological Bulletin* 109 (1991). pp. 5-24.

Courville, J., N. Vézina and K. Messing. "Comparison of the Work Activity of Two Mechanics: A Woman and a Man." *International Journal of Industrial Ergonomics* 7 (1991). pp. 163-74.

Cox, T., M. Thirlway and S. Cox. "Occupational Well-being: Sex Differences at Work." *Ergonomics* 27 (1984). pp. 499-510.

Doyal, L. "Promoting Women's Health," in *Health Promotion Research: Toward a Social Epidemiology.* Bernhard Bandura and Ilona Kickbusch (eds.). Copenhagen: World Health Organization Regional Publications, European Series No. 37, 1991.

Dumais, L., K. Messing, A.M. Seifert, J. Courville and N. Vézina. "Make Me a Cake as Fast as You Can: Forces For and Against Change in the Sexual Division of Labour at an Industrial Bakery." *Work, Employment and Health* 7 (1993). pp. 363-82.

Eichler, M. "Non-sexist Research: A Metatheoretical Approach." *Indian Journal of Social Work* 53 (1992). pp. 329-41.

Elias, R., and F. Cail. "Effets du stress psychosical en informatique: résultants et moyens de prévention." *Cahiers de notes documentaires, Paris, INRS* 122 (1986). pp. 67-73.

Enquête Santé Québec. "Et la santé, ça va?" Québec: Enquête Santé Québec, 1988.

Hamilton, Alice, and Harriet Hardy. *Industrial Toxicology, Third Edition.* Acton, MA: Publishing Sciences Group, 1974.

Harmon, D.K., M. Masuda and T.H. Holmes. "The Social Readjustment Rating Scale: A Cross-cultural Study of Western Europeans and Americans." *Journal of Psychosomatic Research* 14 (1970). pp. 391-400.

Hartmann, H., and B. Reskin. *Women's Work, Men's Work: Sex Segregation on the Job.* Washington, DC: National Academy Press, 1986.

The Health of Canadians: Report of the Canada Health Survey. Ottawa: Statistics Canada and National Health and Welfare, 1981. Catalogue 82-538E.

Holmes, T.H., and R.G. Rahe. "The Social Readjustment Rating Scale." *Journal of*

Psychosomatic Research 11 (1967). pp. 213-8.

Hunter, A.A., and M.C. Manley. "On the Task Content of Work." *Canadian Review of Sociology and Anthropology* 23 (1986). pp. 47-71.

Ilfeld, F.W. "Further Validation of a Psychiatric Symptom Index in a Normal Population." *Psychological Reports* 39 (1976). pp. 1215-8.

Jessell, J.C., and L. Beymer. "The Effects of Job Title vs. Job Description on Occupational Sex Typing." *Sex Roles* 27 (1992). pp. 73-83.

Kaplan, G.A., R.E. Roberts, T.C. Camacho and J.C. Coyne. "Psychosocial Predictors of Depression: Prospective Evidence from the Human Population Laboratory Studies." *American Journal of Epidemiology* 125 (1987). pp. 206-20.

Kohn, J.P., and G.H. Frazer. "An Academic Stress Scale: Identification and Rated Importance of Academic Stressors." *Psychological Reports* 59 (1986). pp. 415-26.

Lacroix, A.Z., and S.G. Haynes. "Gender Differences in the Health Effects of Workplace Roles," in *Gender and Stress*. Rosalind Barnett, Lois Brenner and Grace K. Baruch (eds.). New York: New York Free Press, 1987.

Loscocco, K.A., and G. Spitze. "Working Conditions, Social Support and the Well-being of Female and Male Factory Workers. *Journal of Health and Social Behavior* 31 (1990). pp. 313-27.

Lowe, G.S. *Women, Paid/Unpaid Work and Sress*. Ottawa: Canadian Advisory Council on the Status of Women, 1989.

McIntosh, D.N., J. Keywell, A. Reifman and P.C. Ellsworth. "Stress and Health in First-year Law Students: Women Fare Worse." *Journal of Applied Social Psychology* 24 (1994). pp. 1474-99.

Mergler, D., C. Brabant, N. Vézina and K. Messing. "The Weaker Sex? Men in Women's Working Conditions Report Similar Health Symptoms." *Journal of Occupational Medicine* 29 (1987). pp. 417-21.

Messing, K., and D. Mergler. "The Rat Fights Back: Inhumanity in Occupational Health Research," in *Re-inventing Biology*. R. Hubbard and R. Birke (eds.). Indianapolis: Indiana University Press, 1995.

Messing, K., and J-P Reveret. "Are Women in Female Jobs for their Health? A Study of Working Conditions and Health Effects in the Fish-processing Industry in Quebec." *International Journal of Health Services* 13 (1983). pp. 635-48.

Messing, K. *Occupational Safety and Health Concerns of Canadian Women*. Ottawa: Ministry of Supply and Services Canada, 1991.

Messing, K., G. Doniol-Shaw and C. Haëntjens. "Sugar and Spice and Everything Nice: Health Effects of the Sexual Division of Labor Among Train Cleaners." *International Journal of Health Services* 23 (1991). pp. 133-46.

Messing, K., L. Dumais, J. Courville, A-M Seifert and M. Boucher. "Evaluation of Exposure Data from Men and Women with the Same Job Title. *Journal of Occupational Medicine* 36 (1994). pp. 913-7.

Murgatroya, L. "Women, Men and the Social Grading of Occupations." *British Journal of Sociology* 35 (1984). pp. 473-97.

Nations, M.K., L.A. Camino and F.B. Walker. "'Nerves': Folk Idiom for Anxiety and Depression?" *Social Science and Medicine* 26 (1988). pp. 1245-59.

Norfleet, M.A., and G.M. Burnell. "Loss Items on the Schedule of Recent Life Events

(SRE): Duration of Psychotherapy." *Journal of Psychology* 124 (1990). pp. 165-8.

Roberts, R.E. "Prevalence of Pschological Distress Among Mexican Americans." *Journal of Health and Social Behavior* 21 (1980). pp. 134-45.

Rousseau, T., and M. Jenicek. "Santé physique, mentale, sociale et handicaps des citoyens seniors, Ville de Saint-Laurent: 1. Santé physique et mentale." *Canadian Journal of Public Health* 68 (1977). pp. 210-8.

Schutt, R.K., T. Meschede and J. Rierdan. "Distress, Suicidal Thoughts, and Social Support Among Homeless Adults." *Journal of Health and Social Behavior* 35 (1994). pp. 134-42.

Siemiatycki, J., S. Wacholder and R. Deward. "Degree of Confounding Bias Related to Smoking, Ethnic Group and Socioeconomic Status as Estimates of the Associations Between Occupation and Cancer." *Journal of Occupational Medicine* 30 (1988). pp. 617-25.

Skov, P., O. Valbjørn and B.V. Pedersen. "Influence of Personal Characteristics, Job-related Factors and Psychosocial Factors on the Sick Building Syndrome." *Scandinavian Journal of Work, Environment, and Health* 15 (1989). pp. 286-95.

Steffey, B.D., and J.W. Jones. "The Psychological Impact of Video Display Terminals on Employees' Well-being." *Stress Management* 4 (1989). pp. 101-7.

Stellman, J.M. *Women's Work, Women's Health: Myths and Realities.* New York: Pantheon Books. 1977.

Strang, D., and J. Baron. "Categorial Imperatives: The Structure of Job Titles in California State Agencies." *American Sociological Review* 55 (1990). pp. 749-95.

Tafari, S., F.E. Aboud and C.P. Larson. "Determinants of Mental Illness in a Rural Ethiopian Adult Population." *Social Science and Medicine* 32 (1991). pp. 197-201.

The Health of Canadians: Report of the Canada Health Survey. Ottawa: Statistics Canada and National Health and Welfare, 1981. Catalogue 82-538E.

Vézina, N., M. Cousineau, D. Mergler, A. Vinet and M-C Laurendeau. *Pour donner un sens au travail: bilan et orientations en santé mentale au travail.* Quebec City: Gaetan Morin, 1992.

Yodfat, Y., P. Shvartzman, V. Soskolne and S. Bronner. "Life Events Readjustment Scale in a Kibbutz." *Israel Journal of Medical Science* 29 (1993). pp. 221-4.

Danièle Kergoat

De la division sexuelle du travail et de ses conséquences sur les conditions de travail

It is now commonplace to consider women's occupational health as a full-fledged research topic within sociology. This was not, however, always the case. This paper outlines some of the changes that were necessary to achieve this paradigm shift. To explore women's work, it was necessary to simultaneously consider professional work and housework, waged work and the family, and to elaborate on the concept of the sexual division of labour. This allowed working conditions to be perceived as "gendered," and allowed women's occupational health to emerge from a spurious universality and to be reborn as a separate concern. Women's occupational health was finally a "legitimate" research project.

Aujourd'hui, en sociologie, la santé des femmes comme objet de recherche à part entière va de soi. Il n'en a pas toujours été ainsi. Cet article montre, à partir d'exemples concrets, ce qu'il a fallu réaliser, en amont, pour rendre cette réalité-là possible: démontrer que la prise en compte simultanée du travail professionnel et du travail domestique, du salariat et de la famille, l'élaboration du concept de division sexuelle du travail … étaient indispensables pour appréhender la réalité du travail. C'est seulement alors que flexibilité du travail et conditions de travail ont pu apparaître comme «sexuées» et donc que la santé des femmes au travail pouvait devenir visible socialement, émerger des brumes de la fausse universalité, et apparaître enfin objet de recherche théoriquement «légitime».

UN ITINÉRAIRE DE RECHERCHE

Ayant commencé à travailler de façon autonome dans les années 1968-1970, c'est-à-dire à une période où, en France, la montée des luttes des ouvriers non qualifiés était spectaculaire et portait sur les cadences, les relations hiérarchiques, les conditions de travail, la santé. «Ne pas perdre sa vie à la gagner» date de cette période post-1968. Du même coup, même si la santé n'était pas mon «objet» principal de recherche, les revendications sur ce thème ne pouvaient que s'imposer à moi : la non-qualification, la place dans le procès de travail, la répétitivité des tâches, etc., étaient des nuisances spécifiques pour les ouvriers spécialisés, tandis que les ouvriers professionnels ou les techniciens, subissant d'autres types d'agression, formulaient d'autres revendications et adoptaient d'autres formes de luttes.

Cela dit, ces travaux portaient sur des usines où la main-d'oeuvre était exclusivement masculine. Pour une raison simple : c'est que les entreprises dont on avait «parlé» en mai 1968 étaient des usines d'hommes; ce ne fut que plus tard, dans les années 1972-1974, que de grands conflits dans des entreprises féminisées des secteurs tertiaire et secondaire apparurent au grand jour et firent l'objet de commentaires dans les médias.

Très vite, l'approche de ces conflits me conduisit à constater la présence d'une aporie : il était impossible, à partir de la conceptualisation offerte par la sociologie du travail, de penser les conflits féminisés et même les pratiques revendicatives des services ou ateliers féminins faisant partie d'une usine mixte. La sociologie les ignorait[1] ou, au mieux, (même cela fut plus tardif) en faisait un chapitre «spécifique» au sein d'un ensemble cohérent censé décrire les comportements des «travailleurs».

La constatation d'une telle aporie aboutit vite à la conclusion qu'il fallait repenser toute la conceptualisation si l'on voulait dépasser ce faux universalisme qui consiste à faire comme si les hommes représentaient l'universel et les femmes, le spécifique. Et ce travail de déconstruction devait être mené en même temps qu'un effort de réagencement, parfois de réinvention, des concepts si l'on voulait sortir les pratiques féminines de l'invisibilité et donc de l'inexistence.

C'est ce souci qui a été à l'origine de la création de mon laboratoire, le GEDISST — Groupe d'études de la division sociale et sexuelle du travail — et de la lutte menée pour qu'il soit un laboratoire propre du Centre national de la recherche scientifique (CNRS) : c'était par là, vouloir faire reconnaître sur le plan politique qu'il y avait une légitimité scientifique à analyser le travail à travers, notamment, la grille des rapports sociaux basés sur la différence sexuelle.

C'est ce travail, tant empirique que théorique, que je veux évoquer maintenant : après une rapide mise au point sur ce que j'entends par «division sexuelle du travail», je prendrai quelques exemples et montrerai comment, dans mes travaux de sociologie du travail, j'ai rencontré constamment, de façon latente ou explicite — même si ce n'était pas l'objet — le problème des conditions de travail et donc, si l'on poursuivait le raisonnement, celui de la santé.

DE LA DIVISION SEXUELLE DU TRAVAIL

Ce phénomène de la division du travail selon les sexes, d'une part la partition travail productif/travail reproductif, et d'autre part la division du travail entre les hommes et les femmes à l'intérieur même du travail productif, est un phénomène universel. Il a toujours existé et il existe dans tous les types de sociétés. Le pas est du coup vite franchi qui consiste à le considérer comme «naturel», et donc comme non susceptible d'interrogation, d'interprétations éventuellement divergentes. La sociologie française — et plus largement les sciences humaines[2] — a fonctionné ainsi jusqu'à ce que le mouvement féministe pénètre le monde universitaire.

La sociologie de la famille, très proche en France de la sociologie américaine, était fonctionnaliste et tenait pour acquis les rôles masculins et féminins : les femmes à la maison, les hommes pourvoyeurs de la famille. Quant à l'école française de la sociologie du travail, extrêmement vivante et productive, elle raisonnait sur un modèle masculin celui des «travailleurs» — et universel — «le salariat», «la classe ouvrière»; tout cela bien implanté dans la tradition française du grand écart : proclamation des Droits de l'Homme et du Citoyen d'une part, exclusion des femmes de la citoyenneté et droit de vote octroyé dans le peloton de queue des pays industrialisés d'autre part. Bref, «tout se passait comme si le rapport capital/travail ne créait de classes que masculines» (Kergoat, 1978).

Mais comme je le mentionnais plus haut, les discours académiques ne pouvaient rendre compte que très partiellement des pratiques féminines au travail. Très rapidement, des questions sont formalisées sur les lieux mêmes du travail — plus exactement sur certains — par les actrices des luttes (groupes femmes entreprises, commissions syndicales femmes). Plus tardivement (à l'exception de quelques rares pionnières), les intellectuelles s'emparent des problèmes en affirmant :

- que les catégories de sexes sont des catégories sociales avant d'être des catégories biologiques, on peut donc les étudier sociologiquement (Mathieu, 1991);
- que si, historiquement, il est vrai que le capitalisme a entraîné la séparation des espaces productif et reproductif, il n'en reste pas moins qu'il faut penser ensemble ces deux espaces-temps si l'on veut comprendre le «sexe du travail». C'est cette seconde affirmation qui fut le fondement de la création du GEDISST : refus des disjonctions classiques travail / non travail, travail salarié / travail domestique; refus, également, de penser à l'identique ces deux procès de travail (Chabaud et al., 1985); remise en cause du concept de travail tel qu'il était utilisé en sociologie du travail (sortir du seul domaine des rapports marchands); affirmation qu'une

telle position épistémologique s'imposait pour comprendre tant les pratiques masculines que féminines au travail.

Je mentionnais plus haut que ce phénomène de la division sexuelle du travail était universel. Certes, mais si l'on en examine les modalités, il faut bien admettre qu'il est — aussi — d'une variabilité absolue dans le temps et dans l'espace : tel travail défini péremptoirement comme masculin sera défini comme féminin dans la même société mais à une autre période historique (par exemple, le métier d'instituteur), dans une même branche industrielle mais dans des usines différentes (Milkman, 1987).

La division du travail peut toujours prendre d'autres formes selon l'état et l'évolution des rapports de force entre les hommes et les femmes.

Cela dit, si les modalités de la division sexuelle du travail sont changeantes, il n'en reste pas moins que cette dernière reste toujours structurée par un principe hiérarchique organisé autour de la notion de valeur du travail (*la valeur du travail masculin reste toujours supérieure à celle du travail féminin*). Quelle que soit la nature concrète du travail, la valeur du premier est surévaluée par rapport au second, tandis que celle du second est toujours comparativement dévaluée. Pour expliquer une telle constante, il faut bien faire appel à la notion de rapport social, et à un rapport social antagonique entre deux groupes sociaux. C'est ce que nous désignons en France, sous le terme de «rapports sociaux de sexe», lesquels s'articulent avec les rapports de classe pour former le treillis autour duquel se nouent les pratiques de genre.

Une première illustration: le foyer de jeunes travailleurs (FJT) et le travail à temps partiel, ou l'effet de boucle de l'exploitation et de l'oppression

Les foyers de jeunes travailleurs sont un lieu précieux d'expérimentation pour qui s'intéresse à la division sexuelle du travail : les garçons et les filles de moins de 25 ans qui y sont hébergés sont égaux devant le travail de reproduction de leur force de travail puisque pour un prix modique, ils sont hébergés, nourris, leurs draps sont blanchis et un minimum d'entretien ménager est assuré. À l'inverse de ce qui se passe dans la grande majorité des familles, garçons et filles sont donc idéalement en situation d'égalité par rapport au travail domestique.

Il est impossible de rapporter ici la problématique et les résultats de l'étude; les lecteurs intéressés pourront se reporter à l'article que nous lui avons consacré (Chenal et Kergoat, 1981). À partir du seul cas des jeunes ouvrières, je voudrais simplement montrer que l'analyse de leurs pratiques envers le travail salarié est indissociable de celle de leurs pratiques (idéelles ou matérielles, passées, présentes ou futures) envers le travail domestique.

L'analyse des itinéraires professionnels et familiaux, celle des discours, l'observation des pratiques, a permis de faire émerger une typologie dont je n'évoquerai ici que les deux termes extrêmes :

- les jeunes filles les plus surexploitées (travail précaire, chômage à répétition, basse qualification, salaire de misère, conditions de travail insupportables, etc.) avaient conscience de cette surexploitation mais l'accompagnaient du sentiment aigu qu'elles ne pourraient jamais s'en sortir; travail ne renvoie qu'à souffrance; le salaire, insuffisant pour une personne, devient dérisoire dès qu'elles ont un enfant. Pour sortir de ce qu'elles perçoivent comme un «destin», elles n'entrevoient qu'une solution: trouver un mari et abandonner l'activité salariée. Et bien sûr, non seulement elles acceptent l'ordre patriarcal, mais d'une certaine manière elles en «rajoutent» en faisant l'apologie du travail domestique et en niant tout rapport de domination hommes/femmes. Le mécanisme ici est clair: un travail salarié insupportable induit à projeter sur le travail domestique une autonomie très largement fantasmée et à faire comme si l'assignation au travail domestique était un choix personnel que l'on pouvait mettre en balance avec le choix d'avoir ou non une activité professionnelle. Si la domination patronale est dénoncée, le mariage reste un idéal;

- un second groupe se caractérisait tout différemment: il est composé d'ouvrières qualifiées travaillant dans de grandes entreprises où une présence syndicale garantissait un minimum de protection et de droits sociaux. Ces femmes, souvent syndiquées, investissaient dans la formation professionnelle, souhaitaient obtenir une promotion (étant réalistes, ces souhaits restaient modestes), disaient aimer leur travail et s'y intéresser. À l'inverse des premières, leurs loisirs n'étaient pas structurés par les relations hommes/femmes, mais par des goûts personnels. Leurs avis étaient tout aussi arrêtés en ce qui concernait la sphère reproductive: pas question de vivre avec un homme, encore moins de se lier par le mariage, pas question non plus d'avoir des enfants; leur volonté d'autonomie et de liberté était constamment mise en avant et il leur semblait impossible de vivre avec un homme sans qu'aussitôt, quel que soit l'homme en question, les rapports de domination ne réapparaissent, tout particulièrement à propos du travail domestique. Elles préféraient donc s'en tenir aux relations amoureuses sans engagement et investissaient dans le travail professionnel. Même si l'on ne peut tirer de conclusion causale de cet exemple (du type: un travail professionnel non aliénant entraîne les femmes à remettre en question les rapports sociaux de sexe), il apparaît bien que le fait que le travail domestique apparaisse soit comme un repoussoir, soit comme un idéal, est à mettre en relation avec le type de travail professionnel imposé/proposé aux femmes.

Une étude postérieure dans le temps sur les femmes et le travail à temps partiel (Kergoat, 1985) a confirmé à mes yeux cette relation profonde entre le travail salarié et le travail domestique, la nécessité d'une circulation constante entre ces deux aires pour comprendre les pratiques féminines envers le temps travaillé; elle a par contre infirmé toute relation unicausale entre la prise de temps partiel et le fait d'avoir des enfants.

Avant d'aller plus avant, il faut préciser bien sûr que ce qui m'intéressait n'était pas ici les règles patronales qui imposent massivement aux femmes la flexibilité de l'emploi à travers le travail à temps partiel (cas, en particulier, du commerce et des services), mais bien les stratégies des femmes face au temps travaillé dans l'univers professionnel et dans l'univers domestique, et quelle que soit la modalité du temps salarial: chômage, temps partiel «choisi» ou imposé, travail à temps complet, inactivité.

Deux conclusions majeures s'imposèrent à l'issue de cette étude:

- qu'il soit demandé par les femmes ou imposé par le contrat de travail, et quelle que soit la diminution du temps de travail salarié par rapport au temps plein de 39 heures, l'effet était immédiat sur la répartition du travail domestique. Les hommes, en effet, ne se considéraient légitimement plus tenus «d'aider» leur compagne, et du jour au lendemain, les femmes se retrouvaient avec la totalité du travail domestique sur les épaules. Et cela en toute bonne conscience des maris et des enfants.
- à revenu familial égal et à nombre d'enfants égal (l'âge de ces enfants étant également pris en compte), celles qui demandaient à passer à temps partiel étaient celles dont le travail était le moins qualifié, le moins intéressant. La «demande» des femmes envers le temps partiel n'était donc pas commandée mécaniquement par le nombre d'enfants et leur âge, mais tout aussi fortement par un décrochage du travail salarié, lié au manque d'intérêt de celui-ci, à sa «déqualification», à l'absence de perspectives professionnelles, à la pénibilité des conditions de travail …

FLEXIBILITÉ DU TRAVAIL ET ÉVOLUTION DES CONDITIONS DE TRAVAIL: DEUX VARIABLES MAJEURES POUR LA SANTÉ DES FEMMES AU TRAVAIL

La flexibilité du travail et son automatisation, les débats théoriques qui les accompagnent (faut-il parler de continuité ou de rupture avec le taylorisme?), tout cela, en Europe, se conjugue, sauf exception au neutre, s'inscrivant bien, au moins en cela, dans la tradition friedmanienne.

Et cependant, l'observation (et parfois même la simple lecture de travaux totalement asexués en apparence: voir, par exemple, Kern et Schumann, 1989) montre que l'on peut dégager deux modèles sexués de la flexibilité (Doniol Shaw et al., 1993; Kergoat, 1992):

- l'un masculin, où l'acte de travail est repensé dans sa globalité. Par conséquent, de nouvelles filières sont créées, des programmes de formation mises en place, de nouveaux diplômes font leur apparition. Bref, même si l'on peut s'interroger sur la longévité du phénomène, une réelle politique qualifiante est pensée pour les hommes;
- l'autre féminin, dont le principe est l'additivité. Les femmes continuent de travailler selon le modèle taylorisé, mais s'y ajoutent de nouvelles impositions telles que gestion des stocks, zéro défaut, réparation des pannes mineures, etc. Cela s'appelle «polyvalence» en langage patronal. Le gain de salaire est en général nul, mais la pression objective et subjective, sur chaque individu(e)[3] est forte : il faut, dans le même temps, mener à bien de nouvelles tâches, le travail se complexifie, tandis que l'on demande à chacun et chacune de s'investir dans son travail (exigence du zéro défaut par exemple).

Cela ne peut qu'entraîner des conséquences sur la santé des femmes: elles qui devaient déjà gérer mentalement travail salarié et travail domestique voient, par ce modèle, s'alourdir les charges psychologiques du travail salarié et ses contraintes physiques. Que ce soit à propos des femmes que l'on raisonne en termes d'additivité n'est pas pour étonner! Ne sont-elles pas habituées à mener de front plusieurs tâches à la fois: préparer le dîner tout en surveillant les devoirs, «profiter» d'une course à faire pour mettre en marche la lessive? Mais n'y a-t-il pas un seuil où les neurones féminins sont saturables? Et que se passe-t-il alors? Sans doute la «déprime» sur le plan individuel; mais quand ces phénomènes atteignent toute une population? Nous y reviendrons tout à l'heure.

La flexibilité croissante des postes de travail, le recours de tous les secteurs à l'automation et à l'informatique, expliquent sans doute pour une large part l'insatisfaction massive et croissante quant aux conditions de travail en France.

Lorsque j'ai commencé à étudier les conditions de travail des ouvrières, aux environs de 1972, je me suis aperçue que rien n'avait changé depuis le constat que Madeleine Guilbert établissait en 1966. L'observation sociologique soulignait la continuité: ghettos masculins, ghettos féminins; travail déqualifié pour les femmes, majoritairement ouvrières au bas des classifications, travaillant à la chaîne et sous contrainte de temps, soumises à de fortes contraintes hiérarchiques; travail parcellisé et atomisé, etc.

Il fallut attendre 1978 pour que ces constats sociologiques soient confirmés statistiquement, avec la mise en chantier, par le Ministère du Travail, de grosses enquêtes quantitatives sur les conditions de travail — ou plus exactement sur les représentations qu'ont les salariés (de tout secteur et de tout niveau hiérarchique) de leurs conditions de travail. Nous en sommes actuellement à la quatrième enquête (1991) et les jugements portés ont évolué si négativement depuis la dernière enquête que l'on a cherché désespérément où était l'erreur méthodologique. Apparemment, il n'y en avait pas: travailleurs et travailleuses, dans le secondaire, dans le tertiaire, dans les usines, les services et la fonction publique, estiment globalement que les conditions de travail vont en se détériorant et que la pénibilité s'accroît. Malgré (ou peut-être à cause de) l'automatisation et l'informatisation, il y a intensification du travail: des horaires plus morcelés et plus instables, des rythmes de travail dépendant de plus en plus de la demande des clients, des délais plus courts, des changements de poste constants, des tâches sans cesse interrompues, des accidents du travail plus graves qu'ils ne l'étaient les années précédentes, etc. Donc, aggravation très sensible, tant pour les hommes que pour les femmes. Pour ces dernières, c'est, semble-t-il, sur les problèmes de temps et de rapports à la clientèle que la situation s'est davantage détériorée.

Et les choses ne semblent pas près de s'améliorer. Le chômage de masse (3,7 millions de chômeurs en France soit plus de 11 p. 100 de la population active) touche davantage les femmes que les hommes, le temps partiel continue de croître (actuellement une femme sur quatre travaille à temps partiel en France), et c'est même la notion d'activité féminine qui est remise en question à travers les débats autour du salaire maternel. Les lois votées dans le cadre de la politique libérale remettent en cause ce qui apparaissait pourtant comme des acquis en France: la retraite à 60 ans, le financement de cette retraite, la santé, diminution des droits syndicaux dans les petites et moyennes entreprises grosses utilisatrices de main d'oeuvre féminine, annualisation de la durée du travail, remise en cause du repos dominical, on pourrait énumérer bien des points encore. Tous les points sur lesquels on sait que les femmes sont plus vulnérables que les hommes; elles sont plus qu'eux exposées à la pauvreté, et la gestion de leur temps travaillé (salarié et domestique) va devenir de plus en plus difficile qu'il s'agisse d'une journée, d'une semaine ou d'une année …

CONCLUSION

Ma conclusion sera simple: il est utile de travailler en termes de division sexuelle du travail et non simplement en termes de «condition féminine», qu'il s'agisse des problèmes de santé ou de tout autre problème.

C'est parce qu'on a montré qu'«être ouvrier» n'était pas «être ou-vrière», et que les différences n'étaient pas explicables en termes de plus ou moins d'exploitation, mais bel et bien en termes de domination, c'est parce qu'on a montré que la division sexuelle du travail faisait partie de l'ossature même de la hiérarchie du travail et plus largement de toute la hiérarchie sociale, c'est parce que le concept de division sexuelle du travail rappelle sans cesse que l'on ne peut faire l'impasse sur le travail domes-tique : c'est pour tout cela qu'une telle approche me paraît utile tant théoriquement que socialement. Je ne suis pas une spécialiste de la santé des femmes, mais l'expérience m'a prouvé que toute interrogation sexuée sur le travail amène à rencontrer les problèmes liés à la santé. L'inverse est tout aussi vrai: parler de la santé des femmes amène, à mon sens, à s'interroger sur les rapports sociaux et la division du travail entre les hommes et les femmes.

NOTES

1. Un exemple parfait d'absence de prise en compte du sexe de la main d'oeuvre est donné par un des livres fondateurs de la sociologie du travail française : G. Friedmann, *Le travail en miettes*, 1964.

2. Il faudrait évidemment réserver un traitement particulier à l'ethnologie. Mais elle-même, si elle prenait en compte la sexuation des travaux productifs et reproduc-tifs, ne les interprétait pas en termes de rapports sociaux entre les sexes.

3. Faut-il le préciser? Il s'agit ici de modèles sociologiques: le modèle dit «féminin» n'est pas imposé aux seules femmes; bien des hommes le subissent également. Et la même chose est vraie pour le modèle dit «masculin». Mais le noyau dur de chaque modèle reprend les logiques sexuées qui aboutissaient à ce que tel atelier, tel travail, tel poste, telle forme d'emploi soient pensés d'abord féminins ou masculins.

BIBLIOGRAPHIE

Agir contre le chômage. *Données et Arguments*. Paris: Syllepse, 1994.

Chabaud-Rychter, D., D. Fougeyrollas-Schwebel et F. Santhonnax. *Espace et temps du travail domestique*. Paris: Librairie des Méridiens, Réponses sociologiques, 1985.

Chenal, O., et D. Kergoat. «Production et reproduction. Les jeunes travailleuses, le salariat et la famille». *Critiques de l'Economie Politique* (nouvelle série) 7 (1981). pp. 118-31.

Collectif. *Le sexe du travail. Structures familiales et système productif*. Grenoble: Presses Universitaires de Grenoble, 1984.

Doniol-Shaw, G., et A. Lerolle. «L'évolution du rapport genre — qualification: question d'identité et de pouvoir». *Cahiers du Gedisst* 7 (1993). pp. 13-26.

Friedmann, G. *Le travail en miettes*. Paris: Gallimard, 1964.

Guilbert, M. *Les fonctions des femmes dans l'industrie*. Paris: Mouton, 1966.

Hirata, H., et C. Rogerat. «Technologie, qualification et division sexuelle du travail». *Revue Française de Sociologie* XXIX (1988). pp. 171-92.

Kergoat, D. «Ouvriers = ouvrières?». *Critiques de l'Economie Politique* (nouvelle série) 5 (1978). pp. 65-97.

— *Les ouvrières*. Paris: Éditions du Sycomore, 1982.

— *Les femmes et le travail à temps partiel*. Paris: Documentation Française, 1985.

— «Les absentes de l'histoire», dans *Ouvriers, ouvrières. Un continent morcelé et silencieux*. Paris: Autrement (série Mutations, no. 126), 1992. pp. 73-83.

Kern, H., et M. Schumann. *La fin de la division du travail?* Paris: Éditions de la M.S.H., 1989.

Mathieu, N-C. *L'anatomie politique. Catégorisations et idéologies du sexe*. (Recueil de textes couvrant une vingtaine d'années de recherche.) Paris: Côté-Femmes Éditions, 1991.

Milkman, R. *Gender at Work: the Dynamics of Job Segregation by Sex during World War II*. Chicago: University of Illinois Press, 1987.

Ministère du travail. *Enquêtes sur les conditions de travail*. Paris: Ministère du travail, 1978, 1984, 1987, 1991.

Thébaud-Mony, A. «La précarité moderne». *Politis-La Revue* 7 (1994). pp. 31-6.

Making Issues

Visible in

Public Policy

Rendre

les enjeux

visibles dans

l'application

des politiques

publiques

Katherine Lippel

Watching the Watchers

How Expert Witnesses and Decision-makers Perceive Men's and Women's Workplace Stressors

Plusieurs juridictions nord-américaines prévoient l'indemnisation des lésions psychologiques reliées à des événements «stresseurs» vécus au travail. Dans une étude antérieure, nous avons examiné l'évolution des règles de droit applicables à ces questions dans 60 juridictions nord-américaines. Souvent, les critères juridiques utilisés pour déterminer l'accès à l'indemnisation tiennent compte du caractère inusité des «stresseurs», de l'importance des événements survenus dans la vie personnelle des individus qui réclament compensation et de la relation entre les événements «stresseurs» et le travail. Notre étude actuelle porte sur la perception des témoins experts et des décideurs chargés d'évaluer l'admissibilité des réclamations, quant au travail et aux expériences de vie des hommes et des femmes. Nous examinons les décisions des bureaux de révision paritaire de la Commission de la santé et de la sécurité du travail, et de la Commission d'appel en matière de lésions professionnelles. Nous cherchons à déterminer s'il existe, dans la perception de ces variables, une différence qui soit en relation avec le sexe de la personne qui réclame une compensation. Nous vérifierons ensuite si une telle différence a un effet sur le sort de la réclamation. Nous présentons ici le cadre juridique de l'étude, la méthodologie appliquée et les résultats préliminaires. Notre conclusion: il existe, au niveau des décisions en appel, une différence entre les hommes et les femmes dans leur accès à l'indemnisation. Cette différence ne peut s'expliquer ni par la prédisposition, ni par les problèmes personnels, ni par la personnalité de la travailleuse réclamante.

Workers' compensation schemes in many North American jurisdictions compensate psychological disability caused by workplace stress. In a previous study we described how legal rules applicable to this issue have evolved in the 60 North American jurisdictions. Legal criteria used to determine eligibility for coverage often include work-relatedness tests that take into account such factors as the "unusualness" of the workplace stressors, the existence of intervening stressors in the claimant's personal life, and links between the stressors and the work environment. We are currently conducting a study in which we examine expert witnesses' and decision-makers' perceptions of men's and women's work and life circumstances as reported in Quebec compensation review and appeals decisions. We seek to determine whether perception of these variables differs depending on claimants' gender and, if so, whether there is a correlation between differences and case outcome. We present the legal framework underlying the study, the methodology applied and preliminary findings. We conclude that there is a gender based difference in access to compensation on the appellate level that cannot be explained either by predisposition, difficult life circumstances or personality.

INTRODUCTION

A policewoman learns she was on the target list of Marc Lépine, the murderer responsible for the "Montreal Massacre." She experiences a disabling anxiety reaction.[1] A sales clerk goes into a depression after a series of conflicts with a new supervisor culminating in a redefinition of work schedules in violation of rules of seniority.[2] A case coordinator is diagnosed with burnout after new compensation legislation has been brought in without proper training for those obliged to apply it.[3] A prison guard cuts down a prisoner who has hanged himself. She goes into shock.[4] A male worker is investigated for sexual harassment. Athough he is eventually exonerated, he is unable to work because of a psychological disability caused by the tarnishing of his reputation.[5] A woman prison guard working in a men's penitentiary is sexually harassed by the prisoners to the point where her state of anxiety prevents her from working.[6] All these people filed claims under Quebec workers' compensation legislation.

Is compensation for psychological disability linked to work-related stress a feminist issue? Stereotypes would have it that work stress is more prevalent in male-dominated work places: executive stress is so well known it has become a marketing tool for everything from long distance phone cards to Clamato juice. Everyone knows that police officers and prison guards are exposed to extreme stress, and their stressful work, along with that of lawyers and ambulance drivers, can be shared weekly by a television-watching public. Television images of women's stress rarely picture the workplace, but rather that of the homemaker who sends everybody off to school and work so that she can finally relax with a cup of tea. In the nineties, féminisme oblige, we now have the occasional television image of the woman executive exposed to stress. But stressful working conditions of waitresses, sales clerks, seamstresses and secretaries are rarely, if ever, seen in the media.[7] Images of overburdened teachers or youth protection workers don't seem to sell fashion, or for that matter situation comedies and drama.

Despite these popular images, stress-related disability is a significant problem for women workers, who are often in occupations providing minimal worker control and maximal external pressures.[8] Electronic monitoring of productivity, invasive supervisors and overburdening without adequate resources, particularly in the helping professions, are often associated with women's work. Ironically, the invisibility of the work may be an additional stressor: recognition for the value and importance of one's work is an effective mitigator of even the most stressful conditions. Not only is the stress of the work invisible to employers, but it is often invisible to the worker, who integrates the negative image of her job. The importance of such jobs is often trivialized.[9]

Access to compensation for disability arising out of workplace stress may also be adversely affected by the invisibility of women's work. In a previous study we were intrigued by the attitude of officials in Workers' Compensation Boards, who seemed particularly prone to stereotyping in their discussion of workplace stress. Over and over again, they spontaneously mentioned prison guards and police officers as being prime targets for stress compensation. When asked whether their secretaries were under stress, many expressed surprise at the question, while quickly answering that their own work, unlike that of their secretaries, was stressful, because they bore the responsibility for the smooth running of the operation (Lippel, 1989; 1990).

In our current study we are analyzing all published and unpublished Quebec review board and appeal decisions in order to determine if there exist gender-based discrepancies in the application of criteria used to evaluate claims for psychological disability attributed to stressful work situations. As we are relying only on the written decisions, information is tainted by the selection process applied by the decision makers themselves. We have nevertheless chosen to examine as many variables as the decision format will allow, including those specific to expert testimony, and those specific to the discourse of the decision makers themselves.

Our project is still in progress, and the objectives of the present paper are to present the framework in which the study is operating, while tracing some paths that appear intriguing in light of what is very preliminary research (97 of some 200 decisions have been analyzed thus far). In previous studies we have examined law as it is applied to compensation claims for stress in American states and in all Canadian provinces (Lippel, 1989; 1990; 1992). Our current study focuses on Quebec law.

In this paper we will first present the medicolegal framework applicable to all compensation claims, with particular emphasis on issues arising when doctors, scientists and lawyers all think they're discussing the same issue. In the second part we will address rules specifically applicable to stress claims. In the third part we will use some of our preliminary findings to examine the impact of this structure on women's claims for stress-related disability.

Research specific to workers' compensation provides insight into the perceptions of decision makers and expert witnesses about men's and women's work. It allows a glimpse, however imperfect, of the way in which a state apparatus views credibility, the role of family obligations, and the importance of women's work. More importantly, it provides tools that will permit better results in the recognition of compensation claims for stress, which in turn may have an impact on prevention. Prevention becomes more of a priority for employers as compensation costs escalate; undercompensation allows government institutions to underestimate danger, thus legitimizing the low priority given to policy development in many jobs occupied by women.

PART 1: WHAT CRITERIA ARE APPLIED TO DETERMINE THE RIGHT TO COMPENSATION?

Compensation claims in no way reflect a true portrait of stressors in the workplace as they only include those cases where workers allege workplace stress to have been debilitating to the point that they are temporarily, or sometimes permanently, unable to work. A worker making a claim for compensation has the burden of proving not only that the working conditions have been a significant factor in the development of the psychological disability, but also that the work events leading up to the disability fall within the framework of the legislative definition of "employment injury": "an injury or a disease arising out of or in the course of an industrial accident or an occupational disease ..."

As with all other workers' compensation claims, these claims are supposedly decided without consideration of fault: A worker who loses a hand as a result of his or her own distraction or clumsiness will be compensated. Theoretically, the same approach applies to claims for psychological disability. All Canadian legislation in this field follows this transactional model[10]: Workers need not prove employer negligence and are covered for their own errors; in exchange they only receive a fraction of the compensation they might have expected from the civil courts in a negligence case. Even those workers who could clearly prove employer negligence are precluded from suing their employer.

Hearings on stress claims, as with other claims, are supposed to determine whether an industrial accident or disease has given rise to the disability. Quebec adjudicators have a very legalistic approach, rather than a teleological one: in light of definitions provided in the *Act Respecting Industrial Accidents and Occupational Diseases*[11] they determine whether the factual demonstration before them justifies recognition of the claim.

Early decisions regarding stress claims were so legalistic that some claims were refused even though the decision maker concluded that the disability was work related.[12] In these cases, adjudicators underlined the importance of the definitions provided in Section 2 of the Act:

> An "industrial accident" means a sudden and unforeseen event, attributable to any cause, which happens to a person, arising out of or in the course of his work and resulting in an employment injury to him.
>
> An "occupational disease" means a disease contracted out of or in the course of work and characteristic of that work or directly related to the risks peculiar to that work.

The worker has the burden of proving that the events leading up to trauma constitute work-related injury under either the definition of industrial accident or occupational disease. To do so, convincing evidence must be shown of three variables:

1. the nature of the work-related events leading up to the disability must be deemed to be sudden and unforeseen (industrial accident) or the disease must be attributable to risks either characteristic of or peculiar to that work (occupational disease);

2. the disability itself, which must be medically corroborated;

3. legal causation: the disability (2) must have as its probable cause the work-related events (1).

Circumstances giving rise to the disability are facts to be proven by the worker's own testimony, as well as that of other witnesses. Employers will often call witnesses to contradict the worker's version of events. Perceptions by the decision maker of the credibility of testimony favouring the worker often determine success or failure of the claim. If the decision maker cannot identify with the worker's experience, it is unlikely he or she will be inclined to look upon the claim favourably. Elastic concepts in law will be interpreted narrowly and controversy arising from the evidence will be resolved against the worker. Global evaluation of the circumstances allegedly giving rise to the disability will directly or indirectly determine the worker's chance of success.

Both the existence of the disability and the causal link between disability and work are seen as issues to be determined in the light of testimony by expert witnesses, most commonly that of doctors. Causation is considered a medicolegal issue: expert evidence addresses issues of epidemiology, disability, diagnosis and treatment; legal reasoning determines whether workplace incidents can be deemed to have made a significant contribution to the disability. Regardless of the nature of the claim, the interaction between law and medicine often leads to confusion because of the interdisciplinary approach and the uniformity of the language applied. This confusion systematically hinders the person who by law bears the burden of proof — in the case of workers' compensation, the onus to establish the legitimacy of the claim lies on the worker. This negative impact is particularly evident in the context of industrial disease claims where evidence is often comprised of both medical testimony and scientific studies often based on principles of epidemiology where scientific certitude is of the essence.[13] Many difficulties arise in this context.

Language itself is a source of difficulty: In compensation law, an event is deemed *probable* if it is more probable than not that it occurred, yet expert witnesses often await certitude before affirming causation. The Supreme Court of Canada discussed the imbroglio created by the interaction between law and medicine in these terms:

> It is not therefore essential that the medical experts provide a firm opinion supporting the plaintiff's theory of causation. Medical experts ordinarily determine causation in terms of certainties whereas a lesser standard is demanded by the law.
>
> As Louisell points out in *Medical Malpractice, Volume 3*, the phrase "in your opinion with a reasonable degree of medical certainty," (which is the standard form of question to a medical expert) is often misunderstood. The author explains that: "Many doctors do not understand the phrase … as they usually deal in 'certainties' that are 100 percent sure, whereas 'reasonable' certainties which the law requires need only be more probably so, i.e., 51 percent."[14]

Legally, a disability is deemed to have been caused by work, in the context of workers' compensation, in cases where the answer to the following question is negative: "Would the worker be suffering from the disability but for the employment event, exposure, or circumstance?" It is sufficient that the employment was a significant factor in the development of the disability, even if it was not the sole, or even the primary cause of the disability.[15] Yet scientists and even doctors are reticent to conclude that a causal relationship exists if scientific studies have yet to demonstrate, with scientific levels of certitude, the existence of the causal relationship. If no epidemiological studies exist, scientists will be unwilling to affirm causation; yet in a legal context their refusal affirms absence of causation, even though no scientific evidence as to the absence of causation may exist.

An examination of the respective objectives of law and medicine facilitates identification, if not resolution, of the confusion. Adjudicators have to make a decision regarding a claim by relying on information available at the time the claim is made. They cannot abstain until scientific knowledge permits certitude: Whether they accept or refuse a claim, someone — either the worker or the compensation fund — bears the cost of scientific ignorance that may lead to an erroneous conclusion. Both civil law and common law systems establish an evidentiary burden of 50-percent-plus-one in cases of a civil nature, as opposed to that applicable to criminal cases, where guilt must be established beyond a reasonable doubt. Law seeks honesty, but it never has the pretension of stating the truth. Professor Terence Ison thus formulated the appropriate question: "The legally relevant question [is] what is the best available hypothesis about the cause of the disease in the particular case?"[16]

Often doctors who testify will comment that it would be unfair to ascribe responsibility for a disability to the employer, because work was not the cause of the disability but only contributed to its development. This attitude can actually lead to misleading testimony, as can be seen by the following testimony by a cardiologist:

> As near as I can tell, the lawyer is primarily concerned with whether there is reasonable cause or suspicion that the work activity is a precipitating event or contributed in any way. It's the fault of the law that says that if there is a contribution there is a certain award. I think that in many instances we can say that there could have been some precipitation or aggravation of the chronic degenerative disease by some kind of work activity. The problem with that is the inequity in making the whole thing compensable.[17]

Multifactorial causation is often present in cases of occupational disease, and this is particularly true when the disability is of a psychological nature. The law clearly provides for compensation in cases where work has contributed to the disability, even though the worker may have been particularly vulnerable because of a personal predisposition. This principle, poetically referred to as the "thin skull rule," applies to both tort law and compensation law. Compensation must be provided if there is evidence of work contribution, even though the worker would not normally have been injured in similar circumstances were it not for personal vulnerability.[18]

In summary, legal practitioners defending workers are continually confronted with multiple sources of frustration. One of the most important is that caused by a double confusion: on the one hand, the reticence of doctors or scientists to infer a causal relation between working conditions and a disability on the basis of scientific rather than legal criteria; on the other hand, the inevitable interpretation of the decision maker, often a lawyer unfamiliar with the multiple meanings of the terms used, that an opinion to the effect that work was a *possible* cause of the disability implies that the expert feels that the best hypothesis is that work *did not* play a role in the development of the disability. This confusion, conjugated with legal reasoning, leads to a refusal of compensation, even though it was legally probable that work did in fact play a role in the development of the disease.

PART 2: COMPENSATION FOR STRESS CLAIMS

All claims for psychological disability are viewed with scepticism by the compensation boards and employer lobbies[19] because psychological disability is so difficult to measure "objectively." When the source of the psychological disability is workplace stress, as opposed to physical pain or organic brain damage, the misgivings are exponential. Not only is the existence of a disease of the mind open to debate ... the very nature of stressors in the workplace is often intangible; their impact is difficult to measure. Evidence of disability is mostly gathered from worker testimony and evaluation by a psychiatrist, or occasionally by a psychologist. These experts often base their opinion on worker-reported versions of the workplace. Critics say that it all seems to be so unscientific — the system is seen to be vulnerable and the recognition of stress claims is said to open the floodgates to fraudulent or unfounded claims. Basically, by assuming workers to be liars or prone to blame the employer for everything, they recommend total exclusion of compensation for chronic stress. An analogy can be made with the most pernicious non-recognition of industrial diseases: If no studies are made of asbestos-related cancers, no claims may be made (Brodeur, 1985; Epstein, 1979). If you can't measure causation, it is non-existent. Of course the whole debate is clouded by the discourse of scientific objectivity: If it can't be measured, who is to say whether it exists or not? Given the choice, a cost-effective system should assume the non-existence of the disease or the disability, or, at worst, ignore work factors in the causation equation.

Although this discourse is still prevalent both in the compensation board milieu and in the literature, judicial action in most American states, and quasi-judicial decisions in some Canadian jurisdictions, have now clearly determined that psychological disability arising from chronic workplace stress is compensable. However, the strength of the anticompensation lobby has had a significant impact on the development of rules applicable only to stress claims.

In most American states, workers' compensation legislation provides access to compensation for those who suffer "personal injury by accident," but courts in many of these states have developed special rules applicable only to claims for purely psychological disability, and most of these judge-made rules provide for more stringent criteria in accepting such claims (De Carlo and Gruenfeld, 1989; Lippel, 1992; 1989). In these states it is not sufficient to demonstrate that workplace stressors actually caused the psychological disability of the worker; it must also be demonstrated that these stressors were of an unusual nature, out of the ordinary. The rule to this effect has rarely been defined in legislation and the meaning of "unusual" is unclear. Unusual for whom? Compared to what standard? To the workers' ordinary life outside the workplace? To her usual work? To the labour market in general? All of these standards have been used, sometimes interchangeably, even though they result in very different conclusions.

An eloquent illustration of this is drawn from an interview with compensation board spokespersons outside Quebec. The board exacted evidence of unusual stress before compensating psychological or physical disabilities related to stress. It applied the rule to mean that stress had to be greater than that usually encountered in the worker's habitual work. In the example given in the interview, it applied the criteria to refuse compensation sought by a fireman for a heart attack occurring during the fighting of a fire, the reasoning being that it was not an exceptional fire. Spokespersons went on to explain that compensation for a heart attack suffered by an accountant during tax period would likely be granted because the habitually unstressful job becomes exceptionally stressful during the period prior to tax-filing deadlines. Other jurisdictions could just as easily apply the same rule to accept the fireman and refuse the accountant: firemen work in jobs more stressful than those of the general workforce.

A further equally vague question requires the worker to demonstrate that the disability arose "out of and in the course of " employment. These terms serve to determine causation. They also, even where the cause of the disability is clear, serve to determine whether the events leading up to the disability are themselves work related.

Canadian jurisdictions have slowly, and often reluctantly, accepted certain compensation claims for psychological disability attributed to workplace stressors. In the beginning, only acute stress claims were recognized as compensable — claims for psychological trauma related to sudden, often violent incidents: witnessing a fatal accident or a violent crime; near escape from an explosion or a train derailment.

Gradual or chronic stress was initially ignored by the compensation system, but in recent years many provinces have revised their position and recognized certain claims. Recently, Manitoba[20] and New Brunswick[21] have specifically excluded chronic stress claims from the gambit of compensation legislation, but several other jurisdictions accept such claims. Saskatchewan was the first Canadian province to adopt a stress-compensation policy, in 1987. Since the late 1980s, two Canadian jurisdictions, Ontario and Quebec, have accepted several claims for psychological disability attributed to chronic or gradual stress in the workplace — the type of stress that wears on the worker over time, resulting eventually in his or her inability to work at all. Often the accumulation of many specific stressful events lead to this result; in other cases, the poisoned atmosphere of the workplace, poor working conditions, overwork, lack of control, ambiguity of the working role or conflict-ridden rapport with a colleague or a supervisor all contribute to the eventual disability.

The medicolegal framework applied to all compensation claims takes on certain peculiarities when stress claims are involved. We shall summarize applicable proceedings in Quebec, although many jurisdictions have analogous structures.

Workers alleging disability arising out of workplace stress must claim within six months of their knowledge that the disability is work related. Claiming involves providing the Compensation Board — in Quebec, the CSST — with a detailed claim form supported by a medical certificate. In the claim form, circumstances surrounding the "event" must be described in some detail, and the worker is asked to specify whether the claim is based on an industrial accident or an occupational disease. An accompanying medical certificate must be provided by a medical doctor;

psychologists, even if they may eventually testify as experts, are not eligible as "physicians in charge of the worker."[22] The certificate must include a diagnosis and an estimate of the duration of the disability. Although the diagnosis is not necessarily restricted to those inventoried in the *Diagnostic and Statistical Manual of Mental Disorders IV* (DSM IV)[23], other diagnoses, such as burnout, are often viewed with great distrust, leading to almost certain refusal by the Commission.

Regardless of the clarity of the claim, if it relates to chronic stress it will almost inevitably be refused by the first-level decision maker. The claimant may request that the decision be reviewed before a tripartite review board of the CSST, called the Bureau de révision paritaire ("review office" or BRP). Appeal of this decision may be filed at an independent Commission, the Commission d'appel en matière de lésions profession-nelles ("board of appeal," or CALP), where a commissioner, sometimes accompanied by a medical assessor, will eventually hear the appeal and render a final decision. Both review and appeal tribunals hold hearings in which the claimant bears the burden of demonstrating that the circum-stances giving rise to the disability may be deemed to constitute an industrial accident or an occupational disease.

Over the years, the notion of accident has been broadened by the tribunals to include circumstances that, at first, don't seem to correspond to the ordinary sense of the word "accident." When physical disability is at stake, tribunals have often accepted claims based on micro trauma: Although each individual irritant is in itself insufficient to cause injury, the cumulative effect has caused the disability. The first cases of repetitive strain injury were often accepted as accidents, even though the legislative definition defines the term to include a sudden and unforeseen event.[24]

When psychological injury results from chronic workplace stress, Quebec tribunals now apply an analogous reasoning: Each individual example of harassment or frustration may be innocuous, but the cumu-lative effect is to cause personal injury or disease judged to be compensa-ble. Recently, some decision makers have accepted stress claims as occupational diseases, "diseases contracted out of or in the course of work and characteristic of that work or directly related to the risks peculiar to that work."[25]

All concepts surrounding this process are elastic. The "fear of opening the floodgates" syndrome has resulted in the introduction of new and fuzzy criteria, which are applied to stress claims but not applied to claims for physical disability. Decision makers in Quebec will look for events that are out of the ordinary, and will not hesitate to make value judgments on the difficulties alleged by the claimant. They will look for evidence of causation in the testimony of the medical experts, who play a particularly important role when the decision-makers cannot actually see the disability. In the absence of epidemiological evidence, they will often fall back on public opinion's perception of stressful work: work done by the executive, the prison guard, the police officer. Wary of false claims, they will often search through evidence regarding a claimant's personal life in order to assure themselves that work, rather than other factors, led to the disability.

PART 3: HOW DOES THIS FRAMEWORK ADVERSELY AFFECT WOMEN?

Traditional legal theory relies on the premise that a statute has a monolithic meaning, and applies to all in the same way. The theory of legal interpretation invites the reader to find the meaning of the act and the intention of Parliament, and to apply them to the factual situation. The idea that vague concepts permit latitude is antithetical to traditional legal principles, as all rely on the fiction that Parliament has provided an answer to the question at hand, and the interpreter must only discover that answer (Côté, 1992). In practice, elastic terms allow discretion, although it is often disguised. Discretion, although not intrinsically dangerous or negative, may give rise to abuse, and notably to discriminatory practices.

Obscure standards often shroud discretion: Rules stated in general terms give the appearance of neutrality while providing latitude to decision makers (Perelman and Vander Elst, 1984; Rials, 1984). When such standards are not legislatively created, but rather emerge mysteriously from judicial discourse, their use deserves even closer scrutiny. The emergence of the unusual stress rule in the United States, and its application in several Canadian jurisdictions, provides illustration of such a phenomenon. Other criteria applicable in the adjudication of stress claims, evolved for the purpose of sniffing out claims the decision maker does not want to compensate while allowing discretion to accept the "deserving claim," also leave open the possibility of discrimination, be it on the basis of class or of sex.

The same preoccupations that gave rise to peculiar criteria (distrust of claimants) may also give rise to research (distrust of neutrality when faced with vague or soft concepts). We have postulated that decision makers allow soft concepts to evolve in order to maintain some shrouded discretion in the adjudication process. It then becomes interesting to examine how this discretion is exercised, by measuring how the vague concepts are applied. We then examine this portrait to determine if our data provide any information on the perception of women's role in the workplace and in society. Because of the structure of the compensation system, decisions of the review boards and the appeals tribunal (BRP and CALP) provide some information on opinions of decision makers and medical experts called upon to evaluate the claims.

There are limits to the utility of such sources (Jeammaud et Serverin, 1992), and it is dangerous to conclude that case law reflects reality. Unions report that women are reticent to claim, and many disabilities related to work are camouflaged as claims for health insurance. Decision makers have been known to draft decisions in such a way as to support their conclusions, leaving out information that would otherwise bring into question the wisdom of the results. They may also quote extensively from experts who justify their conclusions while referring only succinctly to those holding an opposing view. Obvious cases may be compensated immediately and thus are not appealed and therefore it is impossible to draw conclusions as to the portrait of stress claims, let alone stress in the workplace, from reading the decisions. Our study can in no way provide accurate information on work stress. But we hope to identify certain characteristics of the decision making process itself. Indirectly we also hope to shed some light on the role of "experts," be they doctors, psychologists or scientists.

To date we have analyzed 97 decisions, representing approximately 50 percent of all decisions preselected for final analysis. The total sample is comprised of all published and unpublished decisions regarding workers' compensation claims for psychological stress rendered by the final appeal tribunal (CALP) between 1985 and 1993, as well as review board decisions (BRP), including all published decisions and several unpublished decisions.

Without having completed our content analysis of all decisions in our sample, preliminary results encourage us to pursue the idea that soft concepts in adjudication are sometimes being used to adversely affect the outcome of claims by women. Initial findings demonstrate a clear discrepancy in outcome, particularly at the Review Board level, based on gender of claimant, as can be seen in Table 1.

Composition of the tribunal is also revealing, as can be seen in Tables 2a and 2b. Women claimants are less likely to succeed before the review boards that are composed primarily of male decision makers. Without further study, it would be simplistic to conclude that there exists a causal relation, as far too many variables have yet to be measured. It is conceivable that the gender of some decision makers is more important than that of others.[26] Other questions arise: Does the nature of the stress cases

Table 1   Outcome of Claim Acceptance According to Gender and Tribunal

Gender	Tribunal	Accepted	Refused	Total
Men	BRP	20	13	33
Women	BRP	5	18	23
Men	CALP	16	9	25
Women	CALP	9	7	16
Total		50 (36m, 14w)	47 (22m, 25w)	97 (58m, 39w)

$X^2 = 8.28$, df $= 1$, p.01: review board (BRP) decisions
$X^2 = 6.39$, df $+ 1$, p.02: review board and appeal tribunal combined

Table 2a   Gender of Decision Makers in Review Board Panel (BRP)

Role	Men	Women	Total
Chair (CSST)(BRP)	30	25	55
Union representative (BRP)	46	8	54*
Management representative (BRP)	50	4	54*

*Information not always available

Table 2b   Gender of Decision Makers in Appeal Panels (CALP)*

Role	Men	Women	Total
Chair	30	10	40*
Medical assessor	19	2	21

*Information not always available

brought before the board differ on the basis of gender? Is there a gender-based distinction in the quality of the representation of the workers? Yet, certain hypotheses may be examined without the answers to these questions.

We are testing several specific hypotheses involving the application of legal rules to the evidence as reported by the decision maker. To evaluate whether and in what way gender has an impact on the outcome of compensation cases, we look specifically to two medicolegal questions: (1) are the factual situations judged to correspond to the legal definition of industrial accident or occupational disease?; (2) is the disability perceived to be related to the work situation described?

These broad concepts provide the framework for decision makers to determine compensability: Given the events alleged and the causal relation between them, is the disability of the worker covered by the scope of the Act? If the answer to this question is in the affirmative, a second series of questions is used to determine whether the facts justify the conclusion that a causal relation exists.

The first question, regarding the legal definition, raises several issues on which opinions may potentially vary according to the gender of the claimant. What constitutes unusual workplace stress that can be attributed to a sudden and unforeseen event? What triggering events are seen to be sufficiently significant to be considered sudden and unforeseen? Are the alleged risks peculiar to that employment, and what type of evidence, epidemiological or otherwise, is needed to demonstrate this? What constitutes work related stressors that are deemed to have arisen out of or in the course of employment, as opposed to stressors intrinsic to relationships with human beings?

As to the second issue regarding work relatedness, several other questions are raised. What impact does the claimant's personal life history and experience have on the recognition of a claim? Of what relevance is the personality of the claimant, and how is credibility determined?

Given that decision makers have developed the criterion of unusual stress as a determinant in the recognition of a claim, it is interesting to see how its application affects women. Claims made by male workers have been recognized under this criterion. Stressful events have been judged to be out of the ordinary in the following circumstances involving claims by men: working with incompetent co-workers (trucker[27] or dynamite technician[28]); being sued for police brutality;[29] being investigated for a sexual harassment complaint;[30] rescheduling of vacation by the employer;[31] having to produce an important report without adequate secretarial resources;[32] being harassed by underlings,[33] a supervisor[34] or colleagues[35] over a period of several months; being exposed to recidivists in the isolation wing of a penitentiary;[36] and working in an isolated environment after having been spurned by work colleagues.[37]

On the other hand, the following examples, drawn from women's work, have been held to be normal working conditions: poisoned relationships with clientele,[38] colleagues or supervisors;[39] compulsory overtime and unfair scheduling practices preventing foreseeable work schedules and violating seniority;[40] intense surveillance by a supervisor;[41] restructuring of work organization without adequate training;[42] overload of responsibility for patients,[43] injured workers[44] or other persons in need;[45] without adequate resources.

Expectations of decision makers regarding what would constitute stressful work seem fairly stereotyped. Some decisions specifically compare the work of the claimant to that of police officers or firefighters,[46] concluding that tense work relations can develop in any workplace, and that they are not peculiar risks in the way that stress is to police work. Even when women occupy roles stereotypically associated with stress, their own cases are often refused as being caused by stress normal to the workplace. Two decisions confirm that sexual harassment of prison guards by prisoners is a normal part of their working conditions.[47] Other cases seem to imply that work is not for the tenderhearted, and that disability resulting from the discovery of a body, apparently a normal occurrence in a penitentiary, should not be compensated.[48] Disability related to the oppressive working environment of the penitentiary is sometimes compensated,[49] sometimes not.[50]

Gender does not completely explain these seeming discrepancies. In our preliminary sample of 97 cases, 14 cases involving women were compensated.[51] Two clearly involved acute stress: One woman was spat upon,[52] another assaulted,[53] and the tribunals agreed these were unusual stressors. Three women under stress because of disciplinary inquiries regarding their behaviour were compensated: a police officer involved in a shoot out;[54] a cashier unjustifiably suspected of fraud;[55] and a teacher accused of assaulting a disabled child.[56] Conflicts with a superior have been deemed to be unusual,[57] in select circumstances, and in certain cases overtones of sexual harassment in the context of conflictual relations with colleagues or supervisors have also been held to be unusual.[58] Surprisingly, of the 13 accepted claims by women, three were accepted as occupational diseases — the poisoned relationship with the supervisor,[59] the change in work organization[60] and the implementation of new technology qualified as peculiar risks of the jobs.[61] Finding a body was eventually deemed to be unusual as it was the prison guard's first experience of that nature.[62] Executive overload leading to depression was also held to be unusual in the case of a woman-owned operation that underwent rapid expansion.[63] These are not simply illustrations of those claims by women that have been accepted in our sample. They describe the totality of the claims sampled and, for the most part, they don't appear to fall into the grey zone where judicial discretion must be exercised. When fuzzy concepts need to be called upon, it appears to be more difficult for women's claims to be accepted.

Stereotypical expectations seem to be widespread and are exacerbated by the fact that epidemiological data are not available on sales work, while they are available for police work.[64] Often the decision makers associate the seeming banality of the circumstances with the credibility of the claimant, giving the impression that she is complaining about nothing. Sometimes this reflects the evidence provided by doctors, whose testimony may be the source of the banality associated with the circumstances.

At other times the value judgments seem to come from the decision makers themselves.

A peculiar category of refusals is that wherein decision makers accept that the claimant is disabled because of specific circumstances, but conclude that the circumstances themselves did not arise out of and in the course of employment. A few illustrations are in order. A police officer learns she was on the target list of Marc Lépine and is diagnosed with an anxiety reaction. Her disability is clearly related to the shock engendered by this information. Her claim is refused: She is on his hit list as a woman in a non-traditional job, not as a police officer. Her claim is refused because "it is well known that the criminal obsession of the killer was related to the fact that some women were working in men's jobs, rather than to the fact they worked as police officers."[65] Her disability is thus not work related. The employer of a sales clerk installs video cameras, focused on the toilet, in the women's washroom, for what seems to be his own libidinous pleasure. A worker discovers videos of herself and the resulting shock is disabling. Her claim is refused because the harassment was not employment related, but related to the fact that she was a woman.[66] Many claims involving harassment or conflict-ridden relationships[67] are accepted, but many are refused as being related to work relationships rather than to work. One may question the validity of the distinction between work-related stress and stress related to working relationships,[68] which appears to be a fine line invented by decision makers, sometimes inspired by psychiatrists, and having no place in the legislation.

The second series of questions, regarding work relatedness in the specific case, allows for discussion by both doctors and decision makers of the worker's personal life circumstances, and his or her personality. Our preliminary findings as to gender-based differences in the relevance or use of these variables are of some interest.

The personal life of the claimant is sometimes discussed: menopause, marital difficulties, or problems with children are all potential intervening variables that conceivably explain psychological disability in a way that allows decision makers to absolve work. Although, thus far in our study, personal life has been raised almost as often, in absolute numbers, for men as for women (nine times for men, from a total of 58 claims; 10 times for women, from a total of 39 claims), preliminary results lead us to believe that the issues regarding claimants' personal lives are not raised by the same people for the same reasons. In our sample, male claimants were most likely to raise their personal lives themselves, primarily to show that their personal lives were going well. In the case of women, the issue of the absence of personal problems was rarely mentioned in the decisions. Thus, six claims involving men and only one claim involving a woman underlined the absence of personal problems; all were accepted.

When personal life problems were mentioned at all, it was either to underline difficulties with a spouse, to raise issues regarding the claimant's childhood, or to mention a death in the family. The employer's expert witness was usually responsible for raising the issue. If we eliminate those statements implying positive family life, only three claims filed by men mentioned personal problems,[69] whereas nine claims by women touched upon difficulties at home or a death in the family. The effect of personal life factors on outcome is also interesting. A man breaking up with his girlfriend during the period of work stress still received compensation (the only case involving a male claimant having marital difficulties),[70] whereas signs of personal difficulties at home often absolve work in the case of women claimants (five of the seven cases involving women with marital difficulties were refused).[71]

Issues surrounding a claimant's personality are often raised, although decision makers rarely base their decision, at least overtly, on such elements. The way these different variables are brought into play may vary on the basis of gender. Preliminary results are intriguing. Of those cases where personality was mentioned as an issue, perfectionism seemed to increase rather than decrease the chances of success for men, whereas this did not seem to be the case when the same comment was made about women. Favourable comments about personality had little effect on outcome, and most of such comments referred to women claimants. Preliminary results can be seen in Table 3.

Table 3 Mention of Personality and Outcome According to Gender

Personality	Mention		Accepted		Rejected	
	Men	Women	Men	Women	Men	Women
Perfectionist	7	4	7	1	0	3
Nervous	3	0	1	0	2	0
Vulnerable or fragile	5	6	3	3	2	3
Positive attribute	2	4	2	2	0	2
No mention	34	19	19	6	15	13
Other	7	6	4	2	3	4
Total mentioned	24	20	17	9	7	12

Previous psychiatric history of the claimant could have a negative impact on recognition of claims; yet, as can be seen from Table 4, this does not explain the low acceptance rate for women's claims. Although the numbers are small, it can be seen that the proportion of successful claims in all three categories of women claimants, whether they have prior psychiatric history, no prior history, or no mention of prior history in the file, is lower than the success rate of men with prior psychiatric history.

Table 4 Mention of Psychiatric History and Outcome According to Gender

History	Mention		Accepted		Rejected	
	Men	Women	Men	Women	Men	Women
Prior history	12	5	9	1	3	4
No prior history	13	9	11	5	2	4
No mention	33	26	16	8	17	18

Anecdotal evidence encourages us to pursue certain questions. Several women claimants have seen their claims refused on the basis of medical evidence to the effect that their personality structure[72] and their desire to be autonomous,[73] to be their own boss or to succeed in their work,[74] were the causes of their disability, and, as such, the disabilities were not compensable. Particularly in the helping professions, when a worker hesitates to say no and falls victim to exhaustion from overwork, she will be told by the courts that her disability is due to her own personality and not to her work.[75] Yet all male claimants in our current sample who were described as perfectionists were compensated.

Although the figures used are small, they do lead us to believe that peculiarities of women claimants' personalities, past psychiatric history or personal lives do not explain the discrepancy between the acceptance rates for male and female claimants. Women's claims are also unsuccessful in those cases where personal life, psychiatric history and personality are not mentioned.

CONCLUSION

So what happened to the workers described in the introduction? The police officer on Marc Lépine's hit list lost her case and it is currently in appeal. The criterion applied to refuse her case? The threats were related to her being a woman in a man's job; therefore they were not work related. The sales clerk in conflict with her supervisor also lost. In rendering the decision, the Board took special care to underline that being a sales clerk was not stressful in the way that police work was; it pointed out that no epidemiological evidence related to sales in department stores was produced during the hearing. Unfair treatment by management and supervisors was judged to be part of normal workplace stressors, to be expected in all work situations. The CSST case management officer lost her case: It was her Type A personality that incited her to answer the phone when injured workers complained that their case officers refused to return their calls; she overworked herself and had only herself to blame. The prison guard who found the prisoner's body was eventually compensated. The Review Board refused her claim because prisoners' suicides were deemed to be normal in a penitentiary. The Appeal Commission accepted her claim, as the body was the first one she had found and therefore was reasonably unexpected. The man investigated for sexual harassment? The investigation was judged to have had serious consequences on the worker's self-image, and on the image others had of him; the ensuing depression was deemed to be work related and he was compensated. The woman prison guard did not receive compensation for the anxiety caused by sexual harassment by prisoners. All agreed that the sexual harassment was real, but concluded that the disability was not caused by a sudden and unforeseen event: Sexual harassment is a usual and expected event in the context of a penitentiary. Furthermore, the fragility of the worker's personality justified her dismissal, because she was not psychologically strong enough to work in a penitentiary.[76]

When we put these comments in perspective, we may draw certain conclusions. The compensation process itself may systemically lead to discrimination against women claimants. Adjudicators and experts filter women's and men's experiences to determine if compensation should be paid. Most medical experts seem uncomfortable with the inevitable uncertainty involved in all claims for psychological disability, and find comforting the idea that all claims should be refused. Yet Quebec law now clearly permits compensation and experts can no longer avoid giving an opinion. The creation of special rules regarding normality, work-related disabilities and causation invite flexibility in adjudication. After all, they originated in order to allow some claims, while holding back the floodgates and permitting refusal when decision makers felt compensation to be inappropriate.

The ideological bent of both the experts and the decision makers is allowed to flourish, because of the fuzziness of concepts surrounding psychological disability and stress, as well as those regarding probability and certainty in the compensation context. Often decision makers or expert witnesses tend to lean towards refusal of a claim when they can find some rational justification to do so, even though acceptance could be just as easily rationalized. Lack of epidemiological evidence relevant to women's work makes access to compensation even more difficult.

Evidence is at this point anecdotal, and certain impressions need to be confirmed. If experts feel that Type A personalities in women, or the presence of women in nontraditional workplaces, demonstrates pathology, it is unlikely they will accept the link between working conditions and disability. Perfectionist personalities in men appear to be viewed as positive traits; in women, they are inappropriate and those women who become exhausted when trying to save the credibility of the system they work for, be it a hospital, a compensation board or a low-cost housing group, will be blamed for their own disability. Several decisions examined to date rely on the argument that the worker was inappropriate for the job in order to refuse stress claims brought by women workers. It seems unthinkable that similar arguments would be used to refuse compensation for a physical accident and we have yet to see decisions refusing claims by men for the same reasons. The "thin skull rule" exists and workers' compensation is still thought to be a no fault system, yet blame appears and disappears in the vagaries of the decisions that apply soft concepts by using evidence provided by psychiatrists — experts in what may be called a soft science. If experts believe that a mother's presence in the workplace is an indication of pathology, there is little likelihood that working conditions will be held responsible for disabilities, particularly if it is assumed that women's mental health is primarily affected by their personal lives. These values may be expressed or left unmentioned in the decisions themselves.

Because of the broad discretion intrinsic to the adjudication process, success of a claim often depends on whether the decision makers can identify with the claimant's perception of events. When they are emotionally sympathetic to the claim, they need not resort to semantics or conceptual gymnastics to justify recognition. When they feel refusal appropriate, for whatever reason, they need only draw upon one of a series of vague concepts to reject the claim. In this context, it is particularly interesting to identify the decision makers. It is too early to make any conclusions, but it is of note that 96 of the 108 assessors at the review board level, representing unions and management, are men. Chairs seem to be more evenly distributed.

Decision makers are more often men than women. The doctors they listen to are also more often men than women and many doctors seem to be particularly wary in their approach to stress claims. Preliminary findings seem to indicate that doctors focus on women's personal lives but seem to ignore those of men. They seem more inclined to speak of childhood trauma and of problems with a father image when speaking of women. For the moment it is impossible to determine whether the bias comes from the doctors themselves, or from the decision makers who chose to quote, or alternatively muffle by omission, doctors' testimony.

Perhaps the most intriguing questions relate to value judgments about what is labeled normal and abnormal. Sexual harassment in a penitentiary is unequivocally normal; investigation of sexual harassment complaints is unequivocally abnormal, as are investigations of police brutality and theft. Power plays by supervisors are sometimes normal, sometimes not. Introduction of new technology is sometimes normal, sometimes not. Even without the naiveté of traditional legal discourse that postulates coherence, one could nevertheless expect similar facts and circumstances to lead to similar results. Yet this does not seem to be the case. Preliminary findings encourage us to pursue the hypothesis that the gender of claimants, and perhaps of decision makers, intervenes to explain some inconsistencies; class may also be a significant variable.

What does seem clear is that systemic discrimination is facilitated when legal criteria are fuzzy, doctors' roles ambiguous and stereotypes uncontrolled. Lack of research on women's work and stress, unequal access to unionization and adequate legal representation, and possible self-effacement by the claimants themselves may all contribute to undermining the quest for compensation.

ACKNOWLEDGEMENTS

I would like to acknowledge the invaluable assistance of Diane Demers, Nicole Filion and Catherine Néron in the preparation of preliminary research used in this paper, the collaboration of the Commission d'appel en matière de lésions professionnelles and the financial support of the Conseil québécois de recherche sociale.

NOTES

1. *Angers et Communauté urbaine de Montréal*, [1991] BRP 518. Over-ruled in appeal: [1994] CALP 1212.

2. *M.C. et S. Canada Inc.*, [1993] BRP 346.

3. *Laflamme et CSST*, [06/07/1987] CALP 60-00213-8608.

4. *Linch et Service Correctionnel du Canada* [1985-86] BRP 174; [1987] CALP 590.

5. *Y. L. et Compagnie M.*, [1993] CALP 986.

6. *Mercier et Service Correctionnel du Canada*, CALP 05083-61-8712.

7. The same may be said for many blue collar jobs, from assembly line work to meat packing.

8. For a review of the literature see Lowe, Graham, *Women, Paid/Unpaid Work, and Stress*, (Ottawa: Canadian Advisory Council on the Status of Women, 1989).

9. Findings of the National Association of Working Women, *The 9 to 5 Survey on Women and Stress*, (Cleveland: National Association of Working Women, 1984), p. 16. As discussed by Lowe.

10. For an overview see Ison (1989), pp. 1 and 163; for an analysis of the transactional evolution of the Quebec compensation system see Lippel (1986).

11. R.S.Q. c. A-3.001

12. See for instance *Gaudreault et Ville de Charlesbourg*, [27/07/1987] CALP, 01577-03-8612.

13. For a discussion of the interplay between law, epidemiology and medicine in the context of compensation see Ison (1989), Lippel (1992), Demers (1992). For a discussion of the interaction of law and science in issues of health and safety in general see Cranor (1993), J. Bertin and M. Henifin (1994).

14. *Farrell v. Snell*, [1990] 2 S.C.R. 311, at 330.

15. Ison (1989), p. 58.

16. Ibid., p. 51.

17. A cardiologist's testimony before the Cardiac Subcommittee of the Statutory Advisory Committee on Medical Care for the Oregon State Legislature, quoted in Milner (1979) at p. 176 note 63.

18. Ison (1989), p. 59. The relevance of this principle in Quebec compensation law was recently reiterated by the Quebec Court of Appeal in the case of *Chaput et Montréal (Société de Transport de la Communauté Urbaine de)*, [1992] CALP 1253 (C.A.).

19. At a conference on the subject held by Southam Publications in Toronto in October 1990, a spokesperson for employers in Ontario stated that business would be "apoplectic" if the right to compensation for stress claims was introduced.

20. S.M 1991-92, c. 36, s.2.

21. *An Act to Amend the Workers' Compensation Act*, [1992] S.N.B., c. 34, s.1, in force since January 2nd, 1993.

22. Term used in the Act to designate the treating practitioner. s. 204ss.

23. *American Psychiatric Association: Diagnostic and Statistical Manual of Mental Disorders*, Fourth Edition, (Washington, DC: American Psychiatric Association, 1994).

24. See for instance *Lisette Dupuis et les Entreprises Queentex Inc.*, [19/04/1988] BRP R-6012 4908; *Suzanne Doyon Bernier et Publications Nord Ouest*, [1988] CALP 604; the leading case on this issue is *Workmen's Compensation Board vs Theed*, [1940] S.C.R. 553.

25. Prison guards and union workers were the first groups to be compensated under this category. More recently, several claims from different walks of life have been accepted, applying the reasoning that the interpersonal conflict, the poor work organization or the introduction of new technology that triggered the disability was a peculiar risk of the workplace, see for instance: *Lambert et Dominion Textile Inc.*,

[1993] CALP 1056; *Cloutier et Commission Scolaire de Portneuf*, [1993] CALP 679.

26. One could speculate that the role of the union representative on the board is to restate the worker's case in terms that will convince the other two Board members. If the representative has difficulty in relating to the claim, it may be that the persuasive function of the position is less effective. The other two members of the Review Board are not expected to have a vested interest in shedding light on the claim. If they misunderstand, this may have less effect on outcome.

27. *Bussières et T.J. Moore Ltée*, [1986] CALP 57.

28. *Castonguay et Frères Ltée et Lehoux*, [1993] BRP 301: over 20 weeks working with dynamite in an urban environment held to be a sudden and unforeseen event.

29. In the following cases, compensation was granted for stress related to law suits, internal investigations or criminal charges brought against claimants, male police officers: *Bergeron et C.U.M.*, [26/11/1986] BRP 9365564; *Gossett et C.U.M.*, [11/12/1989] BRP 60193051, 60334440; and a female police officer: *Gauthier et Ville de Longueuil*, [1991] BRP 63.

30. *Y. L. et Compagnie M.*, [1993] CALP 986.

31. *Dupiré et Agriculture Canada*, [1991] BRP 204.

32. *Gagnon et Commission Administrative des Régimes de Retraite et d'Assurances*, [1989] CALP 769.

33. *DeBellefeuille et Ministère de la Justice du Québec*, [31/07/1986], BRP 9315968.

34. *Gravel et Ministère des Anciens Combattants*, [1990] BRP. 249; see also *Lafleur et Syndicat des Employés de la Commission Scolaire Régionale de Tilly*, [03/10/1985] BRP 8643222; *Anglade et Communauté Urbaine de Montréal*, [17/06/1988] CALP 60-00247-8209.

35. *P.D. et Ville de F.*, [1993] CALP 997.

36. *Dumas et Ministère du Solliciteur Général*, [1990] BRP 329.

37. *Langevin et Ministère du Loisir Chasse et Pêche*, [03/03/1993] CALP 18032-62-9003.

38. *Gauthier et Société d'Habitation Chambrelle*, [1986-87] BRP 1049; *Mercier et Service Correctionnel du Canada*, CALP 05083-61-8712.

39. *Langevin et Centre d'accueil Louis-Dupuis*, [1993] BRP 387; *April-Roberge et Hôpital Laval*, [1986-87] BRP 894; *Lavoie et Hôpital d'Amqui*, [1992] CALP 200; *Laforce et Clinique Médicale La Tuque Enr.*, [1986-87] BRP 630.

40. *M.C. et S. Canada Inc.*, [1993] BRP 346.

41. *Entreprises J.M.C. 1973 et Béraldin*, [1991] CALP 54; *Lalonde-Giroux et Bendex Avelex Inc.* [31/08/1987] BRP 60059203.

42. *Desmeules et Ville de Montréal*, [1992] BRP 416; *Laflamme et CSST*, [06/07/1987] CALP 60-00213-8608.

43. *Langevin et Centre d'Accueil Louis-Dupuis*, [1993] BRP 387; *April-Roberge et Hôpital Laval*, [1986-87] BRP 894.

44. *Laflamme et CSST*, [06/07/1987] CALP 60-00213-8608.

45. *Bibeau et Villa Marie-Claire Inc.*, [1992] BRP 155; *Gauthier et Société d'Habitation Chambrelle*, [1986-87] BRP 1049.

46. *M.C. et S. Canada Inc.*, [1993] BRP 346, at 350: "il n'y a pas de preuve épidémiologique démontrant qu'un syndrome anxio-dépressif est une maladie caractéristique des fonctions occupées par la travailleuse (vendeuse au service de ventes par catalogue)."

47. *Raymond et Service Correctionnel du Canada*, [16/01/1992] 15225-60-8911; *Mercier et Service Correctionnel du Canada*, [17/04/1991] CALP 05083-61-8712.

48. *Linch et Service Correctionnel du Canada* [1985-86] BRP 174; this decision was reversed in appeal, because it was the worker's first such experience: *Linch et Ministère du Solliciteur Général du Canada*, [1987] CALP 590.

49. *Loukil et Seradep Inc.*, [1986-87] BRP 113, where the male penitentiary worker was compensated for a depression related to the depressing atmosphere of the penitentiary. See also *Dumas et Ministère du Solliciteur Général*, [1990] BRP 329; *Brunelle et Service Correctionnel Canada*, [31/03/87] CALP 63-00042-8607; *Linch et Ministère du Solliciteur Général du Canada*, [1987] CALP 590. Only the Linch case involved a woman claimant.

50. *Claude et Service Correctionnel Canada*, CALP 01142-60-8610; *Mercier et Service Correctionnel du Canada*, CALP 05083-61-8712; *Raymond et Service correctionnel du Canada*, [16/01/92] CALP 15225-60-8911. All these cases involved women.

51. Only thirteen claims were involved; one claimant's claim was confirmed, thus she is represented twice in the statistics.

52. *Lessard et S.T.C.U.M.*, [1991] BRP 460.

53. *Lemousy et Hôpital Rivières des Prairies*, [1988] CALP 573.

54. *Gauthier et Ville de Longueuil*, [1991] BRP 63.

55. *Guitar-Prieur et Miracle Mart*, [1989] CALP 738.

56. *Cloutier et Commission scolaire de Portneuf*, [1993] CALP 679; ten of her sixteen colleagues testified to corroborate her allegations regarding harassment by their supervisor.

57. A secretary working for a union was compensated for disability related to harassment by a superior, whose persistent criticism was held to be an abnormal working condition in *Béliveau-St.-Jacques et Conseil Central de Sherbrooke*, [09/02/1989] BRP 60183128. In *Blagoeva et Commission Contrôle d'Énergie Atomique*, CALP 15883-60-8912, a highly educated inspector of nuclear facilities was compensated after persistent conflict with a new superior left her disabled; see also *Cloutier et Commission Scolaire de Portneuf*, [1993] CALP 679.

58. In *Leduc et Les Aliments Claude Dufour Inc.*, [1993] BRP 199, taunting comments of a sexual nature and inappropriate threats of dismissal by a new supervisor were held to be unusual stressors. See also *Leduc et Les Centres d'Accueil du Haut St Laurent, Bureau de révision*, [30/10/1984] BRP 8518466; *Béliveau-St.-Jacques et Conseil Central de Sherbrooke*, [09/02/1989] BRP 60183128. Ironically, recognition of harassment as a work injury has led employers to claim that civil claims for damages brought to the courts or to the Human Rights Commission, are precluded by virtue of the exclusionary rule intrinsic to workers' compensation: see *Fédération des Employées et Employés de Services Publics Inc. et Confédération des Syndicats Nationaux (CSN) et Louisette Béliveau St-Jacques et al.*, (1991) R.J.Q. 279, Quebec Court of Appeal; an appeal to the Supreme Court of Canada is currently pending.

59. *Cloutier et Commission Scolaire de Portneuf*, [1993] CALP 679.

60. *Leclair et Pavillons Bois Joly Inc.*, CALP 10713-62-8812.

61. *Lambert et Dominion Textile Inc.*, [1993] CALP 1056.

62. *Linch et Ministère du Solliciteur Général du Canada*, [1987] CALP 590.

63. *Soubigou et Maloso Inc.*, [1988] CALP 977.

64. Both the decisions of *M.C. et S. Canada Inc.*, [1993] BRP 346, a saleswoman in conflict with colleagues and supervisors, and *Langevin et Centre d'Accueil Louis-Dupuis*, [1993] BRP 387, involving a caseworker underline the absence of epidemiological data. On the penury of epidemiological data relating to women and work see Lowe (1989), p. 13.

65. "Il est connu que l'obsession criminelle du tueur était beaucoup plus relative au fait que certaines femmes exerçaient des 'fonctions d'hommes' plutôt qu'au fait que certaines femmes exerçaient des fonctions de policiers," *Angers et Communauté Urbaine de Montréal*, [1991] BRP 518, at page 520. Over-ruled in appeal: [1994] CALP 1212.

66. Case related to the author by the lawyer of the claimant; she won her appeal at the review board level.

67. See for instance *Lambert et Dominion Textile Inc.*, [1993] CALP 1056; *Béliveau-St.-Jacques et Conseil Central de Sherbrooke*, [09/02/1989] BRP 60183128.

68. See for instance *Desmeules et Ville de Montréal*, [1992] BRP 416; *C. et S Canada Inc.*, [1993] BRP 346.

69. In one of the cases marital difficulties arising out of the workplace stress were alleged, as the worker and his wife were having problems since he was accused of sexual harassment: *L.Y. et Compagnie M.*, [1993] CALP 986.

70. *Bouchard et Sureté du Québec*, [1988] CALP 701.

71. See for instance *C. et S. Canada Inc.*, [1993] BRP 346.

72. *Laflamme et CSST*, [06/07/1987] CALP 60-00213-8608.

73. *Claude et Service Correctionnel du Canada*, CALP 01142-60-8610.

74. *Bibeau et Villa Marie-Claire Inc.*, [1992] BRP 155.

75. *Bibeau et Villa Marie-Claire Inc.*, [1992] BRP 155; *Laflamme et CSST*, [06/07/1987] CALP 60-00213-8608; *Gauthier et Société d'Habitation Chambrelle*, [1986-87] BRP 1049. A surprising exception is the decision in Soubigou where a woman administrator, having overworked herself in a new business she had opened, was compensated for burnout.

76. This case (Mercier), as well as the case of *Claude et Service Correctionnel du Canada*, CALP 01142-60-8610, which also refused compensation to a woman working in a penitentiary should be compared with *Loukil et Seradep*, where the male penitentiary worker was compensated for a depression related to the depressing atmosphere of the penitentiary. See also *Dumas et Ministère du Solliciteur Général*, [1990] BRP 329; *Brunelle et Service Correctionnel du Canada*, [31/03/1987] CALP 63-00042-8607. The same psychiatrist testified in both the Mercier, Claude and Brunelle decisions, alleging either that the worker was not ill or alternatively that the worker did not have what it takes to work in a penitentiary, being too sensitive. In the case of Brunelle, a man, his testimony did not affect the decision to recognize the claim. Even those women who occupy such stereotypically stressful employment seem to have difficulty in getting compensation.

REFERENCES

American Psychiatric Association. *Diagnostic and Statistical Manual of Mental Disorders*. Fourth Edition. Washington, DC: American Psychiatric Association, 1994.

Bertin, J., and M. Henifin. "Scientists Talk to Judges: Reflections on Daubert v. Merrell Dow." *New Solutions* 4 (1994).

Brodeur, Paul. *Outrageous Misconduct*. New York: Pantheon Books, 1985.

Côté, Pierre André. *The Interpretation of Legislation in Canada*. Second Edition. Cowansville, Quebec: Éditions Yvon Blais Inc., 1992.

Cranor, Carl F. *Regulating Toxic Substances: A Philosophy of Science and the Law*. New York: Oxford University Press, 1993.

De Carlo, Donald T., and Deborah H. Gruenfeld. *Stress in the American Workplace: Alternatives for the Working Wounded*. Pennsylvania: LRP Publications, 1989.

Demers, Diane. "La preuve médicale-une arme à deux tranchants pour le travailleur en matière de maladie professionnelle," in *Développements récents en droit de la santé et sécurité au travail*. Cowansville: Éditions Yvon Blais Inc., 1992. pp. 1-21.

Epstein, Samuel S. *The Politics of Cancer*. San Francisco: Sierra Club Books, 1979.

Ison, Terence. *Compensation for Industrial Disease Under the Workers' Compensation Act of Ontario*. Discussion paper produced for the Industrial Disease Standards Panel, Toronto, September 1989.

— *Workers' Compensation in Canada*. Second Edition. Toronto: Butterworths, 1989.

Jeammaud, Antoine, and Évelyne Serverin. "Évaluer le droit." *Recueil Dalloz Sirey* 34 (1992). pp. 263-8.

Lippel, Katherine. "Compensation for Mental-Mental Claims Under Canadian Law." *Behavioral Sciences and the Law* 8 (1990). pp. 375-98.

— *Le droit des accidentés du travail à une indemnité: analyse historique et critique*. Montreal: Éditions Thémis, 1986.

— "L'incertitude des probabilités en droit et en médecine." *Revue de droit de l'Université de Sherbrooke* 22 (1992). pp. 445-72.

— *Le stress au travail: L'indemnisation des atteintes à la santé en droit québécois, canadien et américain*. Cowansville: Éditions Yvon Blais Inc., 1992.

— "Workers' Compensation and Psychological Stress Claims in North American Law: A Microcosmic Model of Systemic Discrimination." *International Journal of Law and Psychiatry* 12 (1989). pp. 41-70.

Lowe, Graham. *Women, Paid/Unpaid Work, and Stress*. Ottawa: Canadian Advisory Council on the Status of Women, 1989.

Milner, F.S. "Heart Disease Due to Occupational Emotional Stress: A Compensable Claim Under Oregon Workers' Compensation Law?" *Environmental Law* 10 (1979).

Perelman, C., and R. Vander Elst (eds.). *Les notions à contenu variable en droit*. Brussels: Établissements Émile Bruylant, 1984.

Rials, S. "Les standards, notions critiques du droit" in *Les notions à contenu variable en droit*. C. Perelman and R. Vander Elst (eds.). Brussels: Établissements Émile Bruylant, 1984. pp. 39-53.

Nicolette Carlan and
Martha F. Keil

Developing a Proposal for a Working Women's Health Survey

Traditionnellement, les femmes n'ont pas fait partie des études portant sur la santé au travail parce que les postes qu'elles occupent sont à bas salaire et considérés comme à faible risque pour la santé, parce que les femmes sont moins souvent représentées par un syndicat et parce qu'elles travaillent dans des milieux plus petits. Jusqu'à maintenant, une seule étude du Comité des normes en matière de maladies professionnelles (CNMP) intitulée «Report to the Worker's Compensation Board on the CGE Lamp Plant Issue», s'est penchée sur les femmes en relation avec la santé au travail. En tenant compte du fait qu'en 1990, en Ontario seulement, 2,5 millions de femmes travaillaient à l'extérieur du foyer, il a été décidé que les problèmes des femmes en matière de santé au travail devraient faire partie de l'ordre du jour du CNMP. On a confié au Dr Gina Feldberg, directrice du Centre des études en matière de santé à l'Université de York, une étude sur la santé des femmes au travail. Cette étude a été financée par l'Agence pour la santé et la sécurité au travail, avec l'appui du CNMP. Un groupe consultatif de femmes représentant divers secteurs académiques, légaux et médicaux, fut formé pour assister à l'exécution de cette étude. Pour déterminer quels problèmes étaient prioritaires pour les travailleuses, le groupe consultatif a suggéré l'organisation d'une série de «focus groups». L'information accumulée lors de ces rencontres servira à rédiger un résumé des inquiétudes des femmes. À plus long terme, cette information orientera le choix des projets retenus par le Comité des normes en matière de maladie professionnelle pour aider les travailleuses.

Women have traditionally lacked representation in occupational health studies because their work is low-paying, is considered non-hazardous, is usually non-unionized and because, in the past, there were only small numbers of women in many workplaces. To date, only one Occupational Disease Panel (ODP) study, "Report to the Workers' Compensation Board on the CGE Lamp Plant Issue," reported on the health experience of women. By 1990, over 2.5 million women worked outside the home in Ontario alone, and it was decided that women's concerns should be placed on the agenda of the ODP. Dr. Gina Feldberg, Director of York University's Centre for Health Studies, was commissioned to carry out the Working Women's Health Study, with funding from the Workplace Health and Safety Agency and with cooperation from the Occupational Disease Panel. An Advisory Group of women from different sectors — including academia and the legal and medical communities — was established as part of the project. The Advisory Group thought it appropriate to set up a series of small focus groups. These groups would establish what problems were important to working women, and collect information to assist in creating a summary of a comprehensive range of women's concerns. Ultimately, this information will be used by the ODP to undertake projects that serve women.

The purpose of this paper is to describe the path taken by a regulatory organization in its attempt to provide service to the women in the workforce. Specifically, we will be describing the involvement of the Ontario Industrial Disease Standards Panel ("the Panel") in the development of a proposal for a provincewide survey of working women's health concerns.

The Panel came into existence as a result of a general workers' compensation reform movement that began in the 1970s and culminated in significant legislative changes in the 1980s. The specific mandate of the Panel is set out in the Workers' Compensation Act. It is authorized:

- to investigate possible industrial diseases;
- to make available findings of probable connections between diseases and industrial processes, trades or occupations in Ontario;
- to create, develop and revise criteria for the evaluation of claims respecting industrial diseases; and
- to advise on eligibility rules regarding compensation for claims respecting industrial diseases.

With this broad a mandate, one might expect that the Panel would have been inundated with requests for investigation from all occupational sectors of the province. However, this has not been the case and, in particular, health issues affecting female-dominated workplaces have not been brought to the Panel's attention.

If one looks at the occupational sectors that have brought their concerns to the Panel, a pattern of characteristics emerge. More tellingly, this pattern also identifies some of the problems inherent in trying to ascertain occupational disease prevalence among working women.

For example, historically in Ontario and elsewhere there were high rates of lung cancer among uranium miners. It is, therefore, not surprising that one of the unions representing miners — the Steelworkers — expeditiously approached the Panel to undertake investigations into mining health hazards.

What was of immense help in conducting these investigations was the Mining Master File, one of the earliest comprehensive data systems for a readily identifiable group of workers. This database contains the working history of all licensed miners in the province between 1956 and 1988 — approximately 90,000 entries in total. As a result, there was an enormous amount of reliable data that could be used as a basis for epidemiological studies and could also be linked with the Canadian Mortality Database.

In addition, many mine employers had pension plans so that retired miners could be traced with a reasonable degree of accuracy and any epidemiological studies would be more complete. The wealth of good data on Ontario miners was complemented by the worldwide availability of comparable studies with comparable findings.

As a result, the Panel was able to compile 22 epidemiological studies which evaluated the rates of lung cancer among Ontario miners. On the strength of this evidence, the Panel recommended that the Workers' Compensation Board (WCB) presume that a miner's lung cancer was a result of his work unless the contrary was proven. If this Report is adopted by the WCB it will mean that it will be easier for miners to have their claims recognized and in turn prevention in the workplace should also be enhanced.

In exploring how regulatory agencies deal with these issues, the characteristics of the mining sector and its working population are worth noting:

- a large, reasonably stable workforce;
- reliable and long-term work history data;
- worldwide comparison data;
- an organized voice for the workers;
- a workplace with many potential and recognized hazards;
- exposure data; and
- good company records and pension plans.

To date, the subjects of the majority of the investigations carried out by the Panel share most, if not all, of the above characteristics.

What this means for the study of health effects experienced by women in the workplace is of concern. Women have historically been excluded from occupational studies because of their relatively small numbers in those workplaces chosen for study. In a recent survey of 1,233 cancer studies published from 1971 to 1990 in eight major occupational health journals, only 14 percent presented analyses of data on white women and only 10 percent on non-white women (Zahm et al., 1994). In a literature review of gastric cancer requested by the Panel itself, almost all the studies excluded women (Stock, 1993). Women are employed in sectors like sales and service which exhibit reduced compliance with government health and safety monitoring programmes (SPR Associates, 1994).

To summarize, women are less likely:

- to work in organized workplaces;
- to work in large workplaces;
- to have pension plans;
- to do paid work;
- to work in an environment where records of the nature and amount of workplace toxins are maintained; and
- to have uninterrupted work histories.

In practical terms, this means that there have been almost no investigations by the Panel on female-dominated workplaces. It also means that any such investigation would have to address significant methodological obstacles.

There has previously been only one Panel investigation into a female-dominated workplace — the Report on the Canadian General Electric (CGE) Lamp Plant Issue (Shannon, 1988). That matter had come to the Panel because of a reported excess of breast and gynaecological cancers among female workers in the Coiling and Wire Drawing Department (CWD) at the CGE Plant in Toronto. In his report on this issue commissioned by the Panel, Dr. Shannon wrote:

> The cancers of *a priori* concern were significantly increased in women in the CWD, but not elsewhere in the plant. The excess was greatest in those with more than five year exposure [in CWD] and more than 15 years since first working in the CWD, with eight cases of breast and gynaecological cancers observed in this category compared with 2.67 expected. Only three cancers occurred in men in the CWD.

This group of women shared some of the characteristics of the miners. They had relatively stable work histories, they were represented by a union and there was some evidence about the nature and extent of the workplace exposures. However, of special interest are the characteristics of these women that differed from the characteristics of the miners. First, the female workforce was only about 1,000 during the study period and there were 12 women suffering from breast and gynaecological cancers. While this may appear to involve a large number of workers, the sample is relatively small when the size of other study populations are considered — for example, there are more than 40,000 workers in the cohort for the INCO mining operations in Ontario. Second, according to the majority of the Panel members there was insufficient evidence about the amount or effect of workplace exposures. Lastly, there were apparently no other worksites with similar exposures to confirm or negate the findings in this study.

As a result of this investigation, the majority of the Panel, as it was constituted at the time, determined that there was insufficient evidence to find a probable connection between work at CGE and these cancer cases, although the majority of the Panel did think that the WCB could consider workers' compensation benefits in some limited way for the women with breast cancer. In summary, the majority of the Panel did not think that there was sufficient evidence to invoke a legal presumption that would simplify the payment of WCB benefits.

In the future, when the Panel is confronted with a possible workplace cluster of serious illness like the cancers at the CGE Lamp Plant, the Panel would like to be able to reach a decision on adequate information and not deny the existence of a relationship because the data is incomplete. This issue did, however, concretely demonstrate the problems arising from studying working women in small numbers and with limited information.

In Ontario, there have been no studies of occupational disease in those female-dominated occupations where cohorts would be numerous enough for adequate information to be gathered. When the question of occupational disease among women was first considered by the Panel, there was some resistance to focusing on one sex as a discrete entity. It was asked why we should study women separately. The answers bear repeating — as does the fact that they are not well known.

While the above statistics demonstrate that women do not figure in what we can call "male" studies and that their "female" work isn't considered hazardous, they do, nevertheless, comprise a significant percentage of the workforce. As of 1990, there were 2,523,835 Ontario women working outside the home. Canadian women's labour participation has grown from 3,680,000 in 1975 to 5,978,000 in 1989 — an increase of over 62 percent (Women's Bureau, 1990).

These facts and figures were a surprise to some Panel members but, in the end, they proved persuasive enough to ensure that women's concerns were placed on the agenda. The question then became how to do this effectively and in a representative fashion.

It was decided to put together an advisory group of women representing workers from different occupational sectors and the academic, legal and medical communities. The purpose of the advisory committee was to determine what those affected thought should be done. In the summer of 1993, a meeting was held with people (mostly women) from unions, management, advocacy groups and the academic and scientific communities. We outlined the Panel's mandate and concern regarding working women to ascertain if there was a consensus on how the agency might properly look into this issue.

There was general support for further work; all the participants agreed that women's concerns in the workplace had not been properly addressed. However, there was not unanimity as to whether the Panel was the proper agency to be responsible for this work. At the meeting, this objection focused on the fact that some of the problems thought to be present in women's work — like soft tissue and repetitive strain injuries — were not within the Panel's mandate. These issues were, however, of tremendous concern to the union representatives.

The Panel was clear that it would not be proceeding with issues outside its jurisdiction. Nevertheless, the Panel's activity in this area continued to be a concern in the employer community. As a matter of interest, we received a letter after the meeting from an employer representative who suggested that the Panel had no authority to conduct this kind of social research investigation and protested any further action on its part. He apparently thought that only traditional epidemiological research could add to our knowledge about occupational diseases.

Philosophical disputes about mandate notwithstanding, there was agreement on several points among all members of the advisory committee. As a starting point, the group decided that self-identification of issues was crucial to an effective exploration of working women's health concerns. This was so for two major reasons. First, because of the lack of work done on women's health issues, it wasn't clear what problems were of importance to working women themselves. Second, because women have traditionally been excluded from decision making, a format which gave them some control over the project seemed important. No one wanted control of the agenda to be dictated by the academic or scientific community without input from working women.

The next question to be addressed was how best to obtain information of a diverse and wide-ranging nature. At this point, it was acknowledged that recessions have a chilling effect on occupational health. Workers are less likely to report problems for fear of losing their jobs. Women, many of them in low-paying and non-unionized jobs, are particularly vulnerable.

As a consequence, it was the advisory group consensus that a survey approach based in the workplace was not apt to be successful. The union representatives were particularly emphatic that workers would feel ambivalent about participating in anything they thought might have adverse employment repercussions.

The exception to the above was the general enthusiasm for using a hospital setting. Because of the large numbers of women in almost every area of hospital work, the diverse nature of the work and kinds of exposures, the fact that hospital workers tend to be unionized, and, lastly, their generally reliable health records, there was agreement that a hospital would lend itself to a general case study or survey of health concerns.

As to the actual mechanics of eliciting a wider range of information, there was little initial support for employing the telephone or mail questionnaire system. The group thought that the response rate would be poor for a number of reasons:

- "double workdays" are a reality for most women and they don't have time to respond while at home;
- there are often language and literacy restrictions to such questionnaires which might skew the responses; and
- without a proper explanation of the possible benefits there is little incentive for the women to respond.

In the end, it was concluded that small focus groups would be an appropriate tool to establish concerns among working women. This would allow for:

- input by the participants and a flexible structure;
- inclusion of non-unionized women in a non-threatening environment;
- inclusion of women whose first language was not English; and
- a diverse sampling of workers.

The first meeting ended on the understanding that the Panel would be seeking a research proposal to undertake the kind of work we had discussed at the meeting. Unfortunately, the enthusiasm and innovative thinking that had come out of the group went into a kind of bureaucratic hibernation as there was no funding to carry on with any of the suggestions for focus groups or research methodologies tailored to the special needs of working women.

However, as a direct result of the meeting, the Ontario Nurses' Association formally asked the Panel to study the issue of health hazards to nurses associated with the use of and exposure to antineoplastic drugs. As a group, nurses share many of the characteristics that allow for a successful epidemiological study: large numbers; good records; opportunity for follow-up; pension plans; known or quantifiable exposures; and a union presence. A study that has been done in the U.S. on this issue could be used for comparison purposes (*Proceedings for the International Conference on Women's Health: Occupation and Cancer*, 1993:33). The Panel has been able to put this specific investigation on the agenda for this year.

The Panel did not simply abandon the issue of working women's health concerns while it sought alternative funding. In the interim, the Panel asked Professor Karen Messing to review methodological questions involving research in women's occupational health and to update her literature review done for Labour Canada (Messing, 1991) and her 1994 report for the Panel (Messing, 1994). Lastly, based on the above, she agreed to identify research priorities for 1994. Professor Messing's work for the Panel confirmed the perceptions described at the working women's health group some six months earlier. Her report explored some methodological issues facing any study of occupational illnesses specific to women or female-dominated workplaces:

- how and when to analyze data by gender;
- how to take into account the different life patterns of women and men;
- how to identify health problems which arise in women's traditional work and for which strategies and methodologies may not yet have been developed;
- how to deal with problems arising from the historical exclusion of women and their work in epidemiological studies;
- how to treat definitions of work and the double workload of most women;
- how to incorporate the treatment of biological alterations which are not treated as pathologies — that is, because the aggressors present in women's work have been understudied, identification of occupational disease is embryonic and may well go unrecognized; and
- how to resolve difficulties in estimating exposure by job title and the fact that men and women with the same job title may perform markedly different tasks with corresponding differences in exposure.

Like many of the women within the working group, the report highlighted musculoskeletal problems and the discrete issues arising from women's anthropometric characteristics (size, shape). Indoor air quality, occupational cancers, stress and cardiovascular effects and menstrual disorders were suggested priorities for research. Lastly, the report noted that several professions dominated by women have been little examined: specifically, waitressing and cleaning.

Happily, the Panel has been successful in facilitating funding from the Workplace Health and Safety Agency, and Dr. Gina Feldberg at York University's Centre for Health Studies has been commissioned to carry out the proposal for the Working Women's Health Survey (Feldberg, 1994). Consequently, a project that had been dormant for some time had to be reactivated immediately in order to receive funding consideration.

Because of the commitment to a consultative approach, we scheduled an immediate meeting of the advisory group. At the meeting, there was much discussion over what kind of data we proposed to collect. Specifically, the group grappled with the issue of whether to include data on race. This particular portion of the discussion merits inclusion because data collection which focuses on disadvantaged groups is not a simple matter. Data can be used in a number of ways, some more desirable than others.

Simply put, members of the committee were concerned that results concerning disease incidence by race would be used to overshadow or diminish the results concerning possible occupational problems. By way of example, over the past 30 years, studies of stomach cancer in various occupations have attributed cancer incidence to ethnicity and diet (individual characteristics) rather than to elements specific to the work environment (occupational characteristics).[1] Recently, a large corporation refused a proposal by the Panel to undertake a feasibility study for a data collection system. The Panel wanted to focus on work exposure and the employer wanted focus on data about diet and lifestyle.

Ultimately, there was general agreement within the advisory group that the benefits of such data for prevention attempts could not be overlooked and that structured analysis could preclude, as much as possible, inappropriate use of the data on ethnicity. For that reason, such data should be collected.

The proposal ultimately accepted by the advisory group enumerated the physiologic, sociologic and economic variables which impinge upon working women's health:
- menstruation;
- lactation;

- sexual and sexist harassment;
- pregnancy;
- underemployment;
- body size and shape;
- degree of worker control over work activity;
- double workdays;
- job security; and
- low pay.

The proposal concluded that survey methodology, developed from a literature review and focus groups, would be the best way of obtaining innovative and comprehensive information about working women's health concerns.

Such an approach could overcome the problems of obtaining data from more standard sources — that is: the traditional emphasis on mortality rather than morbidity; exclusion of self-reporting and self-perception from standard indices; non-recognition of women's unique health and disease status in the categorization or clarification of disease; the requirement for large sample sizes; and presumptions about the nature of hazardous work.

The proposal sets out a three-pronged survey technique:

- a series of focus groups;
- a telephone or mail questionnaire; and
- case studies or epidemiological analyses.

The proposal incorporates an assumption that work-related health concerns span a broad physiologic and psychological range. A series of focus groups conducted throughout the province of Ontario with women who work in a wide variety of occupational settings can systematize women's perceptions about their health. Focus groups in which the interviewer uses a schedule with the same, open-ended questions but allows for clarification or follow-up questions are best suited to obtain relevant data. With this format, there are fewer presumptions made about what the participants do or do not understand and ambiguous responses can be sorted out immediately. This kind of approach would encourage inclusion of women whose first language may not be English and would not exclude women based on education or literacy levels.

The information obtained from the focus groups can then be divided into three categories:

- the typical response, which is defined as one that recurs and has no substantial refutation in other interviews;

- the unusual or atypical remark which is not repeated often enough to be considered reflective of the interviews;
- the rare comment that contradicts the majority of views.

In order to assure representative input, two distinct kinds of focus groups were proposed:

MIXED GROUPS: This kind of group includes representatives from the "key areas" in which women work. These areas can be defined geographically; by work site/setting; by industrial category; or by sort of work done. Relying on contact through unions, the researchers will attempt to assemble groups which include representatives of the varied tasks women perform. This approach recognizes the interaction between health problems, working environments and the variables of age, race, class, ethnicity, ability and geographic location. Accordingly, efforts will be made to diversify representation in the groups.

CONCENTRATED GROUPS: This is a series of concentrated groups in which only one work area, or a series of closely interrelated work areas, are represented. These groups would allow for closer analysis of specific concerns. As well, they allow for analysis of the influences of such variables as work environment, age and ethnicity — because the type of work studied will be constant, the influence of other variables will emerge.

The focus group study includes the advisory committee as a resource in finding participants. While their involvement is essential, union locals cannot provide as comprehensive a selection of female workers as male workers due to the larger number of women in non-unionized settings. Accordingly, there will be a need to rely on individual contacts and community groups.

While it is anticipated that the focus groups will supply detailed and qualitative data, further information is necessary. Notwithstanding the limitations of the survey format, it can open up the process for more statistical analysis. Accordingly, the second prong of the proposal suggests a mail-back questionnaire. While this traditionally has a lower response rate than a telephone survey and makes more literacy demands, it is markedly more economical. This was, in the end, a consideration.

To make the questionnaire as user-friendly as possible, multi-language forms were proposed. In addition, there will be four contacts with the participants:

- a covering, explanatory letter that accompanies the questionnaire along with a stamped return envelope;
- a reminder card a week after first contact;
- a repeat mail-out to non-respondents of the first questionnaire; and
- a last mail-out to non-respondents.

As with the focus groups, questionnaires will be mailed out in such a way as to be representative of employment type, geographic location, class, race and other variables. They will include questions about:
- employment history, status and work conditions;
- demographics;
- health history and recent health experiences; and
- perceptions of the impact of work on health.

Finally, the sample designs for the mail-out will involve union members, public sector organizations and private sector employers. We recognize that outworkers and those in small businesses will be missed but responses from those in similarly situated work are expected.

The last prong of the proposal outline suggests case studies. The focus groups and surveys will provide a broad base of information on women's self-identified concerns. Case studies can focus the investigation more narrowly and provide in-depth assessment where there is reason to suspect a relationship between occupation and disease. The case studies can involve more detailed interviews, systematic review of practitioner records and health data and review of work sites. They can also be epidemiological studies examining the interrelationship between work-related exposures and the onset of disease. Of necessity, the structure of the case studies will be determined by the nature of the response to the focus groups and the questionnaires.

From this reasonably brief description, the authors hope to have shown how their approach addresses the methodological problems faced by those endeavouring to obtain valid information about working women. Again, the usefulness of the advisory group cannot be overemphasized, nor can the benefits involved in having the stakeholders assist in formulating and agreeing to the process. To illustrate this, an additional problem was noted by the employer representatives on the advisory committee. When discussing groups to target for the focus groups, community representatives were understandably concerned about the women in the most vulnerable situations — such as non-unionized women with language barriers or outworkers — since their working conditions are so hard to determine. The employer representatives noted, however, that outworkers (people working at home in cottage industries) are not covered under the Workers' Compensation Act. They did not feel that any project funded by compensation money — in effect, paid for by employers whose workers are covered under the Act — should include these workers. It was not possible to secure additional funding specifically to include workers not covered under workers' compensation. However, the proposal was refined so that categories of workers who are covered corresponded approximately to those not covered. While this is not an ideal solution, it makes allowances for the problem and addresses it up front. As everyone knows, problems in data collection are much better dealt with by confronting them directly at the stage of study planning.

In conclusion, the Panel is excited by this venture and the opportunity to participate in a working women's health survey that specifically addresses women's problems and is mindful of women's considerations. At some point, not too far in the future, we hope to be able to discuss the results of this project and the new directions it has established for specific investigations by the Panel into women's occupational diseases.

NOTES

1. Roger Rickwood of the Federally Regulated Employers, Transportation and Communication. Letter to the Industrial Disease Standards Panel (ISDP), June 24, 1993.

REFERENCES

Feldberg, Gina. "Proposal to Develop a Province-wide Survey of Working Women's Health Concerns." Prepared for the Ontario Industrial Disease Standards Panel, March 1994.

Industrial Disease Standards Panel. *Report to the Workers' Compensation Board on the CGE Lamp Plant Issue.* Toronto: Ontario Industrial Disease Standards Panel, November 1988.

Messing, Karen. *Occupational Health Concerns of Canadian Women.* Ottawa: Labour Canada, 1991.

— "Women's Occupational Health: Critical Review and Discussion of Current Issues." Prepared for the Ontario Industrial Disease Standards Panel, March 1994.

Proceedings for the International Conference on Women's Health: Occupation and Cancer, 1993. p. 33.

SPR Associates Inc. *Highlights of the 1994 Survey of Occupational Health and Safety and Joint Health and Safety Committees: A Benchmark of the Internal Responsibility System.* Prepared for the Ontario Workplace Health and Safety Agency, November 1994.

Shannon, H.S., et al. "Cancer Morbidity in Lamp Manufacturing Workers." *American Journal of Industrial Medicine* 14 (1988). pp. 281-90.

Stock, S.R. "Gastric Cancer and Occupation: A Review of the Literature." Report for the Ontario Industrial Disease Standards Panel. Toronto, 1993.

Women's Bureau. *Women in the Labour Force: 1990-91 Edition.* Ottawa: Women's Bureau, Labour Canada, 1990.

Zahm, S.H. et al. "Inclusion of Women and Minorities in Occupational Cancer Epidemiological Research." *Journal of Occupational Medicine* 36, 8 (August 1994). pp. 842-7.

Joan M. Stevenson

Gender-fair Employment Practices

Developing Employee Selection Tests

L'adoption de normes pour la sélection des employés pour des professions impliquant la manutention ou d'autres tâches requérant de la force physique s'est généralisée depuis deux décennies, en partie à cause de l'arrivée des femmes dans des emplois non traditionnels. Au Canada, le droit d'exiger certaines caractéristiques physiques est soumise à un ensemble de principes idéalistes. Pourtant, à l'intérieur de chaque clause, subsistent des pièges qui compromettent l'équité entre les sexes. Ainsi, lorsqu'on évalue les exigences spécifiques d'un emploi, on risque de se baser sur la façon dont les hommes exécutent les tâches manuelles, ou de prescrire une procédure fixe, ce qui, souvent, désavantagera les femmes. En principe, les tests devraient pouvoir révéler à la fois les forces et les faiblesses relatives des femmes. Ces dernières performent mieux, en général, dans l'accomplissement de tâches complexes, mais sont désavantagées lorsque le travail implique la force des membres supérieurs. Malheureusement, la procédure de validation compilée a souvent les résultats en une mesure unique, sous-estimant ainsi la variance rélevée par les tests. Lorsqu'on utilise ces tests pré-embauche, la note de passage peut être fixée plus ou moins haut, selon qu'on veuille minimiser les «faux positifs» ou les «faux négatifs»; le choix fait a alors un impact dramatique sur les femmes. En fait, tout test de sélection basé uniquement sur des variables de force ou de rapidité d'exécution favorise un nombre disproportionné de personnes d'un sexe. Plusieurs employeurs préfèrent utiliser de tels tests, plutôt que d'adapter les caractéristiques des tâches ou des postes de travail. Les recherches futures devront se concentrer sur la validation des batteries de tests pour tenir compte des caractéristiques des femmes et sur l'amélioration des processus d'utilisation de ces tests.

Selection standards for manual handling (and other professions requiring physical strength) have become more common in the last two decades, perhaps in conjunction with the entry of women into non-traditional jobs. In Canada, the requirement for certain physical characteristics for certain occupations are regulated by a set of idealistic principles. However, these principles contain numerous pitfalls that jeopardize gender fairness. In evaluating job demands, there is the danger of incorporating a male approach to manual handling, or of dictating the manner in which certain tasks must be done; both approaches often put women at a disadvantage. Test battery items have the potential to show women's strengths or weaknesses in comparison to men. Factors such as the ability to practise complex skills and the extent of upper body work are both critical to the performance of women. Statistical procedures used to validate tests often pool the genders, thus giving a false evaluation of the amount of variance contained in the selection test. In pre-employment testing, cutting scores can be selected by controlling false negatives or false positives, a practice which has a tremendous impact on women. In fact, any selection test which is based solely on strength- and speed-based variables will always disproportionately favour members of one sex over the other. Many employers are looking at selection tests rather than examining the ergonomics of the work or the work station. Future research, then, should be directed toward the validation of test batteries on women and improved implementation procedures.

INTRODUCTION

The struggle of women to enter non-traditional roles has been researched by feminists, sociologists and historians, and many examples have been given of patriarchal barriers to integration. Rather than address political or societal barriers, this paper will concentrate on physical factors which inhibit women's entry and integration into non-traditional roles. In particular, this paper will focus on current legislation on fair employment practices and implementation of employee selection tests to women.

Selection standards and/or fitness requirements have been in place for decades in all male professions. In some manual materials handling trades such as lumber mills, steel factories or manufacturing plants, the physical conditions of work were such that it was survival of the fittest and workers quit if they were not able to cope. In professional trades such as police work, firefighting or the military, physical requirements and fitness standards were sufficiently arduous that only the upper half or quartile of men could pass the pre-selection test (although maintaining this standard was not required). For example, the Ontario Provincial Police had a height and weight requirement and demanded a rigid fitness and performance level at the Police Academy of those who wished to enter the profession. None of these earlier physical and fitness standards were based on *bona fide* occupational requirements (Wilmore and Davis, 1979).

In the 1970s, the State of California ruled that women must be admitted to the police force. This caused a flurry of concern about both the physical abilities of women to handle job demands and to preserve the safety of society and other police officers. Now, two decades later, it is interesting that, in a domestic quarrel, which is considered to be a risky situation for police officers, a common practice recognized as an effective strategy to defuse the situation is for a female police officer to stand in front and communicate while the male officer stands behind and observes (Campbell, 1993). Despite the proven advantages of hiring female officers, society is slow to accept women as important and equal.

Other professions also have been slow to respond to equal access. For example, in firefighting the barriers are more overt in that this profession is looking to selection standards to solicit physically powerful recruits. Despite the fact that a number of males belonging to ethnic minorities and women passed the selection tests, the City of Toronto was pressured by a *Toronto Star* article into accepting the top ranked Caucasian males (Taylor, 1993). It is interesting that firefighters support selection standards to control job entry but resist the imposition of physical skills maintenance standards to remain firefighters. In a study of Chicago firefighters, one-third of the 40- to 60-year-old men had aerobic fitness levels of 0.6 oz/lb/min (33.5 ml/kg/min) which is below that of the average woman (Sothmann, 1993a; 1993b).

In manual materials handling jobs, there is concern that there will be a reduction in productivity and an increase in musculoskeletal injuries if women enter certain trades (Blue, 1993). In terms of productivity, many jobs were designed to be accessible to male lifting capacity, using normative lifting data from Snook et al. (1991) and Ayoub et al. (1980). As for injury prevention, only one study by Chaffin and Park (1973) determined that a low ratio of operator strength to job demands was related to an increased risk of injury. Messing et al. (1991; 1994) and Lortie (1987) found no gender differences in accident data but both point out that their results were inconclusive since neither jobs nor types of illnesses were the same for men and women. Kumar and Mital (1992) wrote a critical review of the literature on worker safety in manual handling tasks, stating that worker safety would be enhanced if task demands were between 30 and 50 percent of an individual's strength. Since the absolute strength of women is less than that of men, Kumar and Mital are indirectly stating a belief in reduced access for women on the grounds of safety. This is an oversimplification of the importance of strength over other measures as a criterion, since men and women often use different lifting techniques and thus require different levels of force during the tasks (Courville et al., 1991; Falkel et al., 1985; Matzdorff, 1987; Vézina et al., 1992; Stevenson et al., 1990).

The ergonomics literature suggests two methods to alleviate problems of mismatch between workers and their jobs: (1) to change the ergonomics of work to suit the person; or (2) find workers with the strength or capacity to perform the job. The development and use of pre-employment selection tests and worker placement programmes belong to a tradition of attempting to hire the right worker for a particular job, thus assuring productivity based on job demands while reducing the possible harmful physical effects of creating a mismatch of worker and job (Chaffin and Andersson, 1991).

LEGISLATIVE REQUIREMENTS

Selection tests are regulated by a subsection of the Canadian Charter of Human Rights under *bona fide* occupational standards for employment. Although a job-demands analysis, a scientific approach and minimal acceptable criteria are required by law, this does not guarantee fair employment practices. Physically demanding jobs are particularly problematic in setting gender-fair standards, because of the disparity in anthropometry, strength and endurance between men and women.

In Canada, federal and provincial jurisdictions each have separate Human Rights Acts and Commissions which handle a number of employment issues including recruitment, hiring, promotion and dismissal (Canadian HRC, 1985). Surprisingly few cases have been adjudicated by Human Rights Tribunals. The most noteworthy to date was the decision in the case of *Action Travail des Femmes vs. Canadian National Railway* (CNR) in 1984. In this case, the selection test consisted of a number of manual tasks that were not part of the current jobs. CNR was forced to commence an affirmative action hiring programme for women as a result of their unfair hiring practices.

The scientific literature contains numerous reports of approaches used in employee screening for police forces, fire departments and the military. Companies involved in manual materials handling may use selection tests developed internally or by consultants, but these are often not reported in the scientific literature. Few selection tests are challenged, since applicants are not aware of possible areas of gender bias. Those companies that have been challenged in court usually remove the selection test for fear of either losing the case or bad publicity. One noteworthy case occurred in 1994 with *Dion vs. Gaz Metropolitain* in which the Appeals court upheld the Quebec Human Rights Commission ruling to order an ergonomic study of the workplace to increase accessibility for smaller workers. These cases highlight some of the pitfalls that can occur in the process of setting selection standards.

OCCUPATIONAL REQUIREMENTS

The steps required to establish *bona fide* occupational requirements are defined in the Canadian Charter of Human Rights (CHSA-S1-82-83, Canadian Human Rights Commission, 1985) and are paraphrased as follows:

1. identification of the occupational requirements or essential components of the job;

2. determination of selection test items;

3. establishment of predictive relationships between occupational tasks and selection tests;

4. determination of a selection standard or cut-off score; and

5. setting the standard at a minimum acceptable level.

It is important for scientists, companies and adjudicators to be aware of gender biases that can be present at any step of the process.

PHYSICAL DEMANDS ANALYSIS

An analysis of the job for which applicants will be hired is a critical first step in creating a selection test (Mostardi, 1990). Factors such as reach, force, frequency, posture and time spent doing various tasks are recorded so that researchers can understand task demands and develop an appropriate test battery. To acquire accurate data, a variety of sources must be used: observation; written documents; supervisor interviews; and operator interviews. If only one resource is used to assess job requirements, perceptions of job demands may be incorrect.

The importance of a detailed job analysis is shown through a study by Wilmore and Davis (1979), who were asked to assist in establishing entry criteria for state troopers in California. Although the objective was to create a physical selection standard, the critical tasks analysis revealed that only three of 16 workplace tasks required physical strength or capacity. In this case, the fairness of a physical selection standard in a profession where many other attributes are essential for success in the job must be questioned. Women will necessarily be underrepresented in professions that use physical selection standards as the only pre-employment screening test.

Numerous pitfalls can jeopardize gender fairness in the physical demands analysis phase. For example, describing job requirements will usually result in documenting strategies for performance by men, since they hold most of the jobs. Many researchers have reported that men and women perform tasks differently (Courville et al., 1991; Grieve, 1984; Stevenson et al., 1990), which is not surprising when one considers obvious anthropometric and strength differences. If the physical demands analysis is not sensitive to permitting technique variations, an inherent gender bias, requiring certain techniques, may be imposed.

IDENTIFICATION OF THE SELECTION TEST ITEMS

The next step in developing selection tests is to identify essential elements which will become part of the selection test(s). Ayoub et al. (1987) chose the most demanding component of a task, on the assumption that if one can perform the most demanding task, then all other components also can be performed. For a lawn mowing task, lifting the mower into a truck was defined as the most demanding task. However, this component may not be essential, may involve poor ergonomics or may be demanding in the opinion of males only. Care must be used in defining the essential elements where only incumbents of one gender are defining the perceived task difficulties. Factors such as task frequency, speed of operation, load and administrative controls all contribute to documenting essential elements.

Other researchers have used generic lifting tasks to represent a family of lifts on the assumption that performance will not vary significantly across lift types or strategies used (Gebhardt et al., 1992; Stevenson et al., 1990). Acting on the knowledge that most manual handling tasks in the military involved lifting, Stevenson et al. (1990) used a maximal lift from floor to 5.4 feet (1.35 metres) to represent a family of lifting tasks. However, a lift to this height definitely required upper body involvement, a component where the strength of women is approximately 50 percent that of men. If the task involved only a lift to waist height, women would have taken advantage of their lower body strength, which is approximately 65 percent of male strength.

Other approaches include soliciting the expert opinion of supervisors (Gebhardt et al., 1993) or workers (Gledhill et al., 1992). One implication of this strategy is that most experts currently in manual handling jobs are men who may judge essential elements or perform tasks differently from women.

Regardless of the approach used, there is no requirement to improve the ergonomics of the job, or its essential elements, prior to establishing a pre-employment screening test. If an employer can argue that ergonomic changes would have caused undue financial hardship, then employee screening for workers capable of performing the present work would be considered reasonable. Stevenson et al. (1990) demonstrated that women benefitted from ergonomic changes to a box lifting task more than men. If true for other tasks, this systemic bias favouring a male strategy of work will place women at a disadvantage until the ergonomics of a task have been improved.

APPROACHES TO TEST DEVELOPMENT

The objective of the scientific approach is to develop a valid strategy to measure essential task elements. Most companies will not allow applicants to enter the plant and perform the actual tasks at a worksite. Therefore, it is necessary to create simulations of the tasks which capture the essential elements. These simulations are then compared to performance on a physical test battery which may include measures of muscular strength and endurance and cardiovascular capacity. For example, to establish minimum physical fitness standards for the Canadian Armed Forces, Stevenson et al. (1992) created operationalized tasks that were designed to be one person tasks for land and sea evacuations, entrenchment digging, low/high crawling and sandbag carrying. Operational task definitions are required to provide consistency of task demands for each subject. It is important to allow freestyle protocols during tasks, where possible. It would appear that women are more handicapped by protocol constraints than men because the tasks are not designed with women's physical attributes in mind. Using one of Ayoub's tasks (1982), Stevenson et al. (1991) showed that protocol restrictions underestimate women's potential more than men's.

A second approach, used frequently in police force and firefighting standards, is to combine discrete tasks into a circuit in order to replicate rescue situations. This type of performance has been evaluated by a predictive physiological test battery (Misner et al., 1989; Brownlie et al., 1985) or by using the circuit scores themselves as the selection test (Davis et al., 1982).

In a third approach, Gebhardt et al. (1990) conducted a study in which the actual tasks were performed and supervisor rating scales were developed to appraise performance. Concern over bias had been raised by Cook (1988) and Arvey (1979) because many supervisors either gave low ratings to minority group members or inflated the ratings of such applicants to show management there was no prejudice in their ratings.

Gebhardt et al. (1992) had some success with supervisor ratings, but correlations to actual performance scores were less than with other strategies. Despite some obvious problems, this strategy could be developed as a useful approach.

The possibility for gender bias to invade the scientific method can also be a result of inadequate science or an attitude which assumes that women will not be able to perform as well as men. Unfortunately, there are numerous examples of each problem. Some studies do not include any women in the sample (Davis et al., 1982; Kamon et al., 1982) and so standards are based on male performance only. Other studies may include a small percentage of women, such as in the U.S. Air Force recruit selection test, but there is no overlap in scores by gender and data are pooled without reporting gender-based relationships (Ayoub et al., 1982). Pooling across genders is an artificial method which can inflate the strength of association (correlation coefficients) between selection test(s) and task performance. For example, Stevenson et al. (1995) reported correlation coefficients of $r = 0.59$ for men, and $r = 0.36$ for women on the ability of the U.S. Air Force screening test called the Incremental Lifting Machine (ILM) to predict performance on a box lifting task. When data were pooled, the correlation coefficient jumped to $r = 0.84$, a false representation of the effectiveness of the ILM to predict performance within gender.

CHOOSE A CUTTING SCORE

The cutting score is the criterion which determines whether a subject passes or fails a selection test. Since task scores for women are less than those for men, there will always be more women failing a physical selection test. Although adverse impact is expected, gender bias may also occur unless researchers are aware of factors which can affect the magnitude of gender differences (Beck, 1976; Guion, 1976; 1982).

Choosing an appropriate cut-off score has been approached in numerous ways. One strategy is to use expert panels or productivity to decide an appropriate performance level. This approach carries the danger of being biased by previous standards based on incumbents who may be exclusively men.

Another approach is to set the cut-off score based on a representative sample of male and female subjects. Stevenson et al. (1992; 1994) used this approach in establishing minimum physical fitness standards for the Canadian Armed Forces. Since all of the test battery items were speed or strength related, there was a great disparity in male and female performance. Hence, placement of the cut-off score at the 75th percentile of the sample meant that about 40 percent of women failed the task performance. The test battery required women to maintain a higher fitness level than their male counterparts. This result was realistic and workable, given the physical nature of the selection criteria.

In setting a cutting score, it is important to choose criteria which are defensible and reasonable. Rhodes and Farenholtz (1992) chose a criteria for the Police Officers Physical Abilities Test based on strength and time to apprehend prisoners. This was a novel idea, but 30 percent of male and 84 percent of female current police officers failed to pass the cutting score. Does this mean that those individuals should be removed as police officers? Perhaps one should question the placement of the pass/fail criteria, which is higher than the minimum level suggested by the Canadian Charter of Human Rights.

Gledhill and Jamnik (1992) helped the Toronto Firefighting Department set up selection criteria for potential recruits. Their approach to choosing a cutting score was novel and effective in that men's and women's scores were ranked based on their relationship to the mean score of the sample. Those performing better than average had an increasingly positive score up to three points (Z-scores). Despite a reasonable approach to developing cut-off scores, there was a flurry in the *Toronto Star* (Taylor, 1993) because some Caucasian male applicants who had higher performance scores were overlooked in preference of women and ethic minorities. Since all applicants passed the cut-off criteria, it may have been a mistake to publish actual raw score values; all were acceptable based on the minimum physical performance criterion. The ensuing controversy in the press forced Toronto City Hall to hire not only their original choices, but also the vocal Caucasian men.

STRENGTH AND SPEED AS SELECTION CRITERIA

Research describing physical differences between men and women can be found in the literature on anthropometry, strength, endurance and flexibility, as well as performance differences in standardized manual handling tasks and actual job-related tasks (Dyer, 1982; Chaffin and Andersson, 1991; Kates et al., 1980). In most cases — except flexibility and high repetition tasks (Courville et al., 1991) — men outperform women when performance is measured by size, load, speed. Typically, gender differences are reported as statistical differences or as a ratio of female to male performance.

It is difficult for researchers to assess what constitutes a reasonable difference in task performance by gender for a selection test. For example, the literature reports female to male ratios for upper body strength from 35 percent to 79 percent, and for lower body strength from 57 percent to 86 percent (Laubach, 1976). The variability in ratios is probably a result of small or nonrepresentative sample sizes and testing protocols. In task performance, the range of female to male ratios are even greater, with ranges of 10 percent to 89 percent for specific physically demanding tasks (Pheasant, 1983). One factor which is critical to note is that there is a natural overlap in scores between men and women. In other words, some women are stronger than some men. If gender overlap is not evident in the sample tested, then this may denote a fairness problem.

Another concern with selection tests is the emphasis on short, simple, maximal effort tests from which inferences are made about endurance and safety (Kumar and Mital, 1992). Ayoub (1991) and Mital (1983) reported that women performed at 50 percent of men's performance for low frequency strength-based lifts but obtained 65 percent of male scores for high frequency endurance-based tests. The fact that women may have better endurance than men may not be obvious in manual handling tasks because fixed weights force women to work at a higher proportion of their capacity.

FUTURE DIRECTIONS IN SELECTION STANDARDS

Selection tests are one strategy employers use to have some assurance that the employee can maintain a certain productivity level while maintaining a reduced risk of injury. Therefore, it is not realistic to argue against some form of pre-employment screening. However, the current approach to selection tests can be described as a task-based approach where the goal is to identify those individuals who can perform a task in its present form. This strategy has the potential for a number of systemic and scientific problems since most incumbents are males in jobs designed for men. Furthermore, validation studies are difficult without sufficient women in the sample. Stevenson et al. (1990) showed that certain lifting-task definitions have a greater impact on women than on men. If tasks have been designed to optimize male performance, this does not necessarily create the optimal task definition for women. Hypothetical optimization curves for men and women lifting 910 pounds (2,000 kilograms) are shown in Figure 1. The optimal performance for men in the figure is not the optimal performance for women. If the figure represented the real situation, an arbitrary cutting score based on male performance would not allow women to demonstrate their optimum potential.

Until gender biases are removed from jobs and scientific procedures it will be difficult to endorse the concept of a common cutting criterion for both genders. Cronshaw (1986), sensitive to the dichotomy between affirmative action hiring programmes and common cut-off criteria, suggested that, given appropriately validated selection tests, top-down hiring on the basis of the test scores within racial and gender subgroups would select the most qualified applicants while allowing the desired representation from the various subgroups (Cronshaw, 1986). In other words, if individuals of different ethnic, racial and gender groups pass the minimum acceptable criteria for physically demanding tasks, then there is no reason to choose the person based only on the test score.

Figure 1   Hypothetical Gender Profiles for an Objective-based Lifting Task

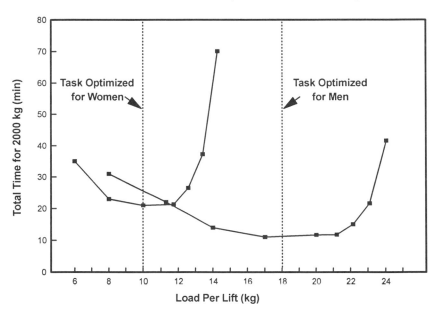

Floor to Shoulder Lifts (Box Width 45.72 cm)

*Right side of both curves from psychophysical data, reported by Ayoub et al., (1980).

Washburn and Safrit (1982) reported increasing concern with the validity of the cut-off scores in the context of the struggles of women and minorities for the right to hold physically demanding jobs. The challenge is to fill the gaps in ergonomic knowledge, as selection standards require extrapolations and interpolations and have implications felt beyond scientific exactitude (Metz, 1985; Ward, 1978; Webb and Tack, 1988). Therefore, it is important to initiate a dialogue among researchers, industry and government to allow the process of developing physical selection tests to proceed toward gender-fair employment practices.

ACKNOWLEDGEMENTS

The author would like to acknowledge the contribution of other members of the Ergonomics Research Group at Queen's University: namely, Tim Bryant, Janice Deakin, Terry Smith and Donna Greenhorn. Research funds for some of studies cited were provided by the Canadian Forces Defence and Civil Institute for Environmental Medicine and the Department of Physical Education, Recreation and Amenities and the Natural Sciences and Engineering Research Council of Canada.

REFERENCES

Arvey, M.A. *Fairness in Selecting Employees.* Don Mills, Ontario: Addison-Wesley, 1979. pp. 5-207.

Ayoub, M.M. "Psychophysical Basis for Manual Lifting Guidelines." Scientific support documentation for the revised *Lifting Equation.* Springfield, VA: National Technical Information Services, 1991.

Ayoub, M.M., A. Mital, G.M. Bakken, S.S. Asfour and N.J. Bethea. "Development of Strength and Capacity Norms for Manual Materials Handling Activities: The State of the Art." *Human Factors* 22, 3 (1980). pp. 271-83.

Ayoub, M.M., B.C. Jiang, J.L. Smith, J.J. Selan and J.W. McDaniel. "Establishing a Physical Criterion for Assigning Personnel to U.S. Air Force Jobs." *American Industrial Hygiene Association Journal* 48 (1987). pp. 464-70.

Ayoub, M.M., J.D. Denardo, J.L. Smith, N.J. Bethea, B.K. Lambert, L.R. Alley and B.S. Duran. *Establishing Physical Criteria for Assigning Personnel to Air Force Jobs: Final Report.* Lubbock, TX: Texas Technical University, 1982. (Air Force Office of Scientific Research # F49620-79-C-0006.)

Beck, R.A. "Determination of Optimal Cutting Scores in Criterion Referenced Measurement." *Journal of Experimental Education* 45 (1976). pp. 4-9.

Blue, C.L. "Women in Nontraditional Jobs: Is There a Risk for Musculoskeletal Injury?" *American Association of Occupational Health Nursing Journal* 41, 5 (1993). pp. 235-40.

Brownlie, L., S. Brown, G. Diewert, P. Good, G. Holman, G. Lane and E. Bannister. "Cost Effective Selection of Fire Fighter Results." *Medicine and Science in Sport and Exercise* 17, 6 (1985). pp. 661-6.

Campbell, M. Personal communication. Kingston, Ontario, Canada. (March 23, 1993).

Chaffin, D., and G. Andersson. *Occupational Biomechanics.* Toronto: John Wiley & Sons, 1991.

Chaffin, D.B., and K.S. Park. "A Longitudinal Study of Low Back Pain Associated with Occupational Weight Lifting Factors." *American Industrial Hygiene Association Journal* 34 (1973). pp. 513-24.

Cook, M. *Personnel Selection and Productivity*. Toronto: John Wiley & Sons, 1988.

Courville, J., N. Vézina and K. Messing. "Analysis of Work Activity in a Job in a Machine Shop Held by Ten Men and One Woman." *International Journal of Industrial Ergonomics* 7 (1991). pp. 163-74.

Cronshaw, S.F. "The Status of Employment Testing in Canada: A Review and Evaluation of Theory and Professional Practice." *Canadian Psychology* 27, 2 (1986). pp. 183-95.

Davis, P.O., C.O. Dotson and D. Laine Santa Maria. "Relationship Between Simulated Fire Fighting Tasks and Physical Performance Measures." *Medicine & Science in Sport & Exercise* 14, 1 (1982). pp. 65-71.

Dyer, K.F. *Challenging the Men: The Social Biology of Female Sporting Achievement*. New York: University of Queensland Press, 1982.

Falkel, J.E., M.N. Sewka, L. Levine and K.B. Pandolf. "Upper to Lower Body Muscular Strength and Endurance Ratios for Women and Men." *Ergonomics* 28 (1985). pp. 1661-70.

Garg, A., and M.M. Ayoub. "What Criteria Exist for Determining How Much Load can be Lifted Safely?" *Human Factors* 22, 4 (1980). pp. 475-86.

Gebhardt, D.L., T.A. Baker and V.A. Sheppard. *Development and Validation of Physical Performance Tests for Dock Workers, Hostler and Driver Jobs in the Freight Industry*. Hyattsville, MD: Human Performance Systems Inc., 1992.

— *Development and Validation of Physical Performance Tests for Craft and Other Positions in the Communications Industry*. Hyattsville, MD: Human Performance Systems Inc., 1993.

Gebhardt, D.L., C.E. Crump, P.J. Russell and B.L. Frost. *Development of Physical Performance Tests and Medical Standards for Pennsylvania State Police Personnel*. Bethesda, MD: University Research Corporation, 1990.

Gledhill, N., and V.K. Jamnik. "Development and Validation of a Fitness Screening Protocol for Fire Fighter Applicants." *Canadian Journal of Applied Sports Sciences* 17, 3 (1992). pp. 199-206.

Grieve, D. "The Influence of Posture on Power Output Generated in Single Pulling Movements." *Applied Ergonomics* 15 (1984). pp. 115-7.

Guion, R.M. "Recruiting, Selection, and Job Placement," in *Handbook of Industrial and Organizational Psychology*. M.D. Dunnette (ed.). Chicago: Rand McNally, 1976. pp. 777-828.

Guion, R.M., and C.J. Cranny. "A Note on Concurrent and Predictive Designs: A Critical Reanalysis." *Journal of Applied Psychology* 67 (1982). pp. 239-44.

Heyward, V.H., S.M. Johannes-Ellis and J.F. Romer. "Gender Differences in Strength." *Research Quarterly for Exercise and Sport* 57, 2 (1986). pp. 154-9.

Kamon, E., D. Kiser and T. Lander-Pytel. "Dynamic and Static Lifting Capacity and Muscular Strength of Steelmill Workers." *American Industrial Hygiene Association Journal* 43, 11 (1982). pp. 853-7.

Kumar, S., and A. Mital. "Margin of Safety for the Human Back: A Probable Consensus Based on Published Studies." *Ergonomics* 35, 7 (1992). pp. 769-81.

Laubach, L.L. "Comparative Muscular Strength of Men and Women: A Review of the Literature." *Aviation, Space, and Environmental Medicine* 47, 5 (1976). pp. 534-42.

Lortie, M. "Analyse comparative des accidents declares par des preposes hommes and femmes d'un hopital geriatrique." *Journal of Occupational Accidents* 9 (1987). pp. 59-81.

Matzdorff, I. "Women at Work in Workplaces Designed for Men: Anthropometry and Ergonomics." *Work and Stress* 1, 3 (1987). pp. 293-7.

Messing, K., J. Courville and N. Vézina. "Minimizing Health Risks for Women who Enter Jobs Traditionally Assigned to Men." *New Solutions: A Journal of Environmental and Occupational Health Policy* 1, 4 (1991). pp. 66-71.

Messing, K., L. Dumais, J. Courville, J. Seifert and M. Boucher. "Evaluation of Exposure Data from Men and Women with the Same Job Title." *Journal of Occupational Medicine* 36, 8 (1994). pp. 913-7.

Metz, B.G. "From Ergonomics to Standards." *Ergonomics* 28, 8 (1985). pp. 1197-204.

Misner, J.E., R.A. Boileau and S.A. Plowman. "Development of Placement Tests for Fire Fighting." *Applied Ergonomics* 20, 3 (1989). pp. 218-24.

Mital, A. "The Psychophysical Approach in Manual Lifting: A Verification Study." *Human Factors* 25, 5 (1983). pp. 485-91.

Mostardi, R.A., J.A. Porterfield, S. King and S. Urycki. "Pre-employment Screening and Health Management for Safety Forces — Methods and Techniques." *The Journal of Orthopaedic and Sports Physical Therapy* 11, 9 (1990). pp. 398-401.

Pheasant, S.T. "Sex Differences in Strength — Some Observations on Their Variability." *Applied Ergonomics* 14, 3 (1983). pp. 205-11.

Rhodes, E.C., and D.W. Farenholtz. "Police Officer's Physical Abilities Test Compared to Measures of Physical Fitness." *Canadian Journal of Sports Sciences* 17, 3 (1992). pp. 228-33.

Snook, S., M. Steven and V.M. Ciriello. "The Design of Manual Handling Tasks: Revised Tables of Maximum Acceptable Weights and Forces." *Ergonomics* 34, 9 (1991). pp. 1197-213.

Sothmann, M. "Empirical Justification of Cut-scores: A Case Study." *Medicine and Science in Sports and Exercise* 25, 5, suppl. 96 (1993).

— "Age Associated Changes in Physical Fitness of Fire Fighters." *Medicine and Science in Sports and Exercise* 25, 5, suppl. 99 (1993).

Stevenson, J.M., D.R. Greenhorn, T.J. Bryant, J.M. Deakin, J.M. Stevenson and T.J. Smith. "Gender Differences in Performance of a Selection Test Using the Incremental Lifting Machine." *Applied Ergonomics*, in press (July, 1995).

Stevenson, J.M., J.T. Bryant, G.M. Andrew, J.T. Smith, S.L. French, J.M. Thomson and J.M. Deakin. "Development of Physical Fitness Standards for Canadian Armed Forces Younger Personnel." *Canadian Journal of Sports Sciences* 17, 3 (1992). pp. 214-21.

Stevenson, J.M., J.M. Deakin, G.M. Andrew, J.T. Bryant, J.T. Smith, J.M. Thomson and J.M. Deakin. "Development of Physical Fitness Standards for Canadian Armed Forces Older Personnel." *Canadian Journal of Applied Physiology* 19, 1 (1994). pp. 75-90.

Stevenson, J.M., J.T. Bryant, G.M. Andrew, L.L. Langley and D.R. Greenhorn. "Self-determined Lifting Styles Compared to Constrained ILM Lifting Protocols." *Journal of Human Movement Studies* 21, 1 (1991). pp. 69-84.

Stevenson, J.M., J.T. Bryant, D.R. Greenhorn, J.T. Smith, J.M. Deakin and B.M. Surgenor. "The Effect of Lifting Protocol in Comparison with Isoinertial Lifting Performance." *Ergonomics* 33, 12 (1990). pp. 1455-69.

Taylor, T. "Burning Issue: New Rules for Hiring to Fire Fighters Up in Arms." *Toronto Star* (31 January, 1993).

Theroux, C. *Canadian Charter of Human Rights*. Ottawa, Ontario: Canadian Human Rights Commission, 1985.

Vézina, N., and J. Courville. "Integration of Women into Traditionally Masculine Jobs." *Women and Health* 18, 3 (1992). pp. 97-118.

Ward, J.S. "Sex Discrimination is Essential in Industry." *Journal of Occupational Medicine* 20, 9 (1978). pp. 594-6.

Washburn, R.A., and M.J. Safrit. "Physical Performance Tests in Job Selection: A Model for Empirical Validation." *Research Quarterly for Exercise and Sport* 53, 3 (1982). pp. 267-70.

Webb, R.D.G., and D.W. Tack. "Ergonomics, Human Rights and Placement Tests for Physically Demanding Work," in *Trends in Ergonomics/Human Factors*. V. F. Aghazadeh (ed.). North-Holland: Elsevier Science Publishers B.V., 1988. pp. 751-8.

Wilmore, J.H., and J.A. Davis. "Validation of a Physical Abilities Field Test for Selection of State Traffic Officers." *Journal of Occupational Medicine* 21 (1979). pp. 33-40.

Yates, J.W., E. Kamon, S.H. Rodgers and P.C. Champney. "Static Lifting Strength and Maximal Isometric Voluntary Contractions of Back, Arm and Shoulder Muscles." *Ergonomics* 23, 1 (1980). pp. 37-47.

Dorothy Wigmore

"Taking Back" the Workplace

Workplace Violence: A Hidden Risk in Women's Work

À cause d'inégalités sociales et structurelles, d'attitudes sexistes, ou de leur position sur les lieux de travail, les femmes sont souvent victimes de violence au travail. Cette violence comprend des abus de pouvoir, des menaces, du harcèlement sexuel, sexiste ou raciste, aussi bien que des assauts physiques. Les études publiées soulignent le cas des infirmières, des enseignantes et des travailleuses sociales, mais le tableau n'est pas complet. Les femmes qui travaillent auprès du public dans des fonctions cléricales d'aide détiennent un pouvoir apparent envers leurs clients, mais aucun contrôle réel. Lorsqu'elles interagissent avec des personnes qui, comme les bénéficiaires de l'aide sociale, ne contrôlent pas eux non plus leur situation, ces travailleuses peuvent devenir la cible de colères déplacées. On attribuera parfois ces épisodes de violence aux comportements des travailleuses, alors que les causes structurelles de ces abus demeureront cachées. On a développé, en Angleterre, une approche utile pour un processus de résolution de problèmes. Les sources potentielles de violence sont détectées à partir d'un examen des facteurs associés aux assauts, à la situation des travailleurs, à leurs interactions, à l'environnement de travail et à la tâche à accomplir, selon une approche non culpabilisante. Ce processus aboutit à une meilleure reconnaissance des problèmes inhérents à l'organisation du travail, aux procédures pour rapporter les événements, à la formation et au soutien du personnel. Des recherches ultérieures devraient porter sur l'évaluation de ces processus de résolution de problèmes, et sur un élargissement des recherches sur la violence. Cela, afin d'inclure ces secteurs peu étudiés, en incorporant les connaissances acquises grâce aux recherches sur la violence contre les femmes dans d'autres contextes.

Because of social and structural inequities, sexist attitudes and the position of women in the workplace, women are often the victims of workplace violence. Forms of violence include: abuse, threats or assaults, including severe verbal abuse and persistent sexual and racial harrassment. Published reports focus on nurses, teachers and social workers, but there are missing voices. Many of those dealing with the public in clerical and support positions have perceived power over others, but no real control. When they deal with people, such as welfare recipients, who also lack control over their situations, workers may become objects of displaced rage. The workers' behaviour may be blamed for violence at work while the structural reasons for on-the-job abuse remain hidden. The British offer a useful framework for a problem-solving process. Potential sources of violence are identified by examining in a non-blaming way factors associated with assailants, workers, the interaction between them, the work environment and the outcome. Responses developed from this process include recognizing problems in work organization, reporting, training and support procedures. Further research should focus on assessing problem-solving measures, widening the scope of research to include the missing voices and incorporating insights from research on violence against women in other contexts.

INTRODUCTION

Violence at work is a serious public health hazard — perhaps one of the most serious in jobs where workers deal with people. It has been minimized, like "family violence," or tolerated as "part of the job." Women, as the caregivers and the front-line service and clerical workers in our society — the people who deal with people — are most at risk for this oft-ignored occupational hazard.

That is the overall picture, pieced together from work done by a few researchers and some unions, and from anecdotal evidence collected from a variety of workers in Canada, the United Kingdom and the United States.[1] In this article I will define and examine some of the evidence about workplace violence, focusing on how it affects women. After describing an analytical approach to the issue, I will discuss a variety of possible solutions and conclude with some recommendations about work to be done.

DEFINING VIOLENCE

Violence is about power and control. It is a process that involves using force or deliberately trying to intimidate someone; the abuser may feel frustration or powerlessness or be fighting loss of control.[2] It is a social problem with structural sources, not a medical or psychiatric issue (Morrison, 1987-1988).

This description will sound familiar to those interested in violence against women and to those concerned with workplace violence. Unfortunately, there is little crossover between the two topics (one exception is Roberts, 1991). The Montreal massacre was not commonly described as an attack against women at work (although those killed or injured were Polytechnic employees or future workers) and workplaces are described as "safe" places for battered women (Kahn, 1991). The recent Canadian report on violence against women continues this separation, limiting workplace violence almost exclusively to a discussion of sexual harassment and ignoring the wide spectrum of other literature, and other definitions, available (Canadian Panel on Violence Against Women, 1993).

This gulf in understanding may partially explain the inconsistent definition of workplace violence.[3] Some authors use the words without defining their meaning; others use different terms and/or limitations (Kushnir Pekrul, 1992; Lipscombe and Love, 1992; Mahoney, 1991; Schniedon, 1992).[4] Some limit their focus to physical assault, or assault resulting in injury,[5] ignoring many of the subtler aspects of violence at work, particularly as they affect women. Others say verbal abuse, including harassment, provides a much more accurate picture of the extent of aggressive behaviour, is a good indicator of the potential for physical assault and improves understanding of the impact of aggression (Lanza and Campbell, 1991). A proposed United Nations Declaration[6] recognizes non-physical abuse or assaults when defining violence against women, and interview-based studies of workplace assaults almost always show that physical injury is just the tip of the iceberg (Poyner, 1989).

In this discussion of workplace violence, I have used the definition developed by the Canadian Union of Public Employees (CUPE), which places the violence in the context of a process that includes actions, causes, effects and responses:

> Violence is any incident in which an employee is abused, threatened or assaulted during the course of her/his employment. This includes the application of force, threats with and without weapons, severe verbal abuse and persistent sexual and racial harassment (Pizzino, 1994).

IDENTIFYING THE PROBLEM
Murder is Definitely Violence

Homicide is the leading cause of occupational death for American women (41 percent of American women killed on the job from 1980-1985 were murdered) and the third most common cause of death for all American workers between 1980 and 1989 (National Institute for Occupational Safety and Health [NIOSH], 1993).

Workplace homicide is so serious a problem that the National Institute for Occupational Safety and Health issued an alert about the topic in September, 1993 (NIOSH, 1993). Its background study showed the risk for women to be highest amongst stock handlers and baggers (eg. in liquor or grocery stores), police and detectives and hotel clerks (Castillo and Jenkins, 1994). The authors postulated that working alone, working in the late evening or early morning hours and exchange of money were key high risk factors. Others agree that robbery is often the original motive in the U.S.; a California study found the highest workplace homicide rates for women in retail and personal services work, where handling money was a key factor (Kraus, 1987).

Gender is rarely considered in studies of murder on the job. A 1992 American review found only six articles and no systematic review of female workplace homicides (Levin, Hewitt and Misner, 1992). Retail trade and service industries are cited most often as being at highest risk. (Food and dairy stores, eating/drinking establishments and gasoline service stations were the most dangerous.) Jobs with the highest risk included sales personnel, service employees (eg. waitresses and grocery baggers), managers and clerical workers. Gunshot wounds were the primary cause of death, although older women were more often stabbed to death. One study examined cases reported to a surveillance system between 1980 and 1985 (Bell, 1991). The highest rates were among working women 65 years of age or older and blacks (killed at 1.8 times the rate of whites). The most frequent time for attacks was between 4 and 5 p.m., but 30 percent were killed between 6 p.m. and midnight and 69 percent between 3 p.m. and 7 a.m.

There may be up to 24 workplace homicides a year in Canada and Quebec, according to the only published study of workplace homicide here (Liss and Craig, 1990). After examining the 84 work-related homicides in Ontario between 1975 and 1985, Liss and Craig confirmed many American findings. The ratio of work-related homicides to all homicides is of the same order of magnitude as in American studies, with a few exceptions. The 11 women killed in the 10 years were 25 percent of all women killed on the job in Ontario. The major job categories posing risk for women were sales and managers/professionals.

Workplace Violence in General

Occupational sectors with the highest risk of workplace homicide usually also have the highest risk of non-fatal injuries from occupational violence

(Hales et al., 1989). However, there is little material about workplace violence in general, except a few American studies of occupational violent crime (OVC) injuries from attack, rape and/or the psychological effects produced by a criminal act. In one study, 21 of 59 injuries were from rape or attempted rape; this study found that retail food industry workers were at highest risk (Thomas, 1992). When Hales et al. (1989) examined Ohio workers' compensation claims from 1983 to 1985, they found rapes were most common amongst grocery store workers (especially those in convenience stores) and real estate employees, but overall OVC rates by gender could not be determined.

The only general report of less physically violent forms of workplace abuse is Stockdale and Phillips' (1989) survey of 800 women and 200 men in England. Those most vulnerable to physical attack were carers, retail outlet workers and professionals who often worked outside the office.

For the most part, though, recent studies and reports about workplace violence have concentrated on experiences in three sectors: health care, education and social work.

Violence in Health care

It would be difficult to find an experienced, practising nurse in Canada today who at some time in his or her career has not been struck, pushed, insulted, threatened, kicked or had something thrown at him or her by a patient. Yet, the extent of the abuse and its ramifications is one of nursing's better kept secrets (McCaskell, 1990).

Assault is an occupational hazard in hospitals[7] and a psychological stressor for health care personnel (Leppänen and Olkinuora, 1987; Sullivan, 1993; Browner, 1987). Reports of patient assault date back to 1889 (Lanza, Kayne, Hicks and Milner, 1991) but only recently has there been a plethora of published stories and studies about nurses' experiences.[8] The British Health and Safety Executive (HSE) reported in 1986 that, amongst health authority workers, nursing staff and ambulance crews were most at risk of assault (HSE, 1986). In the early 1980s, UK and American studies began to concentrate on mental health facilities[9] and, more recently, hospital emergency rooms.[10] Those studies included some investigations of long-term care facilities and pediatric units (Bollinger and Edwards, 1989).

In Canada, where 95 percent of nurses are female (Statistics Canada, 1993a), nurses have studied their own work. When the British Columbia

Nurses' Union (BCNU) commissioned a study in 1991, 72 percent of the 505 respondents had been abused or threatened within the previous five years and 22 percent had been injured; 8.2 percent had experienced more than 100 separate incidents. Verbal abuse was almost universal and 83 percent had been grabbed, 79 percent hit, 68.5 percent threatened with physical violence, 62.5 percent kicked and 51 percent had faced "mental harassment" (BCNU, 1991a).

B.C. nurses had 651 successful violence-related workers' compensation claims from 1986 to 1990 — a figure which comprises 11 percent of all their accepted time loss claims in those years (Gawthrop, 1991; BCNU, 1991b). Between 1985 and 1989, nurses, nurses' aides and orderlies were paid for 7633 "days lost" due to violence on the job (a doubling of their rates in that time), compared to 936 for law enforcement officers, who are usually viewed as being at high risk of attack (BCNU, 1992). Next door in Alberta, the picture is similar: Its compensation board accepted 130 claims in 1992 from nurses for acts of violence resulting in injuries, compared to 56 from police officers (Brasen, 1993).

Verbal abuse was most common in a Saskatchewan survey (Kushnir Pekrul, 1992), affecting 81 percent of the 720 registered nurses working in clinical patient settings. Fifty-four percent had experienced physical abuse in the previous 12 months; patients were usually responsible.

In Manitoba, more than half of the province's 10,000 registered nurses answered their union's 1987 questionnaire (Manitoba Association of Registered Nurses, 1989). In acute care facilities, 31 to 44 percent of respondents had been subjected to verbal abuse. That figure rose to 59 percent in extended/personal care work and was more varied in community agencies. Physical abuse was much less common in community agencies but rose dramatically in acute care and extended/personal care.

The situation is no better in Ontario, where several studies have been done (Roberts, 1991; Lechky, 1994a; *The ONA News*, November 1992). In a 1991 survey of 800 Ontario nurses, 59 percent reported having experienced physical assault during their careers, 35 percent in the previous 12 months and 10 percent in the previous month (Nurse Assault Project Team et al., 1992). Ninety-two percent experienced harsh or insulting language on the job. Patients were responsible for most physical assaults, while harsh and insulting language came most often from patients, patients' families and physicians. Male nurses reported an average of 3.3 assaults in the previous year, compared to 2.1 for female nurses.

After these results were published, the Ontario Nurses Association asked the Ontario government to examine non-supervisory nurses' compensation claims for violence-related injuries. Only accepted claims were used for the 1987 to 1989 study period, and it was found that male rates were 13.9 per 1000 while female rates were 1.4 per 1000 (Liss, 1993). This was 54 and six times higher, respectively, than rates for men and women in the entire Ontario labour force. Most nurses were "struck by" people. The Ontario study could not determine if nurses filed claims about verbal harassment as well, or if the Board accepts those claim types.

Health care workers are often subjected to sexual harassment and assault.[11] The findings range from one in six Ontario nurses being sexually assaulted at work (Phillips and Schneider, 1993), to 26 percent in the BCNU survey (1991) who had to deal with sexual advances, to 39 percent of the Saskatchewan respondents reporting sexual harassment (Kushnir Pekrul, 1992). Patients and physicians are usually the culprits. In a violence survey at an Ontario hospital, nurses wrote "reams" about sexual harassment by doctors, even though they were not asked about it (Lechky, 1994a). Seventy-seven percent of female Ontario doctors responding to a survey reported having experienced sexual harassment by a patient at least once in their career (Phillips and Schneider, 1993).

Violence in Social Work

Books have been written about violence in social work (see Owens and Ashcroft, 1985; Brown et al., 1986). Schultz (1987) says social workers are seen as system critics, making them vulnerable at times of stress, not just because of who they are or what they do but because of what they represent. He found types of physical violence, verbal threats and property damage varied, depending on where the respondents worked. For example, 25 percent of social workers in correctional settings reported knife attacks. Verbal threats were common in all work settings but most pronounced in correctional institutions.

There are few published reports from Canada, where 72 percent of social workers are women (Statistics Canada, 1993a). When the Alberta Union of Public Employees (AUPE) surveyed 1,111 social service and institutional workers in 1985, 30 percent had been physically assaulted, 42 percent physically threatened and 61 percent verbally threatened (AUPE, 1986). In late 1993, a union representative said that, in the Alberta Department of Family and Social Services, there were 59 "security-related incidents" in the second quarter of 1993, compared to 51 in the first three months of the year (COHSN, October 4, 1993).

CUPE analyzed the responses of its Ontario social service workers (70 percent of whom are female) to the union's national survey and found that 65.2 percent of surveyed workers had been subjected to at least one aggressive act at work in the previous two years (CUPE, 1993). Forty-eight percent of workers reporting acts of aggression said that they had been subjected to more than three such incidents in the previous two years. Verbal abuse, including death threats, was most common, but workers were also struck, scratched, hit, kicked and grabbed.

Like nursing staff (see Lechky, 1994b), social workers often must return to work with the individual who assaulted them. Unless action is taken against assailants, where warranted, this may appear to condone their actions. This no-win situation becomes an additional stressor for workers (Wigmore, 1995).

Violence in Education

Education is the third major sector where violence has been recognized as an occupational hazard. The issue is important in England, where the government has issued an education sector guideline (Health and Safety Commission, 1990).

In Canada, 70 percent of teachers and related workers are female (Statistics Canada, 1993a). In 1990, the Manitoba Teachers' Society (MTS) looked at violent events during the previous 15 months amongst members who taught kindergarten to grade 12 (MTS, 1990). Seven percent of respondents had been physically assaulted and almost 40 percent had been abused in some way. A 1993 update showed increased rates of violence (MTS, 1993). The current discussion in Ontario about "zero tolerance policies" to deal with school violence reflects either an increasing concern about the topic and/or an increased incidence. One reason it's on the agenda is work done by the Ontario Teachers' Federation (Robb, 1993a).

Violence Against Other Workers

There's one striking feature in all the above-mentioned reports. Except for some union work, studies and reports deal almost exclusively with professionals, ignoring the experiences of those who work with them in support positions, those shown to be at risk in the OVC studies and others who work with "the public." Women do many of these jobs (in 1989, women comprised 46 percent of Canadian sales workers [Shea, 1990]; and in 1991, 88 percent of bank tellers and cashiers were women [Statistics Canada, 1993a]).

There is a socially accepted incongruity between the position of, and respect accorded to, "professionals" at work and violence.[12] But the story is different for those lower in the hierarchy, who have less control, prestige and voice, especially if they are women (CUPE, 1990). Their stories, like those of nurses, until recently have been heard only at union workshops or (especially for the non-unionized) informal settings. This is partly a result of the sometimes overt, sometimes subtle, condition of their employment: Violence is a part of the job (Wigmore, 1995).

For example, a recent review of violence in health care focuses on nurses and physicians (Jones, 1985). The people they work with are rarely mentioned (eg. nurses' aides, orderlies) or are totally ignored (eg. dietary, cleaning, clerical and reception staff).[13] Liss (1993) agrees that other health care workers are at risk for workplace abuse but says nurses appear to be the victims in the majority of incidents. To support this statement, he cites three studies of American psychiatric hospitals. The experience in those hospitals may be atypical, however, and may not be relevant for hospitals in Canadian settings in particular.

We know that other health care workers face violence on the job:

- BC nurses' aides and orderlies file more than twice as many accepted compensation claims as do nurses for violence-related "injuries" (Britt, 1992). Acts of violence or force accounted for nurses' aides and orderlies' second highest category of wage loss claims in 1989 (Gawthrop, 1991). These claims numbered slightly more than all accepted provincial hearing loss claims and half all successful BC mining sector claims (Statistics Canada, 1991);

- 64 percent of 328 Nova Scotia CUPE members working in 19 homes for the elderly were verbally abused and one-third suffered work-related stress (CUPE, 1990), and the 399 accepted violence-related compensation claims in 1992 were more than 10 percent of provincial health care "accidents" (Pizzino, 1994);

- a Finnish study of health care personnel's psychological stressors refers to a study showing cleaners and social workers were attacked at the same rate (Stymme, 1981);

- the only published English-language study of nursing home nursing aides (according to Statistics Canada [1993a], 83 percent of Canadian "nursing attendants" are women) calls for attention to reducing abuse of these workers, saying the only similar study (about student nurses) also found high assault rates (Lusk, 1992); and

- several authors (Lavoie et al., 1990; Jones, 1985; Convey, 1986; Rix and Seymour, 1988) report that nursing assistants are assaulted more than staff nurses, although in some American public and psychiatric institutions, nurses were more likely to be injured than aides, orderlies and all other staff combined (Rosenthal et al., 1992).

Some of the "missing voices" have work similar to the wide spectrum of service and public sector jobs held by CUPE members. Therefore, a recent survey of the union's members and locals offers some insight into the experiences of these "missing voices" (Pizzino, 1994). Some 1421 individuals (at least 72 percent female) responded to the survey. Sixty-one percent had been subjected to an aggressive act in the past two years and 55 percent of this group reported at least three attacks. Verbal abuse was most common (69 percent), followed by being struck with an object, hit, grabbed, scratched, kicked and slapped. Death threats comprised 20 percent of the verbal abuse; 60 percent was comprised of threats of injury.

Without a collective voice, non-unionized women's experiences are difficult to hear and must be pieced together from disparate studies. For example, in addition to the OVC studies, there is a British document about violence in bank work (HSE, 1993). The presence of these and other "missing voices" shows we have an incomplete picture of workplace violence and increases the odds that jobs at risk are ignored when activities are designed to prevent violence or deal with it when it occurs.

RISK FACTORS
A Framework for Identifying Risk

Something else is missing in most North American work about violence on the job — a comprehensive framework to analyze and address problems (Messing, 1991).[14] It is important to look beyond the horror stories and limited descriptions of "occupation" or job title to more exact descriptions of activities — or "exposure" profiles — especially when investigating women's occupational health issues (Messing, 1991).

Fortunately, a useful framework for doing so is available in British government-sponsored materials about workplace violence.[15] Like others who have studied the problem of workplace violence,[16] the Health and Safety Executive (HSE) in Britain says working with "the public" is the key risk factor[17] but that it is misleading to try to compare the size or seriousness of the risk in different sectors when developing solutions (Poyner and Warne, 1986). One HSE study showed that "… rather than simply reporting on the problems of violence in a variety of organizations, it would be more valuable to identify those aspects of the problem which were common across a wide range of organizations" (Poyner and Warne, 1988). The starting point for doing this in Britain is a five-element analytical framework (Table 1), developed by bipartite committees established by the HSE and based on a key public health principle: Attempt to find solutions whether or not the cause of the problem is known (Poyner and Warne, 1988).

Table 1 Factors in Developing an Exposure Profile — The British Elements (Poyner and Warne, 1988)

Assailant: personality; temporary conditions (eg. drugs, alcohol, illness, personal stress); presence of negative/uncertain expectations; age and maturity (particularly immaturity in children); people with dogs
Employee: appearance (eg. physical build, uniforms); health (stress, other illness, overwork); age and experience; gender; personality and temperament; attitudes; expectations
Interaction: must involve direct contact (not necessarily physical contact, as in nursing, but contact that occurs when someone believes that the worker, or the system the worker represents, is being unfair or unreasonable)
Work environment: the total context of the job (ie. details of work and features of the organizational culture and physical environment: relationships between workers and co-workers and managers; working alone; job location (local service means people are more likely aware of local issues and tensions); handling cash; waiting (eg. bus queue, waiting areas); time of day (eg. after school hours, minor assaults on bus crews by children rise to a peak); territory (where people involved feel most comfortable/threatened); privacy
Outcome: physical injury; attempted injury; threats with a weapon; verbal abuse; angry behaviour

In the following sections I will use these elements to briefly analyze some of the available literature, particularly findings specifically mentioning women or women's work. A selection of other materials is referenced only.

The Assailant

Attitudes such as homophobia, sexism and racism affect how we deal with other people. Most workplace assailants are men (Newhill, 1992). For example, male patients do not treat female doctors primarily as physicians. According to a 1993 study, "the vulnerability in their sex seems in many cases to override their power as doctors" (Phillips and Schneider, 1993). Women in less powerful positions may be at least as vulnerable. Other important factors are covered in studies about health care (Lipscomb and Love, 1992; Keep and Glibert, 1992; Lavoie et al., 1990; Rix, 1987) and social work (Stockdale and Phillips, 1989; Newhill, 1992).

The Employee

Employee gender is a logical risk factor, but the link between violence and gender seems to depend on the kind of interaction involved in the work. Men are physically assaulted more frequently in some settings (eg. in psychiatric units, as orderlies) (Rosenthal et al., 1992). However, the British exposure profile and studies of violence elsewhere indicate that, in general, women are more likely to be assaulted at work than men. The attitudes that lead to attacks on women in the street or in their homes don't stay there. The "public" carries these attitudes into the places women work — welfare and municipal offices, hospitals and elder care facilities, retail stores, banks and libraries. Undervalued work by those in subordinate and powerless positions only reinforces sexist attitudes (Rebick and Kaufman, 1991).

Health care researchers have found links amongst position in an administrative hierarchy (Lanza et al., 1991; Rix and Seymour, 1988), lack of, or inadequate, training (Rosenthal et al., 1992) and expectations of dire consequences (Dubin, 1989). It is understandable that women fear violence in our society — a majority of Canadian women have been sexually assaulted at least once (Statistics Canada, 1993b).

Problematic Interactions

The British HSE's list of problematic interactions includes: giving a service; caring; education; money transactions; delivery/collection; controlling; and inspecting (Poyner and Warne, 1988). Health care studies link violence to routine health care contacts such as feeding, bathing, restraining and the administration of medication (Lanza et al., 1991; Keep and Glibert, 1992; Lipscombe and Love, 1992). Few studies have looked at interactions in sufficient detail (for example, how much time is spent in each of the above activities?) to have a complete picture of these risk factors in specific settings.

The Work Environment

General work environment factors contributing to an increased risk for a cross-section of British workers (most of them women) included: cutbacks; lack of security; poor office layout; workplace policies (for example, working alone); aggressive and sexist behaviour being the norm at work; and toleration of threatening behaviour as "part of the job" (Stockdale and Phillips, 1989). CUPE members report similar problems

(CUPE, 1987); their additions to the list include management attitudes, such as lack of support and dismissal of staff concerns, and prevalence of the attitude that violence is "part of the job."

"Inadequate staff levels" is at, or near, the top of many lists that examine the causes of increasing workplace abuse rates (CUPE, 1991b; Robb, 1993b, c; Hobbs, 1991). Health care work environment factors that increase risk include: working at certain times of day (Lipscomb and Love, 1992); long waiting times (Hobbs, 1991); staff shortages; department overcrowding; availability of drugs and hostages; and using the emergency department for psychiatric and medical clearance of patients with alcohol and drug abuse.[18] It should be noted that emergency department "victimization" is different from abuse of workers in long-term care, chronic care or psychiatric settings (Mahoney, 1991). Nurses working in the former area are more likely to be abused during night and evening hours while in-patient nurses are more likely to be victimized during high-activity times. Verbal abuse and threats or intimidation were higher during 12-hour shifts in all departments.

"Working alone" was the most commonly cited factor in the reported incidents of sexual harassment of female Ontario doctors (Phillips and Schneider, 1993). Combined with fear of the outcome of sexist attitudes, it is often a top concern for women workers (Pizzino, 1994).

The Outcome

The effects of workplace violence — from death to physical injuries to psychological trauma — may appear either immediately or some time after an assault, and may last for months.[19] As is common with the after-effects of domestic violence, coping mechanisms often include denial (Lanza, 1983; Flannery et al., 1991). Nurses tend to minimise their emotional reactions to assault, which may then affect work performance, interactions with co-workers and/or family and job satisfaction (Lanza, 1983). This is likely not unique to nurses.

CONTROL, POWER AND VIOLENCE

Some of the links between power, control and workplace violence include:
- people who behave in a violent way may be in settings or situations where they have little or no control over their own lives (eg. chronic care units) and/or are facing people they perceive have power (eg. nurses, unemployment office clerks) (Morrison, 1992);

- after an attack, assaulted workers may initially feel loss of a sense of control. This is more difficult for women to deal with, perhaps because most attacks on them seem to be "unprovoked" (Engel and Marsh, 1986);
- women admitting to feelings of vulnerability support stereotypes about women's incompetence. Therefore such feelings may be suppressed by female caregivers, who believe they should convey strength (Chinn, 1986);
- workers do not control the organization of their workplace, and the employers who do have control often refuse to acknowledge valid concerns and/or make changes to reduce/prevent violence.

Women at risk of workplace attack are often caregivers and/or front-line workers dealing with the "public," and are often subordinate to (usually) male bosses. Hierarchical organization and sexism is reinforced when patients are moved after a supervisor or (usually male) doctor is assaulted, while (often female) personal care workers reporting abuse are not believed, are blamed for the incidents or are ignored (CUPE, 1991b; Lechky, 1994b).

Roberts says institutional failure to respond to violence against nurses reflects the power dynamic within the male-dominated health care system (Roberts, 1991). The nurse's role is that of nurturer and subordinate caretaker (linked to her role as woman), and she is overseen by mostly-male physicians and administrators. Caretaking partly involves maintaining order — including the balance of power — so that things run smoothly. Assaults upset this order and force nurses to try to deal with the conflicting roles of victim and caregiver, and with their self-image; in the process, they may blame themselves (as do battered women) — self-blame goes with the assigned role.

Women in other subordinate roles in health care settings and in other workplaces may be in a similar position. "Perceived control" is a common state for those who work with the public, where front-line workers and others often seem to be able to determine what people can and cannot do, when and how. But these workers really have little control over the situation; they have not designed their work environment and have little or no say in the policies, priority-setting and budgets that frame the limits of their work. The real rule-makers are hidden from the public, and sometimes from the workers, literally and figuratively. At the same time, the workers interact with people who may be unhappy or disturbed for many reasons and who see the (mostly women) workers doing their job as part of "the system." In short, two sets of people are trying to deal with situations over which they have little control. This powerlessness, which is common, is not conducive to problem-solving (Mahoney, 1991).

RESPONSES TO THE PROBLEM

> Violence is ... a complex but analyzable process, the understanding of which calls not so much for the assigning of labels as for an approach that is rational, systematic, structured according to phases, topological, research-based, and inter-disciplinary. And this understanding should be only an aid to society's efforts to deal with the problem (Agudelo, 1992).

General

Violence at work is not necessarily a random or accidental event (Hales et al., 1989) and is often associated with an organization's main purpose (Poyner and Warne, 1988). Therefore, preventive or control measures are an integral part of managing and work organization.

The best general approach is the public health one used for other occupational health and safety hazards: identify the problem and solve it, with a preventive focus that involves those affected in the process. The British approach does this: It requires the identification of risky jobs/ work situations (using the five elements), a decision about what action to take and monitoring of the decision's effects (Poyner and Warne, 1988). This problem-solving strategy is not victim-blaming, tries to avoid creating new hazards and is most effective when it is specific to the situation (Poyner, 1989).

Common Responses to Avoid

The following are common responses to workplace violence and must be avoided.

Underreporting

> My own encounters with nurses discussing issues of violence, both physical and psychological, have convinced me that violence is an issue of mammoth proportions for nurses. However, just as family violence is privatized, violence in the personal and work lives of nurses is silenced and denied (Chinn, 1991).

Many workplace attacks go unreported unless they produce relatively serious physical injuries, especially when women and/or the less powerful are involved. This reinforces the status quo (Roberts, 1991) and undermines attempts to understand and deal with workplace violence, especially for less-obvious forms of assault.

Most estimates of underreporting come from the health care sector. Sixty-three percent of nursing staff completing a questionnaire after a physical attack also completed an incident form about the assault (Convey, 1986). Liss (1993) estimated the number of assaults that could or should be compensated in Ontario is between 2000 and 5290 every year — 20 to 50 times current levels. Citing her own and others' work, Lanza (1991) says underreporting ranges from three to 300 percent.

Lanza's explanations of underreporting in a health care setting, which may apply elsewhere, include: the definition of assault varies and many victims believe it should be reported only if it is "sufficiently severe"; there are various opinions about the patient's degree of intent to harm; staff is inured to assault ("assaults are so common here"); staff characteristics make reporting difficult (eg. peer pressure to not report, and different kinds of reporting based on gender of the person assaulted); there is fear of blame and/or excessive paper work involved in reporting assaults and not enough time to do so (Lanza, 1991).

Other reasons for underreporting include: the victim is a woman (Corea, 1985); bad experience(s), or knowledge of others having a bad experience, reporting an assault; concern about consequences for the assailant (eg. N.S. workers fear violent residents will be given Haldol, which sedates them but changes them into "zombies" [CUPE, 1991b]); financial worries, especially if workers' compensation claims are contested or not allowed[20]; and minimization of the gravity of attacks (eg. attacks are called "incidents" or severity is downplayed if no physical injury occurs) (Roberts, 1991; Rosenthal et al., 1992; Engel and Marsh, 1986).

It's My/Your Fault

An obvious parallel between abuse of women elsewhere and in their workplaces is victim-blaming. Even those who know better blame themselves (Atkinson, 1993). Lanza and Carifio (1991) showed women were blamed more often than men in situations involving verbal threats and in severe "assault." She suggests traditional coping methods are used in severe assault (ie. more stressful events), including "violence is a man's domain," "men protect women," and, if things go wrong, "women are to blame."

Blame takes several forms. Roberts (1991) points to the potential for blaming victims when forms ask: "What could you have done to prevent this incident?" Almost half the nurses in one survey believed they could predict violence; the difficulty with this mistaken understanding is that, if you fail, you are more likely to feel responsibility or guilt (Ryan and Poster, 1991). Prediction is linked to fear; it is a myth that fear leads to assaults, at least amongst nurses. Blaming the victim (ie. saying she was afraid) contributes to the positive effects of violence for the patient (Morrison, 1987-88).

Another form of blame is rarely acknowledged (Morrison, 1987-88) but becomes apparent after reading most articles about how to respond to workplace violence. Behavioural solutions (eg. de-escalation), in particular, assume women always can respond appropriately to potentially violent situations and ignores the presence of many other workplace hazards and their effects. It is victim-blaming to expect even the best-prepared woman to respond perfectly each time she is in a situation that may lead to workplace abuse, especially if she is in an understaffed, overworked, powerless position.

Good Ideas Badly Executed

Steps employers adopt too easily (eg. security devices or personal defence courses) often raise questions and don't really solve problems (Poyner, 1989). Plexiglass shields and "better" guns may give a false sense of security, feed a "siege" mentality and make things worse. Other inappropriate responses include incomplete or ineffective application of basically good ideas.

Guidelines, programmes and policies are useful but must be up-to-date and easily available to staff (Leiber, 1992). In one study (Johnson, 1988), social workers' guidelines tended to reframe old problems as solutions and did not provide a framework to analyze assaults or attempt any comprehensive risk assessment (workers tend to blame themselves rather than situational factors). There were no provisions for evaluation or collating and analyzing reported incidents. There was also far too much concern for a bureaucratic approach (Poyner, 1988). This may be reflected in the language used in guidelines: Some British health care workers talked about guidelines written in a language that bore no resemblance to their practical work situations (Poyner, 1988).

Many recommended responses to potential violence are behavioral (eg. de-escalation, better training, security devices) or make the worker responsible for taking all kinds of precautions (Stevenson, 1991). Nurses are told their "skilled response" will have the most direct effect among the many forces influencing the likelihood of violence in an emergency department (Bjorn, 1991). This ignores organizational and other factors, pretends nurses have more control than they really do and may lead to victim-blaming after an assault.

Training is often seen as *the* solution, especially after an attack (Poyner, 1988). It may be inadequate, however. In one study (Health and Safety Commission, 1986), only 16 percent of the 12 percent of British health care workers who received training in the prevention of workplace violence found it useful. Work practices taught in training may require changes once workers return to their jobs. "But what happens is staff get back to the workplace and they only have 10 minutes to do a whole list of chores. It just negates all of it [the training workshop]" (Pilon, 1987).

Responses to Encourage

The following responses to workplace violence encourage understanding of the issue and change.

Define Violence Inclusively

The definition of violence used in a workplace is key. Inclusive definitions recognize non-physical violence such as verbal abuse, sexual and racial harassment and the possibilities of institutional sources linked to work organization. They recognize that violence is a process, not an isolated incident (Agudelo, 1992).

Design and Implement Comprehensive Workplace Programmes

Comprehensive programmes start from an inclusive definition of violence and a policy incorporating management's commitment to prevent violence on the job. They have specific procedures about work environment requirements, security measures, how to deal with potentially violent events and attacks, training, restraint procedures, post-incident support (including debriefing and counselling for witnesses and those attacked), other follow-up, evaluation, making changes, etc.[21]

Too often, programmes are presented as having all the correct answers from the start, with no need for evaluation and changes (Poyner, 1989). The truth is that evaluation and follow-up procedures are part of effective comprehensive programmes. Such programmes work best with complete worker involvement and when there is evident enforcement of the programme and its policy (CUPE, 1991a).

Report Attacks

Incident or report forms provide a standard way to document assaults; they also make it easier to analyze events, if they provide the right kind of information and are used in a tracking system. When one hospital used incident reports to flag patient charts (and institute certain measures when patients were checked in), violent incidents decreased by 92 percent in one year (Drummond et al., 1989). There is some discussion about the information that forms should include, the effectiveness of the forms and their uses in a preventive context (Eisenberg and Tierney, 1985; Turnball, 1993; Gentry and Ostapiuk, 1989). In general, it is important to avoid formats that give set answers (eg. for "contributing factors") which may be irrelevant to certain situations and that have no space to fill in the "Other (specify)" category. HSE documents provide several examples. CUPE (1994) has a useful one-page version with copies for various parties, including the joint health and safety committee.

Provide Support

Medical help, counselling and other support are often considered essential for women who are assaulted at home or on the street but have been ignored in many workplaces where workers face abuse (Engel and Marsh, 1986; Leiba, 1992). For example, although social workers in particular know the value of individual counselling or group work for clients, in a 1987 study no agency had "trauma leave" and few offered counselling or related services to their employees (Schultz, 1987).

Much of the nursing, social work and union writing about workplace violence emphasizes the need for post-assault counselling and health care. Responses to assault vary and some are consistent with post-traumatic stress syndrome — in those cases, longer-term help may be needed (Whittington and Wykes, 1992). Support should include medical care, legal advice, information about rights and benefits such as filing charges, workers' compensation, counselling and peer support programmes.[22] Victim-blaming almost vanished in one workplace where an assaulted staff support programme was in place (Flannery, 1992).

Provide Training

Training is *part* of a comprehensive approach to workplace violence. In one study, the overall staff injury rate decreased when a "critical mass" of health care workers used techniques in which they were trained; individual compliance with training was linked to a lower violence-associated injury rate (Carmel and Hunter, 1990). Individuals also become more competent and confident about dealing with a range of situations (Rosenthal et al., 1992; Paterson et al., 1990). Training must include more than information, be integrated and well-balanced and be rigorously evaluated (Poyner and Warne, 1988; Paterson et al., 1990). Regular updating and refresher courses are needed. "Train-the-trainer" approaches are often useful (Health and Safety Commission, 1990).

Important training programme ingredients include: identifying causes of violence and aggression and the magnitude of the problem; learning how to evaluate/anticipate/recognize potential problems; analyzing personal and interactional skills; dealing with specific situations (eg. emergencies, "sundowning"); studying the use of restraints and medication (when, how, who); integrating all aspects of the programme; demonstrating methods of debriefing, support and follow-up after an incident; and clarifying the rights of workers and patients/clients/residents.

Recognize the Importance of Work Design/Organization

> ... although there is a need for some training of staff to cope with difficult customers, and there will be many ways in which security devices can help protect staff, the most satisfactory solution to problems of violence is through the *redesign of the work itself and the way in which staff have to deal with the public* [emphasis added] (Poyner, 1989).

The British materials show the possibility and importance of getting to the root of one of the major factors behind an assault — the work environment (Poyner and Warne, 1988; Hobbs, 1991; Poyner, 1988). One aspect of the work environment that affects the potential for violence is the physical design, which can be analyzed according to the following elements: privacy; colours; lighting; noise level; layout (eg. isolation, dead ends); amount of available space; presence of materials to reduce boredom and frustration; presence or absence of potential missiles and other weapons; presence of shatterproof glass/plastic (where needed); and the reduction of separation between workers and patients/clients/residents (within limits). CUPE documents also have useful recommendations.

How work is done can also change. Work organization topics to address include: control issues for workers and patients/clients/residents, especially work pace and time required to interact with people; and demand issues related to staffing levels and staff — patient/client ratios, working alone, hours of work, etc. For example, Alzheimer patients tend to become more excited, confused and aggressive as the sun sets. This "sundowning syndrome" often coincides with shift changes. A gradual changeover or calming activities would benefit both potential assailants and all workers, rather than new leaving staff to cope (Lewis, 1993).

Cover the Legal Angles

Legal measures — regulation, enforcement, collective agreements — are resisted in many jurisdictions and workplaces. For example, health care regulations about worker health and safety, which included requirements for dealing with violence, have been held up for years in Ontario despite a 1987 bipartite committee agreement. The much-mutilated draft 1993 version left out the sections about violence, for "financial" reasons among others (Ontario Ministry of Labour, 1993).

But some jurisdictions *are* taking action. British Columbia's recent regulation defines violence in such a way as to include threatening statements or behaviour, requires a risk assessment and development of policy and procedures, sets out rules for responding to incidents and requires workers be given training and information (WCB, 1992). Saskatchewan added a vague section about "violent situations" to its legislation in 1993, requiring employers in prescribed workplaces to develop and implement a "policy statement" to deal with potentially-violent situations (Occupational Health and Safety Act, 1993).

The only available American government documents are the Cal/OSHA (1993) health care guidelines and a two-page guideline for public sector health care facilities issued by the New Jersey Department of Labor (1991). (The New Jersey guidelines include a requirement that "safe staffing levels" be maintained.) The California Emergency Nurses Association has written and is pressing for legislation to deal with violence in emergency departments (Keep and Glibert, 1992).

In Europe, aside from the HSE, Sweden recently changed its laws to update a violence regulation originally implemented in 1983. The ordinance includes background and suggested measures, questions, etc. It requires many of the programme components listed earlier and states that workplaces must be "positioned, designed and equipped in such a way as to avert, as far as possible" the risk or threats of violence. It also requires that "cash-in-transit" operations be organized and conducted in a manner that protects workers (Swedish National Board of Occupational Safety and Health, 1993).

Unions recommend that workers demand enforcement of guidelines and regulations/laws by employers and government agencies. Suggested strategies include using the right to refuse (especially if expected to work alone) and filing grievances and workers' compensation claims for all attacks, whether physical or psychological. They also have prepared and won contract language to establish joint health and safety violence sub-committees and anti-violence programmes.[23]

Enforcement *is* possible. The British Columbia WCB gave Vancouver's University Hospital 28 days to ensure a safe level of staffing on its psychiatric ward and to ensure that the workers knew of the changes being made (COHSN, 1992). This occurred after a nurse (who had complained for months and had been attacked) and a nursing aide each used their right to refuse because they would be alone at several points during their 12-hour shifts.

Assailants can be charged. There are precedents for charging psychiatric clients (Ryan and Poster, 1991). A B.C. nurse successfully pressed an assault charge against a patient in a psychiatric unit (Dramer, 1993). The Sudbury and District Children's Aid Society provides up to $250 for an assaulted employee to get outside legal advice and may provide more later (Children's Aid Society of the District of Sudbury and Manitoulin, 1993). A 1990 Calgary General Hospital draft policy allowed staff to charge patients who abuse them (*Calgary Herald*, 1990). An American nurse successfully charged a doctor with assault and battery when he struck her on the forearm and told her to "turn on the [goddam] suction" (Creighton, 1988).

RESEARCH ISSUES

We need a common definition of violence that includes verbal abuse, harassment and institutional violence for use in research, legislation, workplace policies and reports. Then we could start to integrate and share information, knowledge and studies of the violence against women and workplace violence. We also need to integrate workplace violence into the musings and discussion of other occupational hazards and ill-health. The issue may offer unique opportunities to make workplace changes and address some important stressors.

We also need to hear from those "missing voices." The HSE's five elements are a useful method to develop exposure profiles, especially in female job ghettos. In doing so, we have to pay attention to several questions: How is gender entwined in the risk factors for workplace violence? Do women work in poorly-designed work areas? How does gender affect the responses of assaulted women and their co-workers, supervisor(s), non-work friends and family? What barriers do women face in dealing with all aspects of abuse at work, including causes, blame, reporting of incidents and addressing of problems? How can we deal with all of these questions in a problem-solving, inclusive way?

Research work should examine solutions and processes for dealing with the issue. It should critically examine "solutions" requiring behaviour changes and compare them with those that affect workplace design and organization. We need information about problem-solving processes that avoid developing a siege mentality and fostering fear, and give workers a way to integrate their experience and knowledge with that gained elsewhere.

CONCLUSION

Women are often the victims of workplace violence because of social/structural inequities/attitudes and because of the work they do. As a society, we must recognize and condemn violence wherever it occurs — behind the closed doors of a private home, on the streets of our cities and towns and in our workplaces. Workplace violence is all the more offensive because it is a public and occupational health hazard that can be prevented and/or controlled.

Women have fought for years, with some success, to bring violence against women out of the closet at home and to "take back the night" on our streets. Now we are talking about the need to "take back" our workplaces, for our individual and collective health and safety.

NOTES

1. This literature review is limited to English-language materials, although work has also been done in other countries. For example, in 1993, Danish academic Eva Hultengren wrote up a participatory research project in: *Bag om volden. Forsknings — og udvuklingsprojekt*, (Nordjyllands Amt, Socialforvaltningen, Amtsgärden, Neils Bohrsvej 30, 9220 Aalborg Ost., Denmark).

2. Agudelo, F., "Violence and Health: Preliminary Elements for Thought and Action", *International Journal of Health Sciences* 22 (1992), pp. 365-76. Agudelo defines violence as "an event that has a motive, that is materialized in different forms, that produces immediate alterations and delayed consequences, and that is oriented toward the attainment of certain goals. Its causes, forms, and consequences can vary, interact and change."

3. The most common terms are abuse, assault and violence. Assault tends to be used to describe physical violence, while abuse is often associated with verbal violence. Some authors use the terms as substitutes for one another. Others talk of aggression. A study about emergency room nurses uses "victimisation" to describe a variety of violent acts and incidents.

4. For a unique definition of assault (unauthorised touching incidents), see: Reid, W.,

M. Bollinger and J.G. Edwards, "Serious Assaults by Inpatients," *Psychosomatics* 30 (1989), pp. 54-6.

5. This is particularly true of those Americans studying "occupational violent crime."

6. United Nations, "Declaration on the Elimination of Violence Against Women," in *Changing the Landscape: Ending Violence — Achieving Equality*, cited in *Canadian Panel on Violence Against Women*, (Ottawa: Supply and Services Canada, 1993), p. 6.

7. Gestal, J.J., "Occupational Hazards in Hospitals: Accidents, Radiation, Exposure to Noxious Chemicals, Drug Addiction and Psychic Problems, and Assault," *British Journal of Industrial Medicine* 44 (1987), pp. 510-20. However, the focus is on physicians dealing with patients who are mentally ill; a malpractice suit is also considered an assault.

8. Based on the number of documents found after searching health, sociology, education and psychological databases and other sources of information for this and related reviews.

9. Morrison, E.F., "The Assaulted Nurse: Strategies for Healing," *Perspectives in Psychiatric Care* 25, 3/4 (1987/88), pp. 120-6; Lipscomb, J., and C. Love, "Violence Towards Health Care Workers," *American Association of Occupational Health News* 40 (1992), pp. 219-28; Bensley, L., N. Nelson, J. Kaufman, B. Silverstein and J. Kalat, *Study of Assaults on Staff in Washington State Psychiatric Hospitals: Final Report*, (Seattle: Department of Labor and Industries, December, 1993); Cahill, C.D., G.W. Stuart, M.T. Laraia and G.W. Arana, "Inpatient Management of Violent Behavior: Nursing Prevention and Intervention," *Issues in Mental Health Nursing* 12 (1991), pp. 239-52; Carmel, H., and M. Hunter, "Staff Injuries from Inpatient Violence," *Hospital and Community Psychiatry* 41, 5 (1989), pp. 558-60; Craig, T.J., "An Epidemiologic Study of Problems Associated with Violence Among Psychiatric Inpatients," *American Journal of Psychiatry* 139, 10 (1982), pp. 1262-6; Lanza, M.L., "The Reactions of Nursing Staff to Physical Assault by a Patient," *Hospital and Community Psychiatry* 34 (1983), pp. 44-7; Lanza, M.L., "Predictors of Patient Assault on Acute Inpatient Psychiatric Units: A Pilot Study," *Issues in Mental Health Nursing* 9 (1988), pp. 259-70; Larkin, E., S. Murtagh and S. Jones, "A Preliminary Study of Violent Incidents in a Special Hospital (Rampton)," *British Journal of Psychiatry* 153 (1988), pp. 226-31; Rosenthal, T.L., N. Edwards and R. Rosenthal, "Hospital Violence: Site, Severity, and Nurses' Preventive Training," *Issues in Mental Health Nursing* 13 (1992), pp. 349-56.

10. Mahoney, B.S., "The Extent, Nature, and Response to Victimization of Emergency Nurses in Pennsylvania," *Journal of Emergency Nursing* 17 (1991), pp. 282-91. Keep, N., and P. Glibert [1990-1991 California ENA Government Affairs Committee], "California Emergency Nurses' Association's Information Survey of Violence in California Emergency Rooms," *Journal of Emergency Nursing* 18, 5 (1992), pp. 433-9; Lavoie, F.W., G.L. Carter, D.F. Danzl and R.L. Berg, "Emergency Department Violence in United States Teaching Hospitals," *Annals of Emergency Medicine* 17 (1990), pp. 1227-33. The *Journal of Emergency Nursing* did a special issue on the topic in October, 1991 (Volume 17, 5). The Emergency Nurses' Association has a position statement on violence in the emergency setting (*Journal of Emergency Nursing* 17, 6 [1991], p. 32A).

11. Although they are important, other studies of sexual harassment/assault were not reviewed; they are beyond the particular scope of this paper. Kushnir Pekrul's review

of the literature (see references) led her to conclude that, although it might be expected, there was little information about sexual harassment in the health care system.

12. An Ontario community college professor concerned with violence in his workplace made this point to the author.

13. It is complicated by the fact no author defines the tasks done or differences amongst nursing staff work. They assume readers know what "nurses' aides," "nursing assistants" and "orderlies" do, that the titles have similar meanings everywhere and that those with these titles do the same kind of work in different workplaces and countries.

14. The U.K. work is rarely referred to in North American materials and some Canadian quarters, so wheels are re-invented and useful problem-solving approaches remain unfamiliar to North Americans. The recent California guidelines for health care and community service workers (see references), is a good example of this omission. Canadian Union of Public Employees (CUPE) is one of the few organizations using the materials extensively.

15. Health and Safety Commission, *Violence to Staff in the Education Sector*, (London: HMSO, 1990); Health and Safety Executive, *Prevention of Violence to Staff in Banks and Building Societies*, (London: HMSO, 1993); Joint Departmental-Trade Union Working Party, *Violence to Staff: Policies and Procedures*, (Glasgow: Social Work Department, Strathclyde Regional Council, 1986), the document also includes an evaluation of incident reports; Department of Health and Social Security, *Violence to Staff: Report of the DHSS Advisory Committee on Violence to Staff*, (London: HMSO, 1988); Poyner, B., and C. Warne, *Violence to Staff: A Basis for Assessment and Prevention*, (London: Health and Safety Executive, 1986); National Association of Local Government Officers (NALGO) Safety Representative, *Violence — A Work Hazard*, (London: NALGO, 1985); Poyner, B., and C. Warne, *Preventing Violence to Staff* (London: Health and Safety Executive, 1988). In earlier documents, the Tavistock Institute authors called the work environment "the situation".

16. CUPE materials, and materials from one of its sister American unions, the Service Employees International Union (SEIU), in a 1993 package entitled, "Assault on the job. We can do something about it."

17. This is true if the source of the exposure is beyond the employer's contractual control, ie. the staff. However, violence at work is also about abuse from co-workers and management. This narrower definition does not invalidate the framework.

18. Lanza, M.L., "The Reactions of Nursing Staff to Physical Assault by a Patient," *Hospital and Community Psychiatry* 34 (1983), pp. 44-7; Atkinson, J. "Worker Reaction to Client Assault," *Smith College Studies in Social Work* 62, 1 (1991) pp. 34-42; Poster, E., and J. Ryan, "At Risk of Assault," *Nursing Times* 89, 23 (1993), pp. 30-3; Wykes, T., and R. Whittington, "Coping Strategies Used by Staff Following Assault by a Patient: An Exploratory Study," *Work and Stress* 5 (1991), pp. 37-48.

19. Kushnir Pekrul, op. cit.; Pizzino, A., *Report on CUPE's National Health and Safety Survey of Aggression Against Staff* (Ottawa: CUPE, 1994), this was part of the union's "Checking violence at work" campaign; McCaskell, L., "Dealing with Nurse Abuse," *Nursing Report* 27 (1990), pp. 25-33; CUPE Nova Scotia Task Force for Homes for Special Care, *Safety Concerns and Working Conditions in N.S. Homes for Special Care*, (Halifax: CUPE, 1990).

20. This is not reported in the literature, but it is clear from my personal experience that this is a common reason for under-reporting other occupational hazards.

21. Lipscomb and Love, op. cit.; Green, E., "When Caring is Your Only Defence: Management of Violent Behaviour," *Journal of Emergency Nursing* 17, 5 (1991), pp. 336-9; Cal/OSHA, Medical Unit, Division of Occupational Safety & Health, Department of Industrial Relations, *Guidelines for Security and Safety of Health Care and Community Service Workers*, (San Francisco: Cal/OSHA, 1993); Children's Aid Society of the District of Sudbury and Manitoulin, *Employee Safety Manual*, (Sudbury: Children's Aid Society, 1993); Ontario Nurses Association, *Violence in the Workplace: A Guide for Members*, (Toronto: Ontario Nurses Association, 1991); Splawn, G., "Restraining Potentially Violent Patients," *Journal of Emergency Nursing* 39 (1991), pp. 316-7.

22. Morrison, op. cit; Health and Safety Executive, op. cit.; Ryan, J., and E. Poster, "When a Patients Hits You," *The Canadian Nurse* (Sept. 1991), pp. 23-5; Dawson, J., M. Johnson, N. Kehiayan, S. Kyanko and R. Martinez, "Response to Patient Assault. A Peer Support Program for Nurses," *Journal of Psychosocial Nursing* 26, 2 (1988), pp. 8-11, 15; Flannery, R.B., P. Fulton, J. Tausch and A.Y. DeLoffi, "A Program to Help Staff Cope with Psychological Sequelae of Assaults by Patients," *Hospital and Community Psychiatry* 42 (1991), pp. 935-8; Lewis, G., "Managing Crises and Trauma in the Workplace: How to Respond and Intervene," *American Association of Occupational Health News Journal* 41 (1993), pp. 124-30; Murray, G., and J.C. Snyder, "When Staff are Assaulted: A Nursing Consultation Support Service," *Journal of Psychosocial Nursing* 29, 7 (1991), pp. 24-9; Flannery, R., "Assaults on Staff," [Response to a letter to the editor], *Hospital and Community Psychiatry* 43 (1992), pp. 286.

23. British Columbia Nurses' Union, *Briefing Paper: Violence in the Workplace*, (Vancouver: B.C. Nurses' Union, 1991); CUPE *Action Kit: Help Check Violence at Work*, (Ottawa: CUPE, 1994); CUPE, *Health and Safety Guidelines: Stopping Violence at Work*, (Ottawa: CUPE, 1987); The Canadian Nurses' Association (50 The Driveway, Ottawa, Ontario, K2P 1E2) has information and materials from across the country.

REFERENCES

"Abuse by ill no longer ignored. Nurses can lay charges." *Calgary Herald* (July 18, 1990).

"B.C. WCB Orders Hospital to Review Staffing Level." *Canadian Occupational Health and Safety News* (August 13, 1992). p. 6.

"Have-a-Say Looks at Health and Safety Issues." *The ONA News* (November 1992). p. 16.

"Physical and Verbal Abuse of Alberta Social Service Workers on the Rise, Union Says." *Canadian Occupational Health and Safety News* (October 4, 1993). p. 2.

Agudelo, F. "Violence and Health: Preliminary Elements for Thought and Action." *International Journal of Health Sciences* 22 (1992). pp. 365-76.

Atkinson, J. "Worker Reaction to Client Assault." *Smith College Studies in Social Work*. 62, 1 (1991). pp. 34-42.

Bell, C. "Female Homicides in United States Workplaces, 1980-1985." *American Journal of Public Health* 81 (1991). pp. 729-32.

Bensley, L., N. Nelson, J. Kaufman, B. Silverstein and J. Kalat. *Study of Assaults on*

Staff in Washington State Psychiatric Hospitals: Final Report. Seattle: Department of Labor and Industries, December 1993.

Bjorn, P. "An Approach to the Potentially Violent Patient." *Journal of Emergency Nursing* 17, 5 (1991). pp. 336-9.

Brasen, T. "Abuse at Work: The Health Care Industry Fights Back." *Occupational Health and Safety Magazine* (May 1993). pp. 7-13.

British Columbia Nurses' Union (BCNU). *Survey on Violence.* Vancouver: BCNU, 1991a.

— *Briefing Paper: Violence in the Workplace.* Vancouver: BCNU, 1991b.

— *The Violent Story* (video). Vancouver: BCNU, 1992.

Britt, B. "Danger on the Job: Violence in the Health Care Workplace." *Canadian Occupational Safety* 30 (1992). p. 21.

Brown, R., S. Bute and P. Ford. *Social Workers at Risk.* London: Macmillan, 1986.

Browner, C.H. "Job Stress and Health: The Role of Social Support at Work." *Research in Nursing and Health* 10 (1987). pp. 93-100.

Cahill, C.D., G.W. Stuart, M.T. Laraia and G.W. Arana. "Inpatient Management of Violent Behavior: Nursing Prevention and Intervention." *Issues in Mental Health Nursing* 12 (1991). pp. 239-52.

Cal/OSHA, Medical Unit, Division of Occupational Safety and Health, Department of Industrial Relations. *Guidelines for Security and Safety of Health Care and Community Service Workers.* San Francisco: Cal/OSHA, 1993.

Canadian Panel on Violence Against Women. *Changing the Landscape: Ending Violence — Achieving Equality.* Ottawa: Supply and Services Canada, 1993.

Canadian Union of Public Employees (CUPE). *Health and Safety Guidelines: Stopping Violence at Work.* Ottawa: CUPE, 1987.

— *Our Workplaces are Not Yet Healthy, Not Yet Safe: Guidelines for Workplace Health and Safety Programmes.* Ottawa: CUPE, 1991a.

— *Violence in Nova Scotia's Homes for Special Care: Report of the Hearings on Violence for the Nova Scotia Homes for Special Care Task Force.* Ottawa: CUPE, 1991b.

— *Survey Results: Violence Against Social Service Workers.* Ottawa: CUPE, 1993.

— *Action Kit: Help Check Violence at Work.* Ottawa: CUPE, 1994.

Canadian Union of Public Employees (CUPE), Nova Scotia Task Force for Homes for Special Care. *Safety Concerns and Working Conditions in N.S. Homes for Special Care.* Halifax: CUPE, 1990.

Carmel, H., and M. Hunter. "Staff Injuries from Inpatient Violence." *Hospital and Community Psychiatry* 41, 5 (1989). pp. 558-60.

— "Compliance with Training in Managing Assaultive Behaviour and Injuries from Inpatient Violence." *Hospital and Community Psychiatry* 41, 5 (1990). pp. 558-60.

Castillo, D.N., and E.L. Jenkins. "Industries and Occupations at High Risk for Work-related Homicide." *Journal of Occupational Medicine* 36, 2 (1994). pp. 125-32.

Children's Aid Society of the District of Sudbury and Manitoulin. *Employee Safety Manual.* Sudbury, Ontario: Children's Aid Society, 1993.

Chinn, P.L. "Violence and the Health Care 'Family.'" *Advances in Nursing Science* 8 (1986). pp. ix-x.

Convey, J. "A Record of Violence." *Nursing Times* (November 12, 1986). pp. 36-8.

Corea, G. *The Hidden Malpractice: How American Medicine Mistreats Women.* Revised Edition. New York: Harper & Row, 1985.

Craig, T.J. "An Epidemiologic Study of Problems Associated with Violence Among Psychiatric Inpatients." *American Journal of Psychiatry* 139, 10 (1982). pp. 1262-6.

Creighton, H. "Physician Liable to Nurse for Assault and Battery." *Nursing Management* 19 (1988). pp. 17-20.

Dawson, J., M. Johnson, N. Kehiayan, S. Kyanko and R. Martinez. "Response to Patient Assault: A Peer Support Program for Nurses." *Journal of Psychosocial Nursing* 26, 2. pp. 8-11, 15.

Dramer, B. "Assault" [letter to the editor]. *The Canadian Nurse* (1993). pp. 6, 10.

Drummond, D.J., L.F. Spar and G.H. Gordon. "Hospital Violence Reduction Among High-risk Patients." *Journal of the American Medical Association* 261 (1989). pp. 2531-4.

Dubin, W.R. "The Role of Fantasies, Countertransference, and Psychological Defenses in Patient Violence." *Hospital and Community Psychiatry* 40 (1989). pp. 1280-3.

Eisenberg, M., and D. Tierney. "Profiling Disruptive Patient Incidents." *Quality Review Bulletin* 11, 8 (August 1985). pp. 245-8.

Engel, F., and S. Marsh. "Helping the Employee Victim of Violence in Hospitals." *Hospital and Community Psychiatry* 37 (1986). pp. 159-62.

Flannery, R. "Assaults on Staff" [response to a letter to the editor]. *Hospital and Community Psychiatry* 43 (1992). p. 286.

Flannery, R.B., P. Fulton, J. Tausch and A.Y. DeLoffi. "A Program to Help Staff Cope with Psychological Sequelae of Assaults by Patients." *Hospital and Community Psychiatry* 42 (1991). pp. 935-8.

Gawthrop, D. "Patient Violence: Why are Health Care Workers Taking a Beating on the Job?" *Guardian* (March 1991).

Gentry, M.R., and E.B. Ostapiuk. "Violence in Institutions for Young Offenders and Disturbed Adolescents," in *Clinical Approaches to Violence*. K. Howells and C. Hollin (eds.). Chichester: John Wiley & Sons, 1989.

Green, E. "Patient Care Guidelines: Management of Violent Behaviour." *Journal of Emergency Nursing* 15, 6 (1989). pp. 523-8.

Hales, T., P. Seligman, S.C. Newman andf C.L. Timbrook. "Occupational Injuries Due to Violence." *Journal of Occupational Medicine* 30, 6 (1989). pp. 483-7.

Health and Safety Commission. *Violence to Staff in the Education Sector*. London: HMSO, 1990.

Health and Safety Commission, Health Services Advisory Committee. *Violence to Staff in the Health Services*. London: HMSO, 1986.

Health and Safety Executive. *Prevention of Violence to Staff in Banks and Building Societies*. London: HMSO, 1993.

Hobbs, F.D.R. "Violence in General Practice: A Survey of General Practitioners' Views." *British Medical Journal* 302 (1991). pp. 329-32.

Johnson, S. "Guide-lines for Social Workers in Coping with Violent Clients." *British Journal of Social Work* 18 (1988). pp. 377-90.

Jones, M.K. "Patient Violence Report of 200 Incidents." *Journal of Psychosocial Nursing and Mental Health Services* 23, 6 (1985). pp. 12-7.

Keep, N., and P. Glibert. "California Emergency Nurses' Association Introduces Prototype State Legislation to Fight Violence in the Emergency Department." *Journal of Emergency Nursing* 18, 5 (1992). pp. 440-2.

— "California Emergency Nurses' Association's Information Survey of Violence in California Emergency Rooms." *Journal of Emergency Nursing* 18, 5 (1992). pp. 433-9.

Khan, B. "Starting a Program Inside the Bureaucracy." *Vis-à-vis* 9, 1 (1991). p. 7.

Kraus, J. "Homicide While at Work: Persons, Industries, and Occupations at High Risk." *American Journal of Public Health* 77 (1987). pp. 1285-9.

Kushnir Pekrul, L. "Nurse Abuse in Saskatchewan: 'Sticks and Stones May Break My Bones, But Names Can Never Hurt Me.'" Central Michigan University, 1992.

Lanza, M.L. "The Reactions of Nursing Staff to Physical Assault by a Patient." *Hospital and Community Psychiatry* 34 (1983). pp. 44-7.

— "Predictors of Patient Assault on Acute Inpatient Psychiatric Units: A Pilot Study." *Issues in Mental Health Nursing* 9 (1988). pp. 259-70.

— "Commentary." *Journal of Emergency Nursing* 17, 5 (1991). pp. 292-3.

Lanza, M.L., and J. Carifio. "Blaming the Victim: Complex (Nonlinear) Patterns of Causal Attribution by Nurses in Response to Vignettes of a Patient Assaulting a Nurse." *Journal of Emergency Nursing* 17 (1991). pp. 299-308.

Lanza, M.L., and D. Campbell. "Patient Assault: A Comparison Study of Reporting Methods." *Journal of Nursing Quality Assurance* 5, 4 (1991). pp. 60-8.

Lanza, M.L., H. Kayne, C. Hicks and J. Milner. "Nursing Staff Characteristics Related to Patient Assault." *Issues in Mental Health Nursing* 12 (1991). pp. 253-365.

Larkin, E., S. Murtagh and S. Jones. "A Preliminary Study of Violent Incidents in a Special Hospital (Rampton)." *British Journal of Psychiatry* 153 (1988). pp. 226-31.

Lavoie, F.W., G.L. Carter, D.F. Danzl and R.L. Berg. "Emergency Department Violence in United States Teaching Hospitals." *Annals of Emergency Medicine* 17 (1990). pp. 1227-33.

Lechky, O. "Nurses Face Widespread Abuse at Work, Research Team Says." *Canadian Medical Association Journal* 150 (1994a). pp. 737-42.

— "Nurses Mobilize to Battle Growing Violence in the Workplace." *Canadian Medical Association Journal* 150 (1994b). pp. 738-9.

Leiba, P. "Learning from Incidents of Violence in Health Care. An Investigation of 'Case Reports' as a Basis for Staff Development and Organisational Change." *Nurse Education Today* 12 (1992). pp. 116-21.

Leppänen, R.A., and M. Olkinuora. "Psychological Stress Experienced by Health Care Personnel." *Scandinavian Journal of Work, Environment and Health* 13 (1987). pp. 1-8.

Levin, P.F., J.B. Hewitt and S.T. Misner. "Female Workplace Homicides." *American Association of Occupational Health News Journal* 40 (1992). pp. 229-36.

Lewis, G. "Managing Crises and Trauma in the Workplace: How to Respond and Intervene." *American Association of Occupational Health News Journal* 41 (1993). pp. 124-30.

Lipscomb, J., and C. Love. "Violence Towards Health Care Workers." *American Association of Health News Journal* 40 (1992). pp. 219-28.

Liss, G. *Examination of Workers' Compensation Claims Among Nurses in Ontario for Injuries Due to Violence.* Toronto: Ministry of Labour, 1993.

Liss, G., and C.A. Craig. "Homicide in the Workplace in Ontario: Occupations at Risk and Limitations of Existing Data Sources." *Canadian Journal of Public Health* 81 (1990). pp. 10-5.

Lusk, S.L. "Violence Experienced by Nurses' Aides in Nursing Homes." *American Association of Occupational Health News Journal* 40, 5 (1992). pp. 227-41.

Mahoney, B.S. "The Extent, Nature, and Response to Victimization of Emergency Nurses in Pennsylvania." *Journal of Emergency Nursing* 17 (1991). pp. 282-91.

Manitoba Association of Registered Nurses. *Nurse Abuse Report.* Winnipeg: Manitoba Assocation of Registered Nurses, 1989.

Manitoba Teachers' Society. *Report of the Task Force on the Physical and Emotional Abuse of Teachers.* Winnipeg: Manitoba Teachers' Society, 1990.

— *Report of Abuse of Teachers in Manitoba Schools.* Winnipeg: Manitoba Teachers' Society, May 1993.

McCaskell, L. "Dealing with Nurse Abuse." *Nursing Report* 27 (1990). pp. 25-33.

Messing, K. *Occupational Safety and Health Concerns of Canadian Women: A Background Paper.* Ottawa: Labour Canada Women's Bureau, 1991. p. 9.

Morrison, E.F. "The Assaulted Nurse: Strategies for Healing." *Perspectives in Psychiatric Care* 25, 3/4 (1987/88). pp. 120-6.

— "What Therapeutic and Protective Measures, As Well As Legal Actions, Can Staff Take When They Are Attacked by Patients?" *Journal of Psychosocial Nursing* 30, 7 (1992). pp. 41-2.

Murray, G., and J.C. Snyder. "When Staff are Assaulted: A Nursing Consultation Support Service." *Journal of Psychosocial Nursing* 29, 7 (1991). pp. 24-9.

National Institute for Occupational Safety and Health (NIOSH). *Preventing Homicide in the Workplace.* Cincinnati, OH: Centres for Disease Control and Prevention, 1993.

New Jersey Department of Labor. "Guidelines on Measures and Safeguards in Dealing with Violent or Aggressive Behavior in Public Sector Health Care Facilities." *New Jersey Department of Labor Official Bulletin* (1991).

Newhill, C.E. "Assessing Danger to Others in Clinical Social Work Practice." *Social Service Review* 66, 1 (1992). pp. 64-84.

Nurse Assault Project Team, Psychiatric Nursing Interest Group, Registered Nurses' Association of Ontario. *Nurse Assault Survey: A Study of Prevalence and Impact of Physical Assault on Nurses' Work Life, With a View Toward Effective Prevention.* Toronto: Registered Nurses' Association of Ontario, January 1992.

Ontario Ministry of Labour. *Regulation Made Under the Occupational Health and Safety Act for Health Care and Residential Facilities.* Toronto: Ontario Ministry of Labour, 1993.

Ontario Nurses Association. *Violence in the Workplace: A Guide for Members.* Toronto: Ontario Nurses Association, 1991.

Owens, R.G., and J.B. Ashcroft. *Violence: A Guide for the Caring Professions*. London: Croom Helm, 1985.

Paterson, B., J. Turnball and I. Aitken. "An Evaluation of a Training Course in the Short-term Management of Violence." *Hospital and Community Psychiatry* 41, 5 (1990). pp. 368-75.

Phillips, S., and M. Schneider. "Sexual Harassment of Female Doctors by Patients." *New England Journal of Medicine* 329 (1993). pp. 1936-9.

Pilon, D. "When Caring is Your Only Defence: The Growing Problem of Coping with Alzheimer Sufferers." *The Public Employee* (Winter 1987). pp. 2-5.

Pizzino, A. *Report on CUPE's National Health and Safety Survey of Aggression Against Staff*. Ottawa: CUPE, 1994.

Poster, E., and J. Ryan. "At Risk of Assault." *Nursing Times* 89, 23 (1993). pp. 30-3.

Poyner, B. "The Prevention of Violence to Staff." *Journal of Health and Safety* 1 (1988). pp. 19-26.

— "Working Against Violence." *Occupational Health* (August 1989). pp. 209-11.

Poyner, B., and C. Warne. *Violence to Staff: A Basis for Assessment and Prevention*. London: Health and Safety Executive, 1986.

— *Preventing Violence to Staff*. London: Health and Safety Executive, 1988.

Rebick, J., and M. Kaufman. "Ending Violence Against Women is a Men's Issue." *Toronto Star* (December 5, 1991).

Rix, G., and D. Seymour. "Violent Incidents on a Regional Secure Unit." *Journal of Advanced Nursing* 13 (1988). pp. 746-51.

Rix, G. "Staff Sickness and Its Relationship to Violent Incidents on a Regional Secure Psychiatric Unit." *Journal of Advanced Nursing* 12 (1987). pp. 223-8.

Robb, N. "Violence at Work: School of Hard Knocks." *Occupational Health and Safety Canada* (September/October 1993a). pp. 42-8.

— "Rough Treatment for Health Care Workers." *Occupational Health and Safety Canada* (September/October 1993b). pp. 55-8.

Roberts, S. "Nurse Abuse: A Taboo Topic." *The Canadian Nurse* (March 1991). pp. 23-5.

Rosenthal, T.L., N. Edwards and R. Rosenthal. "Hospital Violence: Site, Severity, and Nurses' Preventive Training." *Issues in Mental Health Nursing* 13 (1992). pp. 349-56.

Ryan, J., and E. Poster. "When a Patient Hits You." *The Canadian Nurse* (September 1991). pp. 23-5.

Schnieden, V. "Violence at Work." *Archives of Emergency Medicine* 10 (1992). pp. 79-85.

Schultz, L.G. "The Social Worker as a Victim of Violence." *Social Casework: The Journal of Contemporary Social Work* (1987). pp. 240-4.

Shea, C. "Changes in Women's Occupations." *Canadian Social Trends* (Autumn 1990). pp. 21-3.

Smith, S. "Take Care, Be Aware." *Community Outlook* (April 1988). pp. 10, 12.

Splawn, G. "Restraining Potentially Violent Patients." *Journal of Emergency Nursing* 39 (1991). pp. 316-7.

Statistics Canada. *Work Injuries: 1987-1989*. Ottawa: Statistics Canada, 1991.

— *Occupation — The Nation*. Ottawa: Statistics Canada 93-327, 1993a.

— *The Violence Against Women Survey*. Ottawa: Statistics Canada, November 18, 1993b.

Stevenson, S. "Heading Off Violence with Verbal De-escalation." *Journal of Psychosocial Nursing* 29, 9 (1991). pp. 6-10.

Stockdale, J., and C. Phillips. "Physical Attack and Threatening Behaviour — New Survey Findings." *Occupational Health* (August 1989). pp. 212-6.

Stymne, I. "Våldsrisker i arbetsmiljön [Risks of Violence in the Work Environment]." *Arbetarskyddsstyrelsen* (Solna, 1981). Cited in: Leppanen, op. cit., 1987.

Sullivan, P.J. "Occupational Stress in Psychiatric Nursing." *Journal of Advanced Nursing* 18 (1993). pp. 591-601.

Swedish National Board of Occupational Safety and Health. *Violence and Menaces in the Working Environment*. Ordinance (AFS 1993:2). Solna, 1993.

Thomas, J.L. "Occupational Violent Crime: Research on an Emerging Issue." *Journal of Safety Research* 23 (1992). pp. 55-62.

Turnball, J. "Victim Support." *Nursing Times* 89, 23 (1993). pp. 33-4.

Whittington, R., and T. Wykes. "Staff Strain and Social Support in a Psychiatric Hospital Following Assault by a Patient." *Journal of Advanced Nursing* 17 (1992). pp. 480-6.

Wigmore, D. "Violence in the Workplace: It Doesn't Have To Go With the Job." *Herizons* 8, 4 (Winter 1995). pp. 26-30, 42.

Workers' Compensation Board (WCB) of B.C. *Regulations: Protection of Workers from Violence in the Workplace*. Vancouver: Secretariat for Regulation Review, 1992.

Wykes, T., and R. Whittington. "Coping Strategies Used by Staff Following Assault by a Patient: An Exploratory Study." *Work and Stress* 5 (1991). p. 37-48.

Joan M. Eakin

The Health and Safety of Women in Small Workplaces

Environ un tiers de la population canadienne sur le marché de l'emploi travaille dans des unités de moins de 50 employés. Ces lieux de travail connaissent un taux plus élevé d'accidents et de problèmes de santé que les milieux plus populeux. Ils présentent des défis particuliers pour qui veut intervenir et amener des changements. Or, les femmes sont «proportion-nellement» beaucoup plus nombreuses dans ces entreprises de petite dimension. L'article explore comment les relations sociales liées au travail dans de petites unités peut avoir des conséquences sur la santé des femmes, à la fois par le niveau d'exposition aux risques, par les façons de détecter les problèmes, de les interpréter et d'y réagir. Après avoir déterminé quelques problèmes généraux de santé et de sécurité dans les lieux de travail de petite taille, en mettant l'accent sur leurs dimensions sociales et organisationnelles, l'article puise dans les recherches ethno-graphiques de l'auteure pour traiter des questions de santé et de genre liées à la présence de femmes comme propriétaires de petites entreprises, à la division sexuelle du travail à l'intérieur et entre les petites entreprises, au rôle des liens familiaux dans ces entreprises, aux relations employé-es-clientèle et enfin, aux différences de genre dans les comportements en matière de santé.

About one-third of Canadian workers are employed in workplaces with fewer than 50 employees. Such workplaces have higher rates of injury and ill-health than do larger workplaces, and present particular challenges by way of intervention and change. A disproportionately large number of those employed in this sector are women. This paper explores ways in which the social relations of work in small workplaces may have conse-quences for women, both in terms of exposure to hazards, and in the ways in which problems are identified, interpreted and reacted to. After identify-ing some general health and safety issues in small workplaces, and emphasizing their social and organizational dimensions, the paper draws on the author's own ethnographic research to discuss health and gender issues related to: (1) women as owners of small businesses; (2) the gender division of labour between and within small businesses; (3) the role of family in small workplaces; (4) the employee-customer relationship; and (5) the gendered nature of health-related behaviour.

INTRODUCTION

About one third of the Canadian labour force works in establishments employing fewer than 50 employees (Thompson, 1995). The small workplace sector is comprised of both independently owned for-profit businesses and non-profit public service organizations. The nature of work in this sector is extremely diverse, ranging from "mom-and-pop" corner stores which may barely support the family members working there to investment holding companies which employ only a few persons but process millions of dollars of assets. In this paper, I will focus on the myriad small industrial and service businesses that constitute the majority of small workplaces: retail trade; repair businesses; restaurants; dry cleaners; printing; manufacturing; health and social service agencies; and the like. Although the definition of "small" varies widely in the literature and in statistics, reference in this paper is generally to businesses with from one to 50 employees.

The small business sector employs a disproportionately large number of women, primarily because it is comprised heavily of social service, retail trade and other service businesses in which women form the majority of workers (Messite and Welch, 1987). For example, 80 percent of the Ontario health and social services employ fewer than 10 employees, and 80 percent of the employees in this sector are female (Armstrong, 1991).

The health issues for women in small workplaces include those identified for workers generally in this sector. Small workplaces are often located in certain high hazard industries (MacKinnon, 1987), and have numerous health and safety problems related to noise, dust and chemical exposure control (Spiegel and Yassi, 1989; Tuskes and Key, 1988; ARA, 1987). Compared to larger businesses, small companies have higher rates of injury and ill-health (Thomas, 1991; MacKinnon, 1987; Rutsohn, 1981).

In addition to these general issues, women's health issues in small workplaces also include those identified for women in general in the women's occupational health literature. For example, Messite and Welch (1987) describe women's occupational health concerns arising from physiological factors (e.g. equipment and standards designed for men, risks related to pregnancy), unrecognized hazards in jobs held predominantly by women (e.g. electronic assembly, hairdressers), and social organizational factors (e.g. the dual home/work responsibilities of women and their implications for health).

The available literature, however, does not focus on how women's health issues are related to the size of the workplace and its particular social and organizational character. In this paper I begin to explore the ways in which the social relations of work in small businesses might have consequences for women's health — in how women are exposed to hazards; in how problems are identified and interpreted; and in the response to problems. First, I shall identify some general health and safety issues in small work settings, emphasizing their links to the social organization and working conditions in small workplaces. Then, drawing on my own ethnographic research with small business employers and employees, I shall suggest some of the health issues confronting women in particular, and the gender issues that may find expression in these workplaces.

THE NATURE OF SMALL WORKPLACES AND IMPLICATIONS FOR HEALTH

The small business sector is difficult to characterize accurately because of its extreme variability and because of the kind of data that are available (Armstrong, 1991). Compared to larger enterprises, small workplaces (particularly those with fewer than 20 employees) are, on average, likely to have employees with lower levels of skill and education, lower pay, higher rates of part-time work, limited benefits, multifunction job categories, and a low rate of unionization (Armstrong, 1991). Small firms are also more likely to include family members (many of whom are unpaid), immigrants (some of whom may be illegally employed) and young entry-level workers (most of whom are inexperienced) (Curran and Stanworth, 1979).

Small businesses are often run by one or more owners, who frequently have established or bought their businesses because they were attracted by the prospect of "being their own boss" (Curran and Stanworth, 1979; Eakin, 1992). Other than the owner, there are often few, if any, supervisory or management level employees. Many owners fulfill all managerial functions themselves, including "pitching in" when necessary on the shop floor. The failure rate of new businesses is very high and financial marginality and instability are major problems for many enterprises. For example, Armstrong (1991) notes that 40 percent of Canadian businesses with fewer than 100 employees go out of business within one year of being founded.

These characteristics have numerous possible implications for occupational health and health promotion. For example, young workers are known to have higher rates of occupational injury than other workers (Industrial Accident Prevention Association, 1987). Immigrants may be at special risk of harm at work for linguistic, literacy and cultural reasons, and may be inhibited from addressing health and safety issues by financial and political insecurity. Part-time work may mean that workers receive less health and safety training and this may reduce their likelihood of being interested in or capable of devoting effort to workplace health. Multifunction jobs may mean that workers are engaged in work with which they have limited experience, which in turn increases their chance of exposure to harm. A low rate of unionization can mean that small workplace employees do not have access to the knowledge, awareness, support and collective control that have been central to the contribution of unions to occupational health and safety (Elling, 1986).

In addition to these sorts of factors, my own research points to how health and safety behaviour (what people think and do about health) in small workplaces is related to the organizational environment and the social relations of work. Qualitative analysis of in-depth interviews with small business owners in a wide variety of industrial sectors illuminated the nature of their perspectives on work and occupational health. This research includes a study of 54 business owners in Calgary (Eakin, 1992) and 78 in Toronto (Shain et al., 1994a). In these studies, when asked to identify what health and safety "problems" there were in their workplaces, many owners responded with a version of "there *are* no problems here." Although this was, in some instances, an indicator of ignorance, more often it reflected a different definition of what constitutes a "problem" (e.g. "Nobody's closed us down yet," "Nothing's killed us yet," "You get used to it."), and the low salience of health issues in the context of often brutal economic conditions and limited managerial assistance (as one owner put it, "Safety? Oh, that's way down the list [of worries].").

In this research, owners' responses to issues of health and safety were also influenced by their social relationships with employees. For example, many owners reported a "one-of-the-boys" authority relationship with their employees. This relationship appeared to contribute to the owners' reported reluctance to "impose" unpopular safety precautions on their employees (I'm not about to *make* the guys wear them [masks]!"), and their tendency to take a "leave it up to the workers" approach to workplace health (see Eakin, 1992). Many of these owners perceived that management intervention in employee health behaviour was paternalistic: they declared themselves unwilling to "babysit" or "welfare" or "mother" their employees. Such a relationship may have been rejected because it was inconsistent with prevailing patterns of labour relations in such workplaces, particularly shared norms respecting individual autonomy.

The key point of this research, and of my present study of small business employees, is that perceptions, attitudes and behaviour surrounding workplace health and safety are inseparable from the relations of work, organizational culture and the fabric of everyday work experience — all of which take a particular form in small workplaces.

A common approach to intervention and change in occupational health and safety has been through the legislation of safety standards and prevention practices. In most provinces, however, small workplaces are, to a varying degree, exempted from health and safety regulations. With over 800,000 enterprises employing fewer than 50 workers in Canada (Statistics Canada, 1992), inspection and enforcement by government agencies is very limited. This means that small workplaces generally have fewer legal obligations regarding health and safety than do larger companies, and that they are unlikely to come into contact with health and safety authorities or services. It also means that small workplaces are less likely to have adequate safety training and education for employees (Heath, 1982), and to have in place any of the organizational structures that have been designed to allow for internal management of workplace health problems such as WHMIS (Workplace Hazardous Materials Information System) or Joint Health and Safety Committees (Tuohy and Simard, 1993).

Even if small workplaces were included in legislation, and their compliance could be enforced, it is not clear that the provisions of the legislation are suited to the small business environment. For instance, the nature of social relations in small workplaces may make it especially difficult for employees to exercise the right to refuse dangerous work or to be reinstated for inappropriate health-related dismissal. Some regulations, such as the recent Ontario requirements for companies to send two members of their Joint Health and Safety Committees for "Certification" training, may be unrealistic for many small workplaces.

Non-regulatory approaches to preventing workplace injury and ill-health in small workplaces are also problematic. Although there is very little research into health promotion in such workplaces, it is widely believed that this sector is "hard to reach" (Eakin and Weir, 1995).

Owners are perceived by health professionals to be "unmotivated" and to lack the knowledge, management skills and financial and human resources to address health problems in the workplace (Evans, 1984). Often, they are considered resistant — even hostile — to intervention and change. Employees are even more difficult to reach, particularly independently of the management in the companies in which they work (Eakin and Weir, 1995).

In general, the characteristics of small businesses and of the social relations within them may compromise the health of those who work there, or make it difficult for them (and others) to improve health-related working conditions. Therefore, small workplaces present a particular challenge to those seeking to understand and address the sources of occupational harm.

Many aspects of small workplaces may affect the health of women more than that of men. For example, unpaid and part-time work in small businesses (with the attendant implications for health and safety) is done predominantly by female family members (Armstrong, 1991).

Although my research in small workplaces has not focused specifically on women's occupational health issues, a number of incidental findings are suggestive of other, less explicit, aspects of working in small work-places that have consequences for women in particular. These aspects include: (1) women as owners of small businesses; (2) the gender division of labour between and within small businesses; (3) the role of family in small workplaces; (4) the employee/customer relationship in small workplaces; and (5) the gendered nature of health-related behaviour in small workplaces.

WOMEN AS OWNERS AND MANAGERS OF SMALL BUSINESSES

Women constitute a growing proportion of small business owners (Adler, 1993). Some of the reasons for this lie in sex discrimination and barriers to the career development of women professionals and managers (Statham, 1993; Adler, 1993), while others lie in the gender issues underlying individual work histories and the occupational division of labour. An excerpt from an interview with the proprietor of a hairdressing salon illustrates these issues:

> I have never worked, but ... I had four kids growing up ... and so I didn't really do anything until the last one pretty well left home. And then I was decided to do something, but you know, I had been out of the workforce for some time and I figured my choices were

getting a job as a clerk at the Bay, or going back to school, or buying my own business and being the boss. And so I decided to buy a business instead and just see how it went.

Such an entry to the labour force has several possible implications. For example, it could be that women such as this one would use their past experience — in this case with family and home work — in running their businesses. In an interview study of business owners in Toronto (Shain et al., 1994b) it was found that women owners in the sample tended to emphasize interpersonal relations and conflict resolution when asked about what they found difficult in their jobs. Many perceived their companies to be "like a family." In contrast to male owners, who were more likely to believe that their employees should "leave their problems at home," the women owners frequently reported that they "take on" their employees' personal troubles. For many of the women in this study, espousal of this "parental" role sometimes appeared to incur emotional strain, and at times even appeared to compromise the interests of the business (e.g. absences or inefficiencies are tolerated to accommodate employees), which in turn caused further stress. Similar gender differences in management style and in coping styles have been noted in the literature (e.g. Stratham, 1993).

The health implications of such "gendered" management behaviour — for the women owners themselves and for their employees — are not known. For instance, do the contradictions between business goals and human relations strain women's mental well-being more than they do men's? How might women's styles of management affect the health of employees (e.g. are different styles more or less likely to draw attention to the occupational health needs of employees)?

High demands and inability to control the nature and flow of work (which has been linked to cardiovascular and other health outcomes by Karasek, 1990; and others) is frequently referred to by the small business owners — both men and women — in my studies. For example, they speak of their frustrations getting bank financing, managing fluctuating demand, being "pushed around" by suppliers, never being able to take time off because they have few, if any, supervisory staff. Women owners may experience even less control over their work than do men, as this excerpt from an interview with the owner of a fast food restaurant suggests:

Ninety-five percent of the sales people for companies are men. Well, one man to another, they seem to be able to strike a bargain, or if there's a sale on, he'll phone and let you know. Where, if it's a lady, they kind of ... sometimes they don't give a woman that much consideration.

It would be interesting to know if and how the experience of female owners or managers in small businesses differs from that of women in larger workplaces, and how this experience relates to health. The difficulties associated with role strain and the exercise of authority in women executives and entrepreneurs has been documented in the literature (Greenglass, 1985). Whether the stress associated with these difficulties is the same or different in small work settings is not known. Is it possible, for example, that the organizational culture (usually male defined, as in Marshall, 1993) in such workplaces is more conducive to "feminization," which in turn could make women's styles of working more compatible with prevailing norms, thereby mitigating the associated stress and conflict?

GENDER DIVISION OF LABOUR

The division of labour by gender is evident in small workplaces. As one owner of a delicatessen remarked, "Young men don't seem to want to deal with that much, with food, you know. So ours is more female employees."

Many of the women in my studies (who may not be representative of all small workplace women) work in establishments that engage their knowledge and experience as women and as homemakers: service; food preparation; caretaking; clothing and household retailing; child and other caretaking.

This division of labour has many possible consequences for women's health. One example is the lack of distinction between what women do at work and what they do at home. "I never get to leave this stuff," commented one waitress, adding, "I go home and do the same thing I do at work, only I don't get paid for it." She observed that she found her work very stressful, but that she felt unable to unwind after work. The lack of differentiation between her paid and unpaid work appeared to diminish the value she attributed to her job, and made her resentful of the work she did at home.

A lack of distinction between workplace and home work may also influence the perception of risk in the workplace. For example, owners in one of my studies (Eakin, 1992) tended to dismiss certain risks because they "could happen anywhere." Ironing burns, falls, rashes from cleaning products were often not perceived as work-related because they were not considered uniquely occupational. The association of the risks with domestic life may have contributed to the tendency to overlook or diminish their seriousness as workplace hazards.

Within small workplaces there is also evidence of a gender division of labour. As a woman co-owner of an automotive repair shop explains, "My partner is a mechanic. So I look after the front and he looks after the back." The distinction between "front" and "back" is common in small businesses. The "front" refers to the interface with the customer (reception) and the paper and telephone tasks of the enterprise, while the "back" refers to the shop floor where production/service tasks are carried out. Although, in small workplaces, employees often rotate between front and back (eg. a production worker "helps out at the front" during lunch breaks), women are more often found in the front. The front, however, is often viewed as marginal to the core business. When describing their businesses and their employees, for example, owners would often not include those who worked in the "front."

The health implications of this are that the health needs of such employees are often overlooked. For example, owners rarely identified health "problems" in the "front." Yet, in addition to the hazards of clerical work, these employees were also sometimes exposed to physical and chemical hazards from other parts of the workplace (e.g. paint fumes in autobody shops) and to customers (e.g. stress, violence). The potential hazards confronting "invisible" workers, such as women in the "front," may be unrecognized in many small workplace settings.

THE ROLE OF FAMILY IN SMALL BUSINESSES

The centrality of family to small business is captured in the familiar notion of "mom and pop" enterprises. A very high proportion of small businesses are either run jointly by members of the same family or employ immediate family or relatives (Armstrong, 1991). There is extensive literature on the family business, but the health implications of the role of family involvement in small business have not been addressed. A few possible links are suggested in my data.

A family-related division of labour is common in small businesses. For example, in many companies "the wife" "does the books," and family members help out in times of labour shortage. The role of such family members is often relatively invisible, especially when the work is part-time, or is done at home or after hours. Often, family members are not paid, which compounds some of the paid/unpaid issues noted earlier. This invisibility, however, also means that their health needs are often not recognized, by others and by family workers themselves. When asked about what affected their health at work, many wives in husband/wife business partnerships referred only to hazards they saw for their husbands. They downplayed their own health concerns, or did not acknowledge them at all.

Because women often enter a particular business to "help out" their husbands, they sometimes find themselves in businesses that are heavily male dominated (e.g. trucking, auto repair). The possible health implications of this arrangement for women need to be explored, both in terms of explicit hazards (e.g. sexual harassment, dangers associated with working with equipment designed for men), and in terms of the psychological consequences associated with being in a male-defined organizational culture (Marshall, 1993). It is also possible that women who work for (or with) their husbands, or daughters who work for their parents, may find themselves less free to leave situations of family or marriage-related abuse because of their subordinate status and economic dependency in the business (Neis, personal communication).

Another example of the possible implications for occupational health of "family" is the observation (Eakin, 1992) that the social norms regarding the owner's role in the management of health and safety (e.g. unwillingness to "impose" certain safety behaviours on employees) may be different with family employees. The owner of a construction company, for example, said that although he did not force his other employees to wear a mask when handling insulation, he insisted that his nephew do so. The fact that owners were also more willing to intervene in the case of "green" (inexperienced) workers may reflect the broader social legitimacy of exercising authority in parent/child and teacher/student relationships.

These examples point to the significance of the institution of family on the social relations of production and workplace health and safety. More generally, they are suggestive of how health and safety behaviour is contingent on the social relations in which they are embedded.

THE SIGNIFICANCE OF THE CUSTOMER IN SMALL BUSINESSES

The customer/client is a focal point of most commercial establishments, large and small. In small workplaces, however, the importance of the customer to the well-being of the company is directly apparent to owners and employees. The customer is a symbolic representation of the goals, success and failure of the enterprise. The needs of the customer (hence the business) are often put above the needs of the employees, by both employers and employees. An example of this is the bar waitress who complained of the heavy smoke in the bar, "I smoke without even smoking!" She did not believe anything could be done about this because "ninety percent of the customers smoke." A particular problem for her was a "regular" who smoked cigars, but to whom the owner had given "carte blanche to smoke" because he was a local patron they did not want to lose. Another example is the owner of a drilling rig construction company who, when asked about health and safety problems at work, spoke first of the compliance of their product with public safety standards. He did not, without prompting, think of the health problems of the metal workers producing the product.

An example specifically relevant to women is the report from a lounge waitress that, when customers get rowdy, the "girls" are assigned to serve them because the customers are believed to be less likely to "punch out" a female server. Here the primary consideration is the management of a business problem (in this case a potentially disruptive client) rather than the safety of the employee.

The preeminence of the client also influences employees' perceptions of risk, as illustrated in the following excerpt from an interview with a hairdresser who had just said that some of the chemicals she works with "cause blindness":

Interviewer: Does it ever bother you to be working with things that cause blindness?

Maya: Well, I don't want to cause that to anybody. No, I'm very careful you know. You usually protect the person with cotton around the face.

Here it can be seen that the employee was oriented to the health risks of her client rather than to the threat to herself as a worker.

These examples only hint at the possible health implications of the role of the customer/client in the small workplace setting. Given the observation that women might be more other-oriented (or "nurturant," as in Statham, 1993) than men, are women in small workplaces inclined to put family and customer health considerations ahead of their own?

GENDER AND HEALTH-RELATED BEHAVIOUR

Another way in which employment in small workplaces may affect women's health is through its influence on health-related behaviour: how women think and act with regard to their health.

Gender differences in health behaviour are widely noted in the literature. With respect to occupational health more specifically, Daykin (1990) has noted differences between men and women in terms of how they conceive of occupational risk, with women tending to overlook or downplay problems or hazards that were not stereotypical (male) industrial risks, like falls or dangerous machinery. Evidence of this gender-related perception of risk is evident in my data. For example, a Korean grocery store cashier recounted how painful she found it to have to stand during her whole shift while working at the cash register. She believed that the male stockroom employee did not "understand" her complaints, but hastened to qualify that her work was not as "hard" as was his.

It is not clear how the nature of small business life intersects with gender differences in how occupational health is conceived. How, for example, does the nature of social relations in the workplace (e.g. informal, flexible, non-unionized, shared jobs) promote or discourage the recognition and legitimization of women's perspectives on occupational health?

In my small workplace studies, health behaviour appears in many forms. For example, a bar waitress protected herself from rowdy, potentially dangerous customers through her relations with other customers. She explained:

> It might even be one of my regulars [customer] that'll say "I think there may be a problem over there." It can be taken out of my hands before it even becomes a problem for me. It's almost like an extended staff ... like they don't want to see their bar become a brawling pit, you know.

This woman talked about how important her customers were to her, and about the attention she devotes to maintaining supportive relationships with them. Clearly, one reason for this is that they help ensure her safety at work. This example illustrates the way in which health behaviours are embedded in everyday work experience and go far beyond conventional notions of what constitutes "health behaviour." This is true for all workplaces regardless of size, but since the nature of working life in small workplaces is different from that in larger firms, the forms of health-related behaviour may vary accordingly.

Effort to redress harmful working conditions is another health behaviour that could vary by workplace size. In small workplaces, where workers are not unionized, and where they often work alone or with few others, the opportunities for collective responses to the problems of work are limited. My current research explores the types of actions small workplace employees take in response to perceived occupational risks. Some leave their jobs, some try to change the work situation, while others (often those who are not in a position to do either of the preceding), might engage in private, individual gestures in an attempt to exert some control over working conditions and resist what they perceive to be assaults on their physical and mental well-being. For example, a domestic worker who resented her employer's indifference and lack of respect towards her, and her mistreatment by the children, retaliated by using the children's toothbrushes to clean the toilets just before quitting! This, she explained, was "just to get even, just to feel better."

These are examples of the diversity of occupational health behaviours, and of possible ways in which gender and small organizational size might intersect in relation to these behaviours. For the most part, however, not much is known empirically about these links.

CONCLUSION

I have argued that the social conditions of work in small businesses are not the same as those in larger workplaces, that these conditions have consequences for the health and safety of workers in general and women in particular, and that health issues are embedded in the daily work experiences of both owner/managers and employees.

Research is needed to identify the nature and magnitude of these problems and to guide our efforts to promote the health of such a large but "hard to reach" group of working women. Priorities should be established that reflect the practical opportunities for intervention and change in the small workplace sector.

For economic and other reasons, the improvement of working conditions in hundreds of thousands of small worksites cannot be achieved through continuous direct provision of professional services to individual worksites. Instead, ways must be found to promote change from within, including: (1) increasing awareness of health issues in such settings (both by increasing awareness of professionally defined problems and by helping workers to articulate local knowledge of occupational risks to health); (2) creating the circumstances and supports necessary for small business owners to develop the will and the means to address health and safety issues (e.g increasing their recognition of legal responsibility and of the links between the health of employees and the "bottom line") (Shain and Eakin, unpublished); (3) developing internal organizational mechanisms for employee participation in the organization of work and in health promotion that are appropriate to and feasible within the small business context; and (4) finding ways of "empowering" small business employees to initiate change in the workplace without incurring the devastating personal consequences of individual action (consequences that are evident in my current study of employees).

In achieving these goals, we need to move beyond rather stereotypical thinking to consider what else, besides financial considerations, "motivates" small business owners to address health issues at work, or "impedes" them from taking effective action. We need to identify forms of participation that are native to small work settings and determine what means of promoting them might be compatible with the particular contingencies of small workplace life. We need to identify existing forms of formal and informal employee control over work within the social structure of small workplaces, and learn more about the kind of support employees need if they, rather than owners (on whom most attention is focused, Eakin and Weir, 1995), are to address health and safety problems in their workplaces.

In taking on these general challenges in small workplace health, researchers must develop a framework that takes specific account of women employees. Paying attention to the perspectives of women and to gender issues in small workplaces could not only further the women's occupational health agenda, but also further understanding of an important emerging concern in the larger field of occupational health — the relationship between health and the social organization of work.

REFERENCES

Adler, N. "An International Perspective on the Barriers to the Advancement of Women Managers." *Applied Psychology: An International Review* 42, 4 (1993). pp. 289-300.

ARA. *A Report to the Occupational Health and Safety Education Authority: Needs Assessment Survey* 1. Toronto: ARA, 1987.

Armstrong, P. "Under 10's: Small Establishments in the Private Sector." Unpublished draft report. Toronto: Ministry of Labour for Ontario, February, 1991.

Curran, J., and J. Stanworth. "Worker Involvement and Social Relations in the Small Firm." *Sociological Review* 27, 2 (1979). pp. 317-43.

Daykin, N. "Health and Work in the 1990s: Towards a New Perspective," in *New Directions in the Sociology of Health*, P. Abbott and G. Payne (eds.). London, New York, Philadelphia: Falmer Press, 1990. pp. 153-64.

Eakin, J. "Leaving it Up to the Workers: Sociological Perspective on the Management of Health and Safety in Small Workplaces." *International Journal of Health Services* 22 (1992). pp.689-704.

Eakin, J., and N. Weir. "Canadian Approaches to the Promotion of Health in Small Workplaces." *Canadian Journal of Public Health* 86, 2 (1995). pp. 109-13.

Evans, J. *Summary Report, Workshop on Improving Occupational Health and Safety at Small Employer Work Sites.* Edmonton, Alberta: Government of Alberta, 1984.

Greenglass, E. "Psychological Implications of Sex Bias in the Workplace." *Academic Psychology Bulletin* 7 (1985). pp. 227-39.

Heath, E. "Worker Training and Education in Occupational Safety and Health: A Report on Practice in Six Industrialized Western Nations." *Journal of Safety Research* 13, 4. pp. 157-62.

Industrial Accident Prevention Association (IAPA). *Accident Characteristics for Small Firms.* Toronto: IAPA, 1986.

Karasek, R., and T. Theorell. *Healthy Work.* New York: Basic Books, 1990.

MacKinnon, B. *Work-Related Injuries and Illnesses: Small Employers 1977-1985.* Edmonton, Alberta: Occupational Health and Safety Division, Government of Alberta, 1987.

Marshall, J. "Organizational Cultures and Women Managers: Exploring the Dynamics of Resilience," *Applied Psychology: An International Review* 42, 4 (1993). pp. 313-22.

Neis, B. Personal communication. Memorial University, Newfoundland.

Rutsohn, P., M. Schoolfield and M. McLeod. "Comprehensive Occupational Health: Is it Beyond the Reach of Small Businesses?" *Journal of Small Business Management* (April, 1981). pp. 52-60.

Shain, M., and J. Eakin. *Health, Safety and the Bottom Line: A Study of the Owner\Operators of Small Businesses.* Toronto: Addiction Research Foundation and the North York Community Health Promotion Research Unit, 1994a.

Shain, M., J. Eakin, H. Suurvali and H. and A. Currie. *Dealing with Substance Abuse in Small Businesses: Results of a Qualitative Study.* Interim Report. Toronto: Addiction Research Foundation, 1994b.

Spiegel, J., and A. Yassi. "Community Health Centre-Based Occupational Health Services for the Small Workplace: An Ontario Study of Employer Acceptability." *Canadian Journal of Public Health* 80, 5 (1989). pp. 355-8.

Statham, A. "Examining Gender in Organizational Relationships and Technological Change," in *Women, Work and Coping.* B. Long and S. Kahn (eds.). Montreal: McGill-Queen's Press, 1993.

Statistics Canada. *Canadian Business Patterns Data Base.* Ottawa: Business Registry Master File, Business Registry Division, Statistics Canada, 1992.

Thomas, P. "Safety in Smaller Manufacturing Establishments." *Employment Gazette* (January, 1991). pp. 20-4.

Thompson, P. *Small Business and Job Creation in Canada, 1992.* Toronto: Canadian Federation of Independent Business, 1995. p. 2.

Tuohy, C., and M. Simard. *The Impact of Joint Health and Safety Committees in Ontario and Quebec: A Study Prepared for the Canadian Association of Administrators of Labour Law.* Toronto: Canadian Association of Administrators of Labour Law, 1993.

Tuskes, P., and M. Key. "Potential Hazards in Small Business — A Gap in OSHA Protection." *Applied Industrial Hygiene* 3, 2 (1988). pp. 55-7.

Pat Armstrong

The Feminization of the Labour Force

Harmonizing Down in a
Global Economy

Bien que la participation des femmes au marché du travail se soit accrue de façon spectaculaire et que les femmes aient fait des gains importants, la plupart restent cantonnées dans les postes les moins bien rémunérés, les moins attrayants et les plus précaires. Alors que les hommes continuent à occuper les meilleurs emplois, beaucoup d'emplois traditionnellement masculins ont disparu. En conséquence, les hommes commencent à investir les domaines traditionnellement féminins et leur travail ressemble de plus en plus à celui des femmes.

Although the labour force participation of women has risen dramatically and women have made some important gains, most remain segregated into the lowest paid, least attractive and most precarious labour force work. While men still dominate the best jobs, many of the traditional male jobs have disappeared. As a result, men are moving into traditionally female areas and more of their work is like traditional female work.

INTRODUCTION

In order to understand the particular social, physical and technical barriers to a safe integration of women into the workplace, it is necessary to first understand where women work and how their work differs from that of men. If we look at such measures as participation rates, the proportion of women in traditional male work and in higher education, the gap in wages between women and men, and job tenure, female and male employment patterns have become increasingly similar in recent years. Indeed, it could be said that the labour force is being feminized.

The increasing similarity with men does not necessarily mean improvement for women, however. Women's and men's labour force experiences have become increasingly similar not simply because some women now have the kinds of good jobs traditionally held predominately by men, but also because the labour force work of a growing number of men has become more like that traditionally done by women and because fewer women have alternatives to labour force work. The restructuring that is part of globalization has created more women's work in the market. At the same time, it has eliminated some men's jobs and altered many of the jobs traditionally done by men in ways that make them more like women's work. This kind of feminization of the labour force does not mean that most women's positions have improved but rather that the position of some men has deteriorated. At least part of the increasing similarity between women's and men's work can be explained in terms of a harmonizing down for some men and greater economic pressure on many women. While some women and men do have good labour force jobs, an increasing number of women and men have bad jobs. Some men are responding to this trend by moving into areas where women have traditionally found their best jobs.

This paper explores these processes of feminization and harmonizing down and the associated risks to women's health. It argues that some women have improved their position in the market but many more women do women's work at women's wages and, increasingly, so do some men. Relying primarily on Statistics Canada data, it focuses on the 1990-92 period, because this has been a period of rapid restructuring. However, the limited nature of the data available for the most recent years means that it is often necessary to look at data for an earlier period in order to develop a picture of overall trends. Even with these data, however, it is difficult to develop a picture of differences among women and men based on location, disability and cultural difference.

LABOUR FORCE PARTICIPATION

The dramatic rise in female labour force participation has been amply documented and widely publicized. The steady rise was halted during the 1990s, however, and female labour force participation rates declined between 1990 and 1992. While women's participation rates were rising rapidly, men's were falling slowly. But over the last two years, the rate of decline in male participation has increased. Although women's participation rates decreased by less than one percentage point between 1990 and 1992, men's rates declined by more than two percentage points. The combination of these trends means that the difference between male and female participation rates is decreasing more rapidly than would be the case if men's rates remained stable. Similarly, women's participation in higher education has been rising much more rapidly than that of men, virtually eliminating the difference between the sexes in terms of education. By 1992, almost 6 out of every 10 women over the age of 15 were counted as part of the labour force and this was the case for just over 7 out of 10 men. In that year, 42 percent of the female labour force and 41 percent of the male labour force had completed postsecondary education at either the university or college level (Statistics Canada, 1990 and 1992a: Tables 1 and 5).

Labour force figures include both those with any kind of job in the market and those seeking paid work. This combination of employed and unemployed in one figure can obscure greater differences between the sexes in employment and unemployment experiences. It can also hide differences between the patterns of young people who are still in school and the patterns of those over age 25, who are more likely to seek full-time labour force work. It is therefore useful to examine more specific patterns for women and men as well as for people of different ages. It is not possible from these data to explore patterns for those from different cultural or racial groups, with disabilities or of different immigration status.

Employment patterns indicate a feminization of the labour force and a deterioration in men's position. By 1992, 46 percent of the employed were female. Of those over 25 years of age, 51 percent of the women and 68 percent of the men were officially counted as employed. Just two years earlier, 53 percent of the women and 72 percent of the men in this age group had labour force work. In this two year period, the proportion of young people with employment declined even more. And the decrease was greater for males than for females.

Higher education did not guarantee a job for men or women. Employment declined for those with postsecondary education, regardless of sex or age. The largest drop was for men with postsecondary diplomas or certificates, with employment/population ratios for this group falling from 81 percent to 75 percent. In other words, between 1990 and 1992 the proportion employed declined for both sexes, but it declined more for men than for women and education provided little protection from job loss.

Not surprisingly, the unemployment rate rose significantly for both sexes during this two year period. The largest increase was for young men. However, the unemployment rate rose faster for adult men than for adult women even though more men than women dropped out of the labour force altogether. Indeed, the number of men between the ages of 25 and 65 who left the labour force was five times the number of women. As a result, the number of women and men without paid work became more similar and more men had interrupted employment patterns that were similar to those of women (Statistics Canada, 1990 and 1992a: Table 1).

By 1992, there were 332,000 fewer people with labour force work than was the case in 1990 and overall job loss was almost five times greater for men than for women. But the loss of full-time work was significantly higher than the figures on the net loss indicate. There were 458,000 fewer people with full-time work but 126,000 more people had part-time jobs. The net figure camouflages the fact that much of the new work was part-time. Because men are more likely than women to have full-time jobs, more of them lost full-time work. And because more of women's work is part-time, women took more of the new part-time work. Women's overall loss seems so much less than that of men because many women found part-time work to replace full-time jobs (Statistics Canada, 1990 and 1992a: Table 1).

Part-time work has been, and continues to be, dominated by women. In 1990, 71 percent of part-time workers were women. While there were 125,000 fewer full-time jobs for women in 1992 than was the case in 1990, there were 69,000 more part-time ones. The proportion of employed women with part-time work increased by over one percentage point, leaving more than a quarter of employed women with part-time jobs (Statistics Canada, 1990 and 1992a: Table 18). Given the large loss in full-time jobs, it is not surprising that the proportion of women employed part-time because they did not want full-time work declined sharply, dropping from 39 percent in 1990 to 31 percent in 1992. Put another way, the majority of women in part-time jobs can be classified as "involuntary" part-time workers and their numbers are growing. Fewer and fewer have a choice about taking part-time rather than full-time work.

Although part-time work was still women's work, a rapidly growing number of men could find only part-time employment. The proportion of men working part-time also grew by more than a percentage point during this two year period, with the number of men employed part-time increasing by 57,000. Half of this growth was for men in the 25 to 44 year age group; that is, among the men who have traditionally been the most likely to want and have full-time work. As is the case with women, the proportion employed part-time who did not want full-time work dropped significantly, decreasing from 19 to 15 percent of those employed part-time. But the proportion of women who had little choice increased twice as fast as the proportion of men. In short, more men and even more women found only part-time work and the majority of both sexes did so "involuntarily."

These figures on part-time work refer to all those who usually work less than 30 hours a week, unless they consider themselves full-time. They leave out all those who work for part of a year and thus they overstate the number of people who have full-time work all year. Statistics Canada does not publish data on part-year work in *The Labour Force Survey*, so it is difficult to examine changes between 1990 and 1992. However, data from the Labour Market Activity Survey show both that large numbers of women and men do not have full-year work and that the differences between the sexes are not great. "Sixty-one percent of all women who worked in 1988 were employed the entire year, compared to 69 percent of the men" (Statistics Canada, 1992c: Table 9). Some of these people work for only part of the week, and thus would be classified as part-time. Others work more than 30 hours a week and thus would be counted as full-time even though they are employed only part of the year. Census data indicate that in 1991, almost 40 percent of the men between the ages of 25 and 65 did not work mostly full-time for 49 weeks or more and this was the case for 60 percent of the women (Statistics Canada, 1993b: Table 2). It is clear, then, that many women and quite a few men did not have full-time, full-year work in 1990. And there is every reason to believe that the figures for 1992 would show that the number of part-year workers of both sexes increased in 1992 as more jobs involved short-term contract or temporary work.

In sum, unemployment and both part-time and part-year employment have been growing for both sexes. Women's job loss was smaller, in part because women captured more of the new part-time work, even though most of the women taking the part-time jobs did not do so by choice. With men's labour market position deteriorating more rapidly than that of women in some areas, women's and men's employment patterns became more similar. Another part of the explanation for women's smaller job loss can be found in the nature of the new jobs that did appear during this period, as will become evident in the next section.

INDUSTRIAL RESTRUCTURING

Over the last three decades, employment in all industrialized countries has grown rapidly in service industries and declined in the others (Akyeampong and Winters, 1993). Between 1990 and 1992, job loss in the Canadian goods-producing industries was 25 times that in the service-producing industries. Put another way, 96 percent of the employment loss was in primary industries, in manufacturing, construction and utilities (Statistics Canada, 1993a: Table A16).

For the purposes of the analysis presented here, this restructuring in employment is important for two reasons. First, most of the jobs in the goods-producing industries are male jobs and most of those in the service producing industries are female jobs. Second, many of the new jobs in the service sector are what the Economic Council terms "bad" jobs — jobs that offer little security, little opportunity for promotion, little economic reward and require few recognized skills (Economic Council of Canada, 1990).

Goods-producing Industries

Given that just over 75 percent of those employed in the goods-producing industries are men, it is not surprising that three-quarters of the full-time jobs lost in the goods-producing industries were men's jobs. Nor is it surprising that it was in these sectors where most of the male job loss occurred. More than four out of five full-time jobs lost to men were in the goods-producing industries. These jobs did not disappear for men because women entered the labour force and took male jobs. Their disappearance was part of a major reorganization of employment in the market, as some operations shut down and others introduced new technologies and work structures.

This is not to suggest that there was no impact on women's jobs in these industries. Almost two-thirds of the women employed in goods-producing industries were employed in manufacturing and women in these industries saw their unemployment rate rise by three percentage points between 1990 and 1992. Significantly more women than men lost jobs in the manufacturing industries (171,000 women compared to 149,000 men), even though women accounted for less than a third of those employed in these industries. Moreover, men took just over half of the new part-time jobs, even though they accounted for only 44 percent of the part-time workers in these industries. As a result, the proportion of men employed part-time in these industries increased by a full percentage point (Statistics Canada 1990 and 1992a). Most of this female job loss would be among immigrant women, given that they account for more than two-fifths of the women working in product manufacturing (Badets and McLaughlin, 1989:40).

Rising male unemployment, then, is to a large extent explained by the decline in the goods-producing industries that men dominate, rather than by competition from women. Indeed, when women and men do compete, it is women who are more likely to lose their jobs. Although many men's jobs in these sectors were not necessarily good jobs in the sense of requiring high levels of education, providing non-repetitive work or offering significant opportunities for promotion, many were covered by strong unions and paid relatively high wages. In fact, most unionized men worked in industries in the goods-producing sector.

Service-producing Industries

Even during the recession of the 1990s, employment continued to grow in the service-producing industries. The very large service sector where more than 70 percent of all labour force workers are employed includes a wide range of jobs, many of which may be considered good jobs according to a number of criteria (Economic Council of Canada, 1991: Chapter 2). But many of them fit the Economic Council's definition of "bad" jobs. Within the service sector, employment is divided into three relatively equal parts: traditional service industries, non-commerical industries and "dynamic" services. And within each of these sectors, there are both "good" and "bad" jobs, although the most attractive work is more concentrated in some industries.

Lower-tier Industries; Traditional Services

In his study *The Quality of Work in the Service Sector*, Krahn (1992:15) shows that by 1989 a third of the service workers were employed in what he terms lower-tier services. Jobs in the lower tier were unlikely to have fringe benefits or to be unionized and were most likely to be done by women and young men. A Statistics Canada survey found that "Workers in the lower-tier services, especially those in non-standard jobs, typically reported lower skill requirements and a greater mismatch between their education and job. They were also more likely to say they were overqualified for their job, and were less likely to agree that their job was good" (Krahn, 1992:16). In other words, they were "bad" jobs.

What is meant by lower-tier industries are the retail trades and commercial personal service industries. Although the kind of detailed data necessary to examine the changes in these industries between 1990 and 1992 is not published annually by Statistics Canada, it is possible to look at trends between 1976 and 1991 and, in this way, get some idea about what may be happening in the 1990s.

Employment grew in the retail trades over this 15 year period but it fell by just over 50,000 jobs between 1990 and 1991. It declined because sales declined. Sales declined because work was reorganized to make each employee work harder and because new technologies replaced workers. In both 1976 and 1991, retail trade accounted for 13 percent of labour force workers (see Table 1).

According to Statistics Canada, "In 1991, youth, adult men and women shared the number of jobs in Retail Trade almost equally," although most of the youth and a third of the adult women had part-time work and this was the case for only five percent of adult men (Statistics Canada, 1992a: Table A6). But these groups did not share equally in the jobs lost and gained. Between 1990 and 1991, 52,000 fewer people had full-time work while 1,000 more had part-time employment in retail. Adult men accounted for almost half of the full-time job loss but they took far more than their share of new part-time work. Men's greater full-time job loss is largely explained by their domination of the full-time workforce and by their distribution within the retail sector, rather than by competition from women. Men, for example, account for 80 percent of those in automotive sales and close to 40 percent of men employed in retail trades work in these trades. Men lost jobs here mainly as a result of restructuring and the recession.

Table 1   Industrial Employment Changes in Canada, 1990-1992

	Full-time	Part-time
Both sexes	-458	+126
Goods-producing industries	-355	+37
Service-producing industries	-102	+90
Agriculture	-1	+5
Other primary industries	-28	+2
Manufacturing	-222	+9
Construction	-117	+20
Transportation	-38	+9
Trade	-86	-6
TradeFinance, insurance and real estate	+7	+2
Service	+23	+86
Public administration	+4	0
Unclassified	n/a	n/a

Calculated from: Statistics Canada, *Labour Force Annual Averages 1990*, Ottawa: Minister of Supply and Services Canada, February 1991; and Statistics Canada, *Labour Force Annual Averages 1992*, Ottawa: Minister of Industry, Science and Technology, February 1993a.

Women were more likely to be found in food stores and in general merchandise stores. Sales remained fairly strong in these retail sectors, although here, too, technology was beginning to have an impact and helped account for the loss of 3,000 full-time jobs for adult women, and 5,000 part-time ones (Statistics Canada, 1992a: Tables 2, 3 and 4).

Commercial personal service industries provide a greater share of the labour force employment than do the retail trades. Jobs in these industries increased from 14 percent of the labour force in 1976 to 17 percent in 1991. Overall employment did not decline in these industries between 1990 and 1991 although full-time employment decreased by 31,000. But all of this job loss was among youth and adult women. Full-time employment for adult men increased by 4,000 while 10,000 full-time jobs for adult females disappeared. Part-time work increased for adults of both sexes, although almost twice as many women found only part-time work (Statistics Canada, 1992a: Tables 2, 3 and 4).[1] And these figures do not include the growing number of workers employed full-time on temporary work contracts. Estimates indicate that 13 percent of those working in these industries have jobs with a specific end date (Krahn, 1991:38). Here, too, the variations in patterns for women and men reflect the segregation and restructuring of the market more than they reflect competition between the sexes for jobs.

Employment, especially for women, has grown significantly in the lower-tier industries since 1976. However, between 1990 and 1991, full-time jobs disappeared and more part-time work appeared. And these were the sectors that already had the highest proportion of part-time work. Adult men's full-time job loss was greater than women's in retail trades but adult men captured more of the new part-time work. In the growing commercial personal service industries, however, more men found full-time work while a large number of women lost full-time jobs. As a result, male and female employment patterns became more similar.

Upper-tier Industries: Noncommercial Services

Over this five year period, employment grew more in the noncommercial services than it did in the commercial ones. By 1991, jobs in health, social services and education accounted for almost a quarter of service sector jobs. If jobs in public administration are included, these services employ a third of all those with service jobs in 1991. These jobs were particularly important for women, given that adult women form the overwhelming majority of workers in these industries and that women have traditionally found many of their best jobs here. Many of the jobs require high levels of formal education and for this reason may be classified as highly skilled (Economic Council of Canada, 1991:93). And women who work in these industries are much more likely than other women to be unionized and are much more likely than other women to benefit from affirmative action programmes (National Union of Provincial Government Employees,

1989). Many of the jobs here fit the Economic Council's criteria for "good" jobs.

Of the new full-time jobs created in health, social services and education between 1990 and 1991 for those over age 25, 56 percent went to women. However, women accounted for more than 70 percent of the adult workforce in these industries. Men, then, captured much more than their share of new full-time work. The picture was different in public administration, however, where more adult women found full-time work and more adult men lost full-time jobs (see Table 2).

Table 2 Employment Change For Adult Women and Men, Service Producing Industries, 1990-1991

Occupation	Full-time		Part-time	
	Men	Women	Men	Women
Total employment	-120	-14	+28	+36
Goods-producing industries	-105	-24	+10	+8
Service-producing industries	-16	+10	+18	+28
Transportation and communication	-19	-3	+3	+3
Trade	-42	-3	+5	-4
Wholesale trade	-18	0	+3	+1
Retail trade	-24	-3	+3	-5
Finance, insurance and real estate	+10	-8	-1	+6
Community, business and personal services	+41	+16	+11	+25
Community services	+14	-13	+9	+8
Amusement and recreation	0	-2	+2	-2
Services to business management	+10	-3	+5	+1
Personal and household services	-1	-2	0	+1
Accomodation, food and beverage services	+1	-6	+1	+7
Miscellaneous services	+3	-1	+2	+1
Non-commercial services	+27	+30	+3	+17
Education	+4	+16	0	+8
Health and social services	+25	+21	+3	+12
Religious organizations	-3	-7	0	-2
Public administration	-5	+7	-1	-2

Calculated from: Statistics Canada, *Labour Force Annual Averages 1991*, (Ottawa: Minister of Industry, Science and Technology, February 1992a).

Women were much more successful than men in acquiring the new part-time jobs appearing in health and education. While 20,000 more adult women worked part-time in these industries, this was the case for only 3,000 more men. All of these part-time jobs for adult men were in health and social services. But adult women account for more than 90 percent of the part-time workers and therefore they got less than their share of new part-time work. In public administration, part-time jobs disappeared for both sexes, although twice as many women as men lost such work. In this industry, men experienced more part-time job loss than their numbers would suggest. And here, too, the figures on part-time work do not include those who work full-time on temporary contracts. Estimates indicate that one in ten jobs in health, education and social service is temporary (Krahn, 1991:38).

In sum, employment increased in health, social services and education, and more of the jobs were full-time rather than part-time. And more of the additional jobs went to women rather than to men. But there are at least two reasons to be cautious about assessing these trends as positive and permanent gains for women.

First, men took a much greater share of the new jobs than their traditional numbers would warrant. Second, new state initiatives are threatening jobs in these industries, eliminating some, privatizing others and transforming others into "bad" jobs in terms of security, wages, responsibility, power and skill. The trend towards privatization was evident between 1990 and 1991, when more three-quarters of the additional work in health and social services did not result from an increase in those paid directly by a government agency. Two-thirds of them were for private paid workers and another 10 percent were for self-employed workers. Only one in five new jobs were government-paid. In education, a quarter of the new jobs were not for state employees and, and if the federal government's proposals for education reform are implemented, even more will be privatized in the future (Human Resources Development Canada, 1994). Private paid jobs are less likely to be unionized, secure and well paid than are state sector jobs. They are more likely to be "bad" jobs. And so are many of the jobs for the self-employed, as we shall see in a later section. It should be noted, however, that the income of these private paid and self-employed workers may still come from tax dollars through state purchased services. The impact of new government initiatives designed to reduce payrolls and increase state control is too recent to examine through labour force data, but there is every reason to believe the impact will be greatest on women, given that they form the overwhelming majority of the workforce here.

Nor is there reason to be optimistic about jobs in public administration. Although women may have captured some of the new work as a result of affirmative action programmes, the segregation of the public administration workforce suggests that male job loss is much more likely to be the result of reorganization than of competition from women. And female job gain is much more likely to to be the result of new taxes which increased the need for clerical workers than of women taking male managerial work (Task Force on Barriers to Women in the Public Service, 1990). Moreover, privatization may mean that men are receiving more public sector work as private sector consultants, a process that is impossible to monitor from labour force survey data. And, finally, further downsizing will doubtless eliminate more women's work and may reduce their opportunities for promotion.

Upper-tier Industries: Dynamic Services

Industries involved with distribution (transportation and communications, and wholesale trade) and with servicing businesses (finance, insurance and real estate, and services to business management) make up the rest of the service sector. The Economic Council classifies them as "dynamic" services because they "are high-value-added industries that, for the most part, have become more and more involved in globally competitive markets" (Economic Council of Canada, 1991:8-9). High-value-added does not necessarily mean "good" jobs, however. While there are certainly some well-paid and challenging jobs here, many of the jobs in distribution involve repetitive work with low educational requirements and many of those who provide services to business do repetitive clerical work. Those who hold the good and bad jobs in distribution industries are mainly men and almost all those who do the clerical work are women. Together, these industries provide employment for almost a third of the labour force.

Being competitive and high-value-added does not necessarily mean creating more jobs either. Full-time employment in the distribution industries declined by 60,000 between 1990 and 1992. Men dominated these industries and over half of the full-time jobs lost were lost to adult men, although a significant number of adult women also lost full-time work. New part-time jobs did appear and men over age 25 took the majority of new part-time work, even though women formed the majority of part-time workers (see Table 2).

Employment did increase between 1990 and 1991 in those industries providing service to business. All of the new full-time work went to men over age 25. Both the number of young people and the number of women employed full-time declined significantly. While 20,000 more adult men found full-time work, 11,000 fewer adult women and 6,000 fewer young people had full-time jobs. The net gain in full-time jobs was very small.

Most of the new work in the "dynamic industries" was part-time. Adult women accounted for more than half of the new part-time workers. Adult men took a third of the new part-time jobs but such men had accounted for less than 20 percent of the part-time workers in 1991. In other words, men gained over adult women and young people of both sexes, although more adult men had only part-time work. The "dynamic" services that are defined by the Economic Council as the leading edge in the global economy did provide a limited number of new full-time jobs for men but they left many women and some men in a worse position in terms of full-time work.

These detailed data on industries indicate some clear patterns. Many full-time jobs disappeared in the goods-producing industries as well as in retail and the distributive trades, but new part-time work appeared. New full-time and part-time jobs were created in education, public administration, health and social services and in those industries providing services to business. Only one of these industries is primarily in the private sector.

Although full-time job loss was greatest for young people, a much higher proportion of adult men than adult women lost work. These men lost work to a large extent because jobs disappeared in the goods-producing industries that men dominate. In some cases, full-time jobs were replaced by part-time ones and more of these new jobs went to men. As a result, male part-time employment became more similar to that of women. In the service-producing industries, adult men lost jobs in retail and in distributive trades, in areas that they dominate. In both industries, men took more than their share of new part-time work. Adult men also took more than their share of new full-time and part-time work in both commercial and non-commercial services — areas where many of the "good" jobs are found.

So, while many men lost full-time jobs or replaced them with part-time work, men were more successful than women in capturing new full-time employment in areas where women traditionally found their best jobs. The only exception to this trend was public administration, where women gained and men lost full-time work and men did not acquire significantly more part-time work. This is the only area where significant numbers of women may be successfully competing with men for jobs; and the jobs in public administration are currently under threat. Most of the increasing similarity in men's and women's labour force work can be accounted for by losses to men that had nothing to do with women. The losses can be explained primarily by the restructuring of the labour force.

OCCUPATIONAL RESTRUCTURING

Men's and women's jobs are becoming more similar because many of the good jobs traditionally dominated by men are not so good any more. It is not possible to do a detailed analysis of changes in occupations for the 1990s because only the Census, carried out every five years, publishes information on very specific occupational categories. But by combining information from a variety of sources it is possible to offer an indication of trends in the managerial, administrative, professional and technical occupations that are often considered the most highly skilled and, therefore, the best jobs (Economic Council of Canada, 1991:93). Between 1990 and 1992, this broad occupational category accounted for all the full-time job growth in Canada and a great deal of the new part-time work (see Table 3).

Table 3 Occupational Employment Changes in Canada, 1990-1992

Occupation	Full-time	Part-time
Both sexes	-458	+126
Managerial and other professional	+80	+30
Clerical	-141	+26
Sales	-1	0
Service	-38	+44
Primary occupations	-19	+5
Processing, machining and fabricating	-180	+4
Construction	-117	+2
Transport equipment operating	-33	+8
Material handling and other crafts	-8	-1
Unclassified	n/a	n/a

Calculated from: Statistics Canada, *Labour Force Annual Averages 1990*, (Ottawa: Minister of Supply and Services Canada, February 1991); and Statistics Canada, *Labour Force Annual Averages 1992*, (Ottawa: Minister of Industry, Science and Technology, February 1993a).

The fact that women took the majority of new jobs in this broad occupational group is often understood to be a sign of real progress. But a more detailed analysis of the many occupations within this category suggests a more complicated trend. For example, the number of women in the managerial and administrative category, an occupational classification that is part of the larger managerial group, increased between 1990 and 1992. At the same time, the number of male managerial jobs decreased. But even this category contains a wide range of jobs, many of which are highly sex-segregated. And not all of them could be considered "good" jobs. A third of the additional work was in what Statistics Canada classifies as "other managers and administrators." This category primarily covers managers in very small enterprises or at junior levels where jobs are the least secure and the least well-paid. Many of the jobs in other management categories were not highly rewarded or full-time.

Census data indicate that the number of men employed as senior managers and other senior officials, another occupational group within the managerial and administrative category, dropped by more than 15,000 between 1985 and 1990. At the same time, the number of women grew by less than 10,000. Clearly, fewer men did this kind of work but they were not all being replaced by women. Much of the male job loss reflected the shut-downs and the flattened hierarchies that are part of the new global strategy. There is additional evidence that demonstrates women were not taking the top male jobs. The average salary for women in such jobs was only $40,633 in 1990, compared to an average of $71,349 for men in these jobs and of $38,648 for all men employed full-time. Equally important, more than one in five of the women gaining new employment in this occupation did not have full-time, full-year work (Statistics Canada, 1993c: Table 1).

Similarly, the largest group within the other managers and administrators category is comprised of sales and advertising management occupations. Women took most of the new work here but the average salary for full-time female managers in this category was close to the average for all women and more than $10,000 less than that for all men who work full-time. Women employed full-time got only 60 percent of what men in the same group earned and close to a third had only part-time work and part-time pay. Obviously, with salaries averaging less than $27,000 a year in 1990 and much of the work part-time, these were not the "good" jobs often associated with the term "management" (Statistics Canada, 1993c: Table 1).

In another group within the managerial and administrative category — financial management occupations — jobs grew for both sexes, although women took more of the additional work. However, over 60 percent of the men taking new work found full-time jobs while this was the case for less than 15 percent of the women. And the salaries of women employed full-time in these occupations were, at $36,728, considerably below that of both all men and of the men in these financial management occupations, who averaged $59,416. Together, these figures suggest that the jobs women got in management were not necessarily the good ones men used to have; rather, they suggest fewer of the "good" jobs men used to have existed.

Research by Boyd, Mulvihill and Myles (1991:428) supports this claim. They conclude that "women rarely are supervisors or managers of men although men rule over both men and women. Census data indicate that the inroads of women into management are primarily at the lower rungs. Both census and survey results also show that gender differences in access to management and supervisory positions are largest in those service industries where women are in a majority." Growth in the service industries has been concentrated in areas where women work, so it is not surprising that women took more of the management jobs.

In the other, professional jobs that make up this broad category, employment increased between 1990 and 1992 for both women and men in proportions that matched their share of jobs in these occupations. But here, too, greater detail suggests more complex processes at work. Men took all the new jobs in natural science and women's employment declined in this male-dominated work. In the female-dominated social sciences, men gained almost as many new jobs as women, taking more than their share of the jobs. In teaching, men took almost half the new jobs even though they made up just over a third of the teachers. And while 80 percent of those in medicine and health occupations are women, men took well over half of the new jobs. In short, more men were moving into women's occupations and more women were doing traditional women's work.

Within each of these professional categories, much of the growth was in the jobs at the bottom of the hierarchy, in jobs traditionally dominated by women. In health, for example, jobs for nursing supervisors and for registered nursing assistants and orderlies declined significantly between 1985 and 1990 while jobs for nursing attendants and for those in related assisting occupations accounted for more than two out of every five new jobs in nursing work. A third of the additional work in the entire health professional category went to technicians, opticians, denturists and nutritionists — those in the "other occupations related to medicine" category. So, for instance, there were eight times as many new jobs for dental hygienists as there were for dentists but both jobs were counted as part of the growth in professional work. Together, the nursing attendants, other assistants and the various technician categories accounted for more than half of the overall job growth in health professions.

Women account for over three-quarters of the workers in these jobs, although men took a significant share of the new work (Statistics Canada, 1993c).

Of course, women increased their share of jobs in such professions as pharmacy, medicine and law. But more women in these jobs did not necessarily put men out of work, given that the overwhelming majority of those working in these professions are self-employed. Moreover, women's movement into these professions has coincided with changes in the work that make it more like women's work. Take pharmacy, for example. By 1986, a majority of pharmacists were women. But the growing number of female pharmacists were employees, rather than employers or self-employed professionals, as small drug stores were taken over by large corporations and as more hospitals hired their own druggists. Work became more repetitive as drug companies increasingly prepackaged the required mix and dosage. Moreover, although there were 3,600 more pharmacists in 1990 than there were in 1985, two-fifths of them did not have full-time, full-year work. Female pharmacists working full-time, full-year made little more than the overall average male wage and more than $14,000 less than male pharmacists, an income that reflects their status as employees (Statistics Canada, 1993c). Similar patterns are becoming evident in medicine and law (Armstrong and Armstrong, 1992; Phipps, 1990).

Certainly some of the new managerial and professional work provides "good" jobs. But the growth in these occupations and the significant increases in women's employment here do not simply indicate absolute gains for women. They also reflect a restructuring that is eliminating many of the good managerial jobs men held and transforming some professional work in ways that make it more similar to traditional women's work. In the process, men's work has become more similar to women's work and more men are taking on jobs in areas traditionally dominated by women.

HOURS OF WORK

Data on hours of work provide another indication of how women's and men's work is becoming more similar, and how some of this similarity reflects a deterioration in jobs for both sexes.

We have already seen that many more of the new jobs are part-time or part-year and that this is increasingly the case in what have often been classified as "good" jobs. More adult men and adult women found only part-time and part-year work and men's share of part-time work has been increasing in recent years. Part-time work not only means less pay and little security, it can also mean working shifts. "About 6 in 10 part-time employees are shift workers, and the majority of them do not have regular schedules" (Sunter, 1993:19). And even though the majority of part-time shift workers were young, adult women accounted for a third of all these workers and a growing number of adult men had such work. Women of all ages were less likely than men to have pre-arranged schedules. Shift work, especially when the hours are irregular, make it more difficult to organize family and social life.

At the same time as more people have reduced hours per week and weeks per year, those with full-time jobs are working longer hours. Between 1975 and 1990, the proportion of full-time workers who worked long hours increased much faster than did the proportion who worked full-time. Although three-quarters of those with long workweeks were men, the proportion with long workweeks rose much more rapidly for women than for men, thus reducing the gap between the sexes.

Traditionally, long workweeks have been most common for the men employed in primary industries where work is very long in some seasons and quite short in others. But the men working in fishing, mining, logging and farming cannot explain much of the recent increase in long work-weeks, given that their jobs have been disappearing. What is happening is that more and more of those in the "good" jobs are working long hours. According to Statistics Canada (Cohen, 1992:10), "the incidence of long workweeks for workers with university degrees (19 percent) was double the rate recorded for workers with other levels of educational attainment" and "climbed considerably for teachers (from 14 percent to 20 percent) as well as for managers and administrators (from 11 percent to 17 percent)." It is not surprising then, that as the number of university educated women, and of women teachers and managers increases, so do women's weekly work hours. And most of these women have another job at home or have had to give up marriage and children in order to accommodate their labour force work (Armstrong and Armstrong, 1994: Chapter 3).

Not only are those in the good jobs working more hours but more of them are working shifts. And the "vast majority of both male and female full-time shift workers felt that they had no control over their work schedules" (Sunter, 1993:18). As Sunter (1993:22) points out, the future is "likely to hold more of the same" as the pressure to be more productive increases and as services are supplied more at the customer's convenience. The new technologies that make it possible to work around the clock and around the world also increase the likelihood that more of those in the "good" jobs will work both long hours and irregular shifts.

SELF-EMPLOYMENT

Self-employment has grown significantly since 1975 and this, too, is often taken as a sign of an increase in "good" jobs (Crompton, 1993:24). But most of the self-employed are "own-account" workers — "that is, self-employed individuals who do not themselves have employees" (Economic Council of Canada, 1991:79). Such workers tend to have either very long or quite short hours and to have lower wages than paid workers. Many have little choice about the kind of work they take and they are not eligible for most benefits (Armstrong, 1989:12-13; Cohen, 1988).

In the past, most self-employed workers were men in the primary sector or in construction, and most worked full weeks. By the end of the 1980s, two-thirds of the self-employed own-account workers were in service industries (Economic Council of Canada, 1991:80). A growing number were women and many of them sewed or sold clothes in their own homes, did wordprocessing or gave massages, looked after other people's children or did housekeeping (Crompton, 1993:25). "Among women, 40 percent worked part-time, and almost two-thirds were in traditional services in 1989" (Cohen, 1988:80). Two out of five of them did clerical work (Cohen, 1988:80). In 1991, women in unincorporated businesses averaged 55 percent of men's average income (Crompton, 1993:31). And most self-employed women were not incorporated.

It is not possible from published Labour Force Survey data to examine the detailed trends in the 1990s but it is possible to get some idea of overall patterns. Between 1990 and 1992, self-employment grew by 56,000 and 57 percent of this increase was in unincorporated businesses (Statistics Canada, 1990 and 1992a: Table 13). According to the Economic Council (1991:79), about 90 percent of own-account self-employed workers are unincorporated. This kind of self-employment declined in primary sector industries and increased in manufacturing, finance and services. Two-thirds of the increase was in the service industries and almost three-quarters of these additional self-employed were women.

While some of these women may be choosing to work for themselves, it seems likely that most of this increase is the result of contracting out to homeworkers or of the transformation of permanent jobs into contract jobs. By 1992, the proportion of women and men with self-employment became more similar, to a large extent because women accounted for most of the new own-account self-employed. More women also incorporated businesses. However, the increase was much smaller than that for unincorporated businesses and much smaller for women than for men.

MULTIPLE JOB HOLDING

The 1990s saw a reversal in the trend towards multiple job holding (Krahn, 1991:40) and an increasing similarity between women and men in terms of holding more than one job. Between 1990 and 1992, the number of men holding more than one job decreased by 18,000 and the number of women multiple job holders increased by 6,000. The number of multiple job holders decreased in manufacturing, construction and transportation as jobs became more difficult to find. And they increased in service industries. In other words, they increased in female-dominated areas and decreased in male dominated ones (Statistics Canada 1990 and 1992a: Table 25). It seems likely that restructuring was making it more difficult for men to find extra work and more necessary for women to take on more than one job, given that more women found only part-time jobs.

Among occupations, multiple job holding increased in the management and professional category, in sales and in service. There may be many reasons for this increase but certainly the fact that much of the job increase was concentrated in part-time employment would be a factor in both encouraging people to take more than one job and in making more than one job available. Much of the growth in part-time work in these areas was for women and this may explain why more of them took more than one job.

WAGES

Wage data provide one of the clearest demonstrations of the central argument made in this paper: that women's gains are at least as much a result of the deterioration of men's jobs as they are the result of real improvements in women's position and that this deterioration is mainly the result of restructuring rather than of competition from women.

When the 1991 wage data were released in 1993, a great deal of attention was paid to the significant decline in the wage gap. Between 1990 and 1991, the female to male earnings ratio increased to 70 percent from 68 percent for full-time, full-year workers (Statistics Canada, 1993d:7). Women's wages were up two percent, even after adjusting for inflation.

But a closer examination of wage differences suggest both that women's gains were not made at the expense of men and that women's gains may be not only limited but temporary. Wage patterns over the last seven decades show major differences in male and female gains, suggesting that the wages for each sex often change independently. So, for example, while male average wages rose by 16 percent between 1930 and 1940, women's average wages dropped by six percent. In the 1950s, when men's wages grew by 44 percent, women's rose by only 36 percent (Rashid, 1993: Table 1). Men's real average annual wage fell for the first time between 1980 and 1990 (Rashid, 1993:18).

It is this drop in male average income that explains a great deal of the decline in the wage gap. Between 1990 and 1991, the average earnings of male full-time full-year workers dropped by $370 while average earnings for females employed full-year, full-time rose by $517 in constant dollars. Wages fell in male-dominated occupations. Men's actual earnings dropped in materials handling and in forestry and logging, areas where very few women work. Women's average earnings fell in agriculture. In all other areas, men's average actual annual earnings increased. And in teaching, social science and health — all female-dominated areas — male dollar increases were significantly more than those of women. For example, males employed full-time, full-year in medicine gained $13,832 between 1990 and 1992 while women in health occupations added an average of $2,109 to their income. Some of the decline in male averages is also explained by the disappearance of jobs for male senior managers, although in the managerial category as whole male average wages rose by $4,538 and those of women by only $2,683 (Statistics Canada, 1992b; 1993d). Overtime hours for hourly paid workers also declined between 1990 and 1991, and men are much more likely than women to have paid overtime (Perspectives on Labour and Income, 1993:64).

In occupations in the natural sciences, women did gain more than men in terms of dollar increases and this has traditionally been a male-dominated field. However, as we have seen, between 1990 and 1992, men took all the new jobs in natural sciences and women's employment declined. Fewer women have these more highly paid jobs. Moreover, women's overall wage increases were largely accounted for by their jobs in the public sector and these are precisely the jobs targeted for cutbacks in new state initiatives.

There are other indications that women's gains were not largely the result of women taking "good" jobs from men. Between 1990 and 1992, the largest decline in the wage gap was for those with zero to eight years of education. These are the people most likely to work in the primary and manufacturing industries — that is, in the areas where men's unionized jobs disappeared and where new part-time work for men appeared. At the same time, the wage gap increased among those with university degrees — that is, among those most likely to have the "good" jobs and among the women most likely to be directly competing with men for such jobs (Statistics Canada, 1993d: Text Table 1).

The decline in male wages has an impact not only on the wage gap but also on women's choices about paid employment. Decreasing male wages, especially when combined with rising male unemployment, means there is even more pressure on women to provide economic support for their families. Even with most women in the labour force, family income went down between 1989 and 1990 (Statistics Canada, 1993e:9). The largest decline was among young couples, female lone-parent families and two-parent families with one earner. But families with two earners barely held their own and those with more than two-earners saw their incomes decline. Most women, like men, had little alternative to labour force employment.

Women's average income increased relative to that of men, in part because women did different jobs from men and in part because male average wages declined. In 1991, 80 percent of those in the 10 highest paying jobs were men and three-quarters of those in the 10 lowest paying jobs were women. And those women who made it into the top 10 paying occupations averaged 61 percent of male earnings (Statistics Canada, 1993f:11). Clearly, women's average earnings did not rise primarily because they took the high paying jobs away from men.

CONCLUSION

Restructuring for a global economy has meant the disappearance of full-time jobs in all but the noncommercial services and services to business. Jobs disappeared in the primary industries, in construction and manufacturing, in the distributive and wholesale trades — in the areas where men dominate. Almost all of the full-time job growth has been in the public sector, in areas where women dominate. Although men suffered more in terms of full-time job loss, they took more than their share of new full-time and part-time work in the female-dominated areas. In other words, some men are moving into women's traditional areas and successfully competing with women there.

Restructuring is not only eliminating many men's jobs and creating many part-time or part-year ones, it is also transforming many of the full-time jobs that remain. Many of the "good" jobs are not so good any more. Hours and shift work have increased, and so has insecurity. Work is intensified, whether or not people have full-time or part-time employment. Those women who have moved into traditional male work frequently find that it has become more like traditional women's work and management strategies in all sectors frequently serve to reduce workers' power while claiming the opposite. According to Boyd, Mulvihill and Myles (1991:428), the growth in the "service economy not only represents female subordination, but also represents its continuation." The feminization of the labour force has not primarily meant "good" jobs for most women; it has meant more women's work for some men.

Moreover, new state strategies are designed to cut jobs in the non-commercial services, in the areas where women have found their best jobs and where affirmative action has been most successful. Without new jobs in these areas, women's position would be worse than that of men. Once new policies are in place, this is likely to be the case. Privatization has primarily served to create part-time or short-term, non-union jobs. And any new jobs in the "dynamic" industries are likely to be part-time or part-year and are likely to go to men.

Women's and men's work has become more similar mainly because fewer people of both sexes have a choice about the kinds of paid work they take and because more of the jobs are "bad" jobs. Job insecurity, less union representation, less opportunity for promotion or skill development, lower wages, more unemployment and underemployment has come with globalization. Education has not protected workers and affirmative action policies are more and more difficult to implement in a declining economy and with more liberal trade practices.

All of these developments have depressing consequences for women's health. Less job security, along with longer and more varied hours, increase stress enormously. So do lower wages for men that reduce the household income and increase the pressure on women to earn. The limited workplace benefits that accompany part-time employment mean more women work when they are sick. Downsizing means that work is intensified and injuries increase. Self-employment often means combining household and wage work in ways that bring workplace hazards into the home and that constantly place demands on women. Women who hold some of the "good" jobs are under considerable pressure to demonstrate that they are at least as good as the men. Many highly educated women are underemployed in jobs that leave them depressed and insecure. New developments in the economy are exacerbating old threats to women's health while creating new ones.[2]

NOTES

1. Commercial personal services include amusement and recreation, personal and household services, accommodation, food and beverage services, as well as miscellaneous services. Not included among the commercial services discussed here are services to business management. They are excluded because they are identified as dynamic

services by the Economic Council (op. cit.) and are not considered part of a third tier that provides "bad" jobs.

2. Another version of this paper appears in *Rethinking Restructuring: Gender and Change in Canada*, Isabella Baker (ed.), (Toronto: University of Toronto Press, 1995).

REFERENCES

Akyeampong, E., and Jo Winters. "International Employment Trends by Industry." *Perspectives on Labour and Income* 5, 2 (1993). pp. 33-7.

Armstrong, P., "Is There Still a Chairman of the Board?" *The Journal of Management Development* 8, 6 (1989). pp. 118-35.

Armstrong, P., and H. Armstrong. "Sex and the Professions in Canada." *Journal of Canadian Studies* 27, 1 (1992). pp. 118-35.

— *The Double Ghetto: Canadian Women and Their Segregated Work.* Toronto: McClelland & Stewart, 1994.

Badets, J., and N. McLaughlin. "Immigrants in Product Manufacturing." *Perspectives on Labour and Income* 1, 3 (1989). pp. 39-48.

Boyd, M., M.A. Mulvihill and J. Myles. "Gender, Power and Post Industrialism." *Canadian Review of Sociology and Anthropology* 28, 4 (1991). pp. 407-36.

Cohen, J. *Enterprising Canadians.* Ottawa: Supply and Services Canada, 1988.

— "Hard at Work." *Perspectives on Labour and Income* 4, 2 (1992). pp. 9-12.

Crompton, S. "The Rennaissance of Self-Employment." *Perspectives on Labour and Income* 5, 2 (1993). pp. 23-6.

Economic Council of Canada. *Good Jobs, ad Jobs: Employment in the Service Economy.* Ottawa: Economic Council of Canada, 1990.

— *Employment in a Service Economy.* Ottawa: Economic Council of Canada, 1991.

Human Resources Development Canada. *Agenda: Jobs and Growth, Improving Social Security in Canada.* Ottawa: Minister of Supply and Services, 1994.

Krahn, Harvey. "Non-Standard Work Arrangements." *Perspectives on Labour and Income* 3, 4 (1991). pp. 36-8.

— *The Quality of Work in the Service Sector.* Ottawa: Minister of Industry, Science and Technology, 1992.

National Union of Provincial Government Employees (NUPGE). *Canadian Women at Work: Their Situation, Their Union Status and the Influence on the Public Sector.* Ottawa: NUPGE, 1989.

Perspectives on Labour and Income. "Key Labour and Income Facts." *Perspectives on Labour and Income* 5, 1 (1993). pp. 64.

Phipps, P. "Industrial and Occupational Change in Pharmacy," in *Job Queues, Gender Queues.* B. Reskin and P. Roos (eds.). Philadelphia: Temple University Press, 1990.

Rashid, A. "Seven Decades of Wages Changes." *Perspectives on Labour and Income* 5, 2 (1993). pp.17-21.

Statistics Canada. *Labour Force Annual Averages 1989.* Ottawa: Minister of Industry, Science and Technology, 1990.

— *Labour Force Annual Averages 1990.* Ottawa: Minister of Supply and Services, 1991.

— *Labour Force Annual Averages1991.* Ottawa: Minister of Industry, Science and Technology, 1992a.

— *Earnings of Men and Women.* Ottawa: Minister of Industry, Science and Technology, 1992b.

— *Canada's Women.* Ottawa: Minister of Industry, Science and Technology, 1992c.

— *Labour Force Annual Averages 1992.* Ottawa: Minister of Industry, Science and Technology, 1993a.

— *1991 Census: Labour Force Activity.* Ottawa: Minister of Industry, Science and Technology, 1993b.

— *1991 Census: Employment Income by Occupation.* Ottawa: Minister of Industry, Science and Technology, 1993c.

— *Earnings of Men and Women.* Ottawa: Minister of Industry, Science and Technology, 1993d.

— *Family Income: Census Families 1990.* Ottawa: Minister of Industry, Science and Technology, 1993e.

— *The Daily* (April 13, 1993f).

Sunter, D. "Working Shift." *Perspectives on Labour and Income* 5, 1 (1993). pp.18-21.

Task Force on Barriers to Women in the Public Service. *Beneath the Veneer.* Ottawa: Minister of Supply and Services, 1990.

Afterword

This book was inspired by a two-part workshop entitled "Social, Physical and Technical Barriers to the Safe Integration of Women into the Workplace." The networking and contacts that provided the impetus for this workshop originated in the Research Round Table on Gender and Workplace Health held in Ottawa, June, 1992. Organized by the office of Freda Paltiel, Senior Advisor at the Status of Women, Health Canada, this Round Table brought together researchers from across the country with an interest in gender, work and health. Presentations reaffirmed the persistence of sex-segregated work, with women concentrated in lower paying jobs, and challenged the notion that women are in these jobs for their health.

The Round Table facilitated the creation of a network of researchers interested in gender and workplace health. It also highlighted regional differences in the extent and quality of research in this area. In collaboration with Donna Mergler at the Centre pour l'étude des interactions biologiques entre la santé et l'environnement (CINBIOSE), University of Quebec at Montreal (UQAM), and Ellen Balka in Women's Studies at Memorial University, they decided to organize the two-part workshop that generated the papers used as a basis for *Invisible*. The workshop would encourage further networking and research on gender and workplace health, and help to address regional disparities in such research.

The first part of the workshop was held at Memorial University in St. John's in August 1993. Very little research on gender and occupational health has been carried out in Newfoundland and Labrador. Funded by contributions from Social Sciences and Humanities Research Council, the Institute of Social and Economic Research, the Women's Policy Office of the provincial government, the Dean of Arts office, Newfoundland Federation of Labour, and the Provincial Advisory Council, the workshop helped to increase awareness of women's occupational health issues in Newfoundland.

The second part of the workshop was held at the University of Quebec at Montreal in May 1994. Funds for this portion were obtained from the National Health Research and Development Program of Health Canada, Conseil Québécois de Recherche Sociale, UQAM, CINBIOSE and the Conseil du Statut de la Femme. We would like to thank Freda Paltiel for getting us started, and all of these organizations for supporting the workshop and publication of this book. We would also like to thank our editor, Lynn Henry at gynergy books, and all of the contributors who diligently and promptly reworked their papers in response to our suggestions and comments. We hope that this is the first of many books from the network of researchers on gender and workplace health.

Barbara Neis

Postface

Le contenu de ce livre a été inspiré par un atelier portant sur les obstacles sociaux, physiques et techniques à l'intégration sécuritaire des femmes dans les milieux de travail. Les contacts et les échanges qui ont conduit à l'organisation de cet atelier provenaient de la table ronde sur la santé des femmes en milieu de travail qui s'était tenue à Ottawa en juin 1992. Organisée par le bureau de Freda Paltiel, conseillère principale sur la situation des femmes, à Santé Canada, cette table ronde avait réuni des chercheures et des chercheurs qui s'intéressaient aux questions de la répartition du travail selon le sexe, la santé, travail et santé, partout au Canada. Le contenu des conférences avait réaffirmé que la division sexuelle du travail perdurait, les femmes étant concentrées dans les emplois de plus faible revenu, et avait contesté le préjugé voulant que la protection de la santé des femmes passe précisément par cette division.

La table ronde avait alors permis la création d'un réseau de chercheures intéressées par les questions touchant la division sexuelle dans l'étude de la santé au travail. Elle avait aussi mis en évidence des différences régionales quant à l'ampleur et à la qualité des programmes de recherche dans ce domaine. Par la suite, nous avons décidé d'organiser l'atelier à l'origine du présent livre. L'atelier devait consolider le réseau et encourager la recherche sur la santé des femmes au travail, et aider à réduire les disparités régionales.

La première partie de l'atelier s'est tenue à l'université Memorial de St-Jean, Terre-neuve, en août 1993. Avant cette date, très peu de recherches avaient été effectuées au Labrador et à Terre-Neuve sur cette question. Subventionné au niveau fédéral par le Conseil de recherches en sciences humaines, et à Terre-Neuve par l'Institute of Social and Economic Research, le Woman's Policy Office, le Provincial Advisory Council on the Status of Women, la Newfoundland Federation of Labour et le bureau du doyen de la faculté des arts de l'université Memorial, l'atelier a permis de sensibiliser les gens aux problèmes de santé des travailleuses de Terre-Neuve.

La seconde partie de l'atelier s'est tenue à l'Université du Québec à Montréal en mai 1994. Le financement de cette deuxième étape est venu du Programme national de recherche et de développement en santé de Santé Canada, de l'Université du Québec à Montréal, du Centre pour l'étude des interactions biologiques entre la santé et l'environnement et du Conseil du statut de la femme du Québec. Nous aimerions remercier Freda Paltiel pour avoir donné le coup d'envoi, et tous les bailleurs de fonds pour leur appui à la tenue de l'atelier et à la publication du présent ouvrage. Nous aimerions aussi reconnaître l'apport de Lynn Henry de gynergy books et celui de toutes les participantes qui ont si patiemment et rapidement retravaillé leur texte en réponse à nos commentaires. Nous espérons qu'il s'agit du premier ouvrage d'une série de publications du réseau de chercheures dans le domaine de la santé au travail et du rôle determinant de la tâche selon l'appartenance à l'un ou l'autre sexe.

Barbara Neis

Contributors/Les auteures

Pat Armstrong has been writing about various aspects of women's work since the early 1970s. She has authored or co-authored such books as *The Double Ghetto: Canadian Women and Their Segregated Work* (McClelland & Stewart), *A Working Majority: What Women Must Do For Pay* (Garamond Press), *Take Care: Warning Signals for the Canadian Health System* (Garamond Press), and *Vital Signs: Nursing in Transition* (Advisory Council on the Status of Women). She is currently the director of the School of Canadian Studies at Carleton University in Ottawa.

Ellen Balka is an assistant professor in Women's Studies at Memorial University. Her educational background includes degrees in geography and environmental studies, women's studies and an interdisciplinary doctorate in the applied sciences. Her research focuses on gender and technological change and has addressed the use of technology assessment as an educational tool with women workers, the use of computer networks in the context of feminist social change, and gender and the participatory design of technology. She has recently begun a project investigating how skill, gender, user involvement and expertise are addressed within two approaches to the design of technology (participatory design and ergonomics). She does her best to enjoy life.

Barbara Beardwood has recently completed her PhD at McMaster University. She is a political sociologist with interests in health care, occupational and environmental health, social policy and movements for change.

Nicolette Carlan is the chair of the Occupational Disease Panel (ODP) for Ontario. The ODP is responsible for the investigation of the association between disease and work and provides advice to the Workers' Compensation Board (WCB) about diseases that should be compensated. The Panel is currently working on issues associated with work exposure to noise, health problems resulting from health care workers' exposures to drugs and problems associated with metalworking fluids. Previously, she was a vice-chair with the Workers' Compensation Appeals Tribunal (WCAT) for a five year term. WCAT is an administrative body that determines final appeals from workers and employers within the Ontario Workers' Compensation system. She has also been assistant director of the Office of the Ontario Ombudsman.

Lucie Dumais détient un PhD en sociologie de la London School of Economics and Political Science, University of London. Elle est associée au CINBIOSE depuis 1990, où elle fait des recherches en santé au travail avec des ergonomes et des biologistes. Ses travaux actuels touchent, premièrement, aux problèmes des femmes au travail, autant dans des emplois traditionnels que nontraditionnels, et, deuxièmement, à des questions de nature théorique et méthodologique relatives à la production scientifique.

Joan Eakin is a sociologist in the Faculty of Medicine at the University of Toronto. She is interested in the social aspects of health, illness and health care. Her research is concerned with the relationship between work and health, and issues of prevention and health promotion in the workplace. Recent work includes ethnographic studies of health-related behaviour in very small workplaces and the social dimensions of work-related back injury.

John Eyles is the ecoresearch chair in Environmental Health and professor of Geography at McMaster University. He has published extensively and his current research interests include environmental and community health.

Susan French is an educator, researcher and consultant with a particular focus on the career paths and quality of life of nurses, and women's health in Canada and countries of the South (Pakistan, for example). She is a professor in the School of Nursing at McMaster University and an associate member of the Department of Sociology and the Hamilton-Wentworth Department of Public Health Services.

Martha Keil graduated from the University of Toronto with a Masters in English. She has been the program coordinator at Ontario's Occupational Disease Panel since March 1993. Prior to this, she held positions at the Office of the Ontario Ombudsman as a researcher and an investigator for the Workers' Compensation Board team. She has compiled extensive research and policy papers on various provincial government subjects and has also developed and taught a series of in-house workshops on report writing and consumer service with an emphasis on plain language, client sensitivity and investigative procedures.

Danièle Kergoat, sociologue, est directrice de recherche au Centre national de la recherche scientifique (CNRS) en France. Elle a publié de nombreux travaux, parmi lesquels figurent *Les ouvrières* (Le Sycomore), *Les femmes et le travail à temps partiel* (La Documentation française) et plus récemment, *Les infirmières et leur coordination 1988-1989* (sous la direction de) (Lamarre).

Katherine Lippel is a lawyer and professor of law in the Department of Law at the Université du Québec à Montréal. She is the author of several books and articles on workers' compensation, including a book entitled *Le stress au travail: l'indemnisation des atteintes à la santé en droit québécois, canadien et américain*(Éditions Yvon Blais). She is currently studying gender based differences in access to compensation and rehabilitation and has recently completed a report on precautionary leave for pregnant workers under the Quebec Health and Safety Act.

Donna Mergler is a professor of physiology in the Department of Biological Sciences at the Université du Québec à Montréal. Her research, carried out with the active collaboration of unions and community groups, focuses on early indicators of physical and mental health deterioration resulting from occupational and environmental hazards. She is the 1995 recipient of the Michel Jurdant Prize for research in environmental sciences which is awarded by the Association canadienne-française pour l'avancement des sciences.

Karen Messing was educated at Harvard and McGill universities and received her PhD in Biology from McGill in 1975. She trained in ergonomics at the Conservatoire national des arts et métiers in Paris and is now a professor of Biological Sciences at the Université du Québec à Montréal. She has published many scientific papers on women's occupational health and is the author of *Occupational Health Concerns of Canadian Women* (Human Resources Canada).

Barbara Neis is an associate professor in the Department of Sociology, Memorial University. She specializes in fishery-related research and has examined gender relations, social movements, technological change, industrial restructuring, fisheries science, management and occupational health within the Newfoundland and Labrador fisheries. She is co-editor of the anthology *Their Lives and Times: Women in Newfoundland and Labrador* (Creative Publishers) and is currently examining the origins and impacts of the Atlantic groundfish crises of the 1990s.

Lynn Skillen is an associate professor in the Faculty of Nursing at the University of Alberta. She holds a BScN and MHSc from McMaster University, an Occupational Health Nursing Certificate and a PhD in Sociology from the University of Alberta. Her nursing experience includes work in northern Canada and Columbia. Since joining the Faculty of Nursing in 1981, she has taught health assessment, occupational health, community health nursing and program planning. Her research interests include the social structures and ideologies underlying work hazards and women's work-related health issues.

Janet Sprout is a graduate student in Community Health Sciences at the University of Manitoba. She is currently employed as an acting manager of the Workplace Services Unit with the Manitoba Workplace Safety and Health Branch. Prior to this, she spent many years as a worker advisor for both the Manitoba and British Columbia Departments of labour, representing injured workers at their Workers' Compensation appeals.

Joan Stevenson is a professor of biomechanics at Queen's University in the School of Physical Education. She has a cross-appointment with the School of Rehabilitation Therapy and is the chair of the Queen's Ergonomic Research Group, which is involved in ergonomic contracts in the areas of selection standards, educational programmes, ergonomic assessments and design combined with human factors.

Susan Stock is an occupational health specialist and epidemiologist at the Occupational and Environmental Health Unit of the Montreal Department of Public Health. She is a researcher and clinician whose primary area of interest is the prevention and rehabilitation of work-related musculoskeletal disorders. She is an adjunct professor in the Faculty of Medicine at McGill University.

Catherine Teiger est ergonome, chercheure au Conservatoire National des Arts et Métiers, France. Elle a participé à de nombreuses recherches en France, autant sur le travail des femmes que des hommes, et au Québec, sur le travail féminin de saisie de données et des services financiers. Elle se consacre présentement à la recherche sur les conditions et les moyens par lesquels on peut développer, chez les travailleurs, leurs capacités à transformer le travail en leur faisant s'approprier des outils ergonomiques d'analyse du travail et de ses effets sur la santé.

Nicole Vézina est ergonome, professeure au département de sciences biologiques de l'Université du Québec à Montréal. Ses travaux ont porté surtout sur les emplois traditionnellement féminins de caissières de supermarché et de couturières, mais aussi dans les abattoirs et usines de transformation des viandes et de la volaille. Elle dirige actuellement deux projets: l'un sur la formation des travailleurs dans les abattoirs visant à réduire à long terme les lésions musculo-squelettiques, et l'autre, sur l'impact de l'organisation du travail sur les contraintes musculo-squelettiques reliées à l'activité de couturière.

Vivienne Walters is the director of the Labour Studies Program and a professor of Sociology at McMaster University. She has a long-standing interest in the social bases of health, with a particular focus on women's health and the links between work and health.

Dorothy Wigmore is an occupational hygienist studying ergonomics at the University of Massachusetts-Lowell. A long-time health and safety activist, her first exposure to the seriousness of workplace violence came from members of the Canadian Union of Public Employees (CUPE). As a health and safety specialist, she has worked for their union, as well as the Manitoba government and multi-disciplinary occupational health centres in Manitoba and Ontario.

Annalee Yassi is an associate professor and the director of the Occupational and Environmental Health Unit in the Department of Community Health Sciences at the University of Manitoba. She is also the director of the Department of Occupational and Environmental Medicine at Winnipeg's Health Sciences Centre. She is a physician specializing in both Occupational Medicine and Community Medicine. She has published extensively and has been involved in numerous occupational and environmental health hazard appraisals.

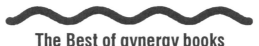

The Best of gynergy books

Each Small Step: Breaking the Chains of Abuse and Addiction, *Marilyn MacKinnon (ed.)*. This groundbreaking anthology contains narratives by women recovering from the traumas of childhood sexual abuse and alcohol and chemical dependency.
ISBN 0-921881-17-7 $10.95

Imprinting Our Image: An International Anthology by Women with Disabilities, *Diane Driedger and Susan Gray (eds.)*. "In this global tour de force, 30 writers from 17 countries provide dramatic insight into a wide range of issues germane to both the women's and the disability rights movements."
Disabled Peoples' International
ISBN 0-921881-22-3 $12.95

Lesbian Parenting: Living with Pride & Prejudice, *Katherine Arnup (ed.)*. Here is the perfect primer for lesbian parents, and a helpful resource for their families and friends. "Thoughtful, provocative and passionate. A brave and necessary book." *Sandra Butler*
ISBN 0-921881-33-9 $19.95/$16.95 U.S.

Miss Autobody: A Play, *Les Folles Alliées,* (translated by Linda Gaboriau). *Miss Autobody* accurately dissects the insidious effects of pornography and misogyny, and splits your sides in the process. "The play reads as that rare piece of blatantly political theatre that works." *Books in Canada*
ISBN 0-921881-25-8 $10.95/$9.95 U.S.

Patient No More: The Politics of Breast Cancer, *Sharon Batt.* "A spectacular book ... carefully researched and thoroughly engrossing ... As exciting to read as a Grisham thriller, it demonstrates that reality is more compelling than fiction." *Bloomsbury Review*
ISBN 0-921881-30-4 $19.95/$16.95 U.S.

The Montreal Massacre, *Louise Malette and Marie Chalouh (eds.),* (translated by Marlene Wildeman). Feminist letters, essays and poems examine the misogyny inherent in the massacre of 14 women at École Polytechnique in Montreal, Quebec on December 6, 1989.
ISBN 0-921881-14-2 $12.95

gynergy books titles are available at quality bookstores. Ask for our titles at your favourite local bookstore. Individual, prepaid orders may be sent to: **gynergy books,** P.O. Box 2023, Charlottetown, Prince Edward Island, Canada, C1A 7N7. Please add postage and handling ($3.00 for the first book and 75 cents for each additional book) to your order. Canadian residents add 7% GST to the total amount. GST registration number R104383120. Prices are subject to change without notice.